PANDEMIC VOICES

Unheard Stories from the Front Lines

Edited by Laura A. Hawryluck, MD, and Nathan D. Nielsen, MD

Pandemic Voices sheds light on previously unheard or overlooked international perspectives of patients and health care and community services workers through unprecedented access to some of the most challenging moments of the COVID-19 pandemic: the innovations, the stories of lives saved, those of lives lost, and the prices paid.

Divided into seven thematic sections, the collection chronicles the experiences from the front lines of the pandemic. It highlights the disruptions faced by medical systems and the innovative adaptations that emerged to simply keep them functioning, as well as the pandemic impacts from locations overlooked by global media. The book delves into the profound effects on health care workers and reveals insights into the strain on health care systems. It amplifies the voices of individuals who faced unique struggles during the pandemic, such as caregivers for children with special needs or individuals battling addiction, in times when resources were basically non-existent in a chaotic landscape. The collection concludes with a reflection on how history will judge our pandemic-era actions, alongside the hard lessons learned on truth, science, and advocacy throughout these challenging years.

In sharing the heartbreaks, the triumphs, and the scars that left none of us untouched, *Pandemic Voices* assesses what we have been through – what went well, what did not – in order to learn and, in time, hopefully to heal.

LAURA A. HAWRYLUCK, MD, is a professor of critical care medicine in the Interdepartmental Division of Critical Care Medicine Program at the University of Toronto.

NATHAN D. NIELSEN, MD, is an associate professor in the Departments of Internal Medicine and Pathology at the University of New Mexico School of Medicine.

Pandemic Voices

Untold Stories from the Front Lines

EDITED BY LAURA A. HAWRYLUCK, MD,
AND NATHAN D. NIELSEN, MD

UNIVERSITY OF TORONTO PRESS
Toronto Buffalo London

© University of Toronto Press 2025
Toronto Buffalo London
utppublishing.com

ISBN 978-1-4875-4934-3 (cloth)   ISBN 978-1-4875-5544-3 (EPUB)
ISBN 978-1-4875-5345-6 (paper)   ISBN 978-1-4875-5242-8 (PDF)

Library and Archives Canada Cataloguing in Publication

Title: Pandemic voices : untold stories from the front lines / edited by Laura
   A. Hawryluck, MD, and Nathan D. Nielsen, MD.
Names: Hawryluck, L. (Laura), 1969–, editor | Nielsen, Nathan D., editor.
Description: Includes bibliographical references and index.
Identifiers: Canadiana (print) 20250131307 | Canadiana (ebook) 20250131374 |
   ISBN 9781487549343 (cloth) | ISBN 9781487553456 (paper) |
   ISBN 9781487552428 (PDF) | ISBN 9781487555443 (EPUB)
Subjects: LCSH: COVID-19 (Disease) – Patients – Medical care – Anecdotes. |
   LCSH: COVID-19 (Disease) – Social aspects – Anecdotes. | LCSH: COVID-19
   (Disease) – Psychological aspects – Anecdotes. | LCSH: Medical personnel –
   Anecdotes. | LCSH: Medical care – Anecdotes. | LCSH: Medical innovations –
   Anecdotes. | LCGFT: Anecdotes.
Classification: LCC RA644.C67 P36 2025 | DDC 616.2/4144 – dc23

Cover design: Val Cooke
Cover image: iStock.com/wildpixel

We wish to acknowledge the land on which the University of Toronto Press operates. This land is the traditional territory of the Wendat, the Anishnaabeg, the Haudenosaunee, the Métis, and the Mississaugas of the Credit First Nation.

University of Toronto Press acknowledges the financial support of the Government of Canada, the Canada Council for the Arts, and the Ontario Arts Council, an agency of the Government of Ontario, for its publishing activities.

   Canada Council   Conseil des Arts
                       for the Arts   du Canada

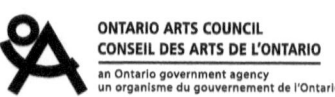

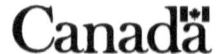

*To all those we have lost.
We will never forget.*

Contents

List of Figures and Tables xiii

Preface xv
NATHAN D. NIELSEN, MD

Part One: Prices Paid

1 My COVID-19 Journey 5
   ANTHONY McDERMOTT, MD

2 Dania: Riyadh Hospital 2020 11
   HASSAN AL-HABEEB, MD

3 Raging Fire: An ICU Physician's Experience as a COVID-19 Patient 14
   KEITH AZEVEDO, MD

4 The Person in the Health Care Worker 19
   RIMA STYRA, MD, MEd, FRCPC

5 COVID-19 on the Front Lines: Mental Health and Resilience 28
   PETER G. BRINDLEY, MD, FRCPC, FRCP

6 Trauma and Trepidation: The Emotional and Moral Toll of Dealing with Sick Patients 31
   MATYAS HERVIEUX, BSc (Hons), DHS, MA, MD, CCFP(EM)

7 Compassion Fatigue: The Palliative Perspective 39
   SONIA MALHOTRA, MD, MS, FAAP, FAAHPM

Part Two: Scarcity

8 The Last Bed: Triage and Triage Avoidance   47
JAMES DOWNAR, MDCM, MHSc, FRCPC, AND
BOJAN N. PAUNOVIC, MD, FRCPC

9 PPE During COVID-19: Scarcity, Science, Logistics,
and Paper Bags   52
STEVE A. McLAUGHLIN, MD, ERIK KRAAI, MD, AND PPE COMMITTEE
OF THE UNIVERSITY OF NEW MEXICO SCHOOL OF MEDICINE

10 OMG, We Are Running Out of Propofol!   61
SCOTT ROACH, PharmD, MBA, AND PREEYAPORN SARANGARM, PharmD,
BCPS, BCCCP

Part Three: Necessity Is the Mother of Invention

11 Anchored in Family: Starting a Business in Health Care Innovation
During COVID-19   69
SABRINA FIORELLINO, JD

12 A Voice from the Operating Room to the Intensive Care Unit:
An Anesthesiologist, Redeployed   77
GIANNI R. LORELLO, BSc, MD, MSc (Med Ed), CIP, FRCPC

13 How COVID-19 Changed the Way We Transported Patients
Between Ontario's Hospitals: Prone Patient Transports   82
ANDY PAN, MD, FRCPC (EM CCM), DRCPSC (PTM), MICHAEL PEDDLE,
MD, FRCPC, DRCPSC, AND RUSSELL MacDONALD, MD, MPH, FCFP, FRCPC,
DRCPSC

14 Transporting Patients: Kilometres to Go to Find a Home   88
BOJAN N. PAUNOVIC, MD, FRCPC

15 When the Going Gets Tough, the Tough Get Going:
A "Hybrid Model" of Paediatric and Adult Critical Care
During the COVID-19 Surge   91
AKASH DEEP, MD, FRCPCH, PHILIP KNIGHT, MD, MBChB, MRCPH, AND
LOUIS SKEVINGTON-POSTLES, BSc, MSc

16 Lessons Learned from COVID-19: Personal Perspectives from a Low- and Middle-Income Country   101
MERVYN MER, MBBCh, DIP PEC (SA), FCP (SA), PULMONOLOGY SUBSPECIALTY, CERT CRITICAL CARE (SA), M MED (INT MED), FRCP (LONDON), FCCP, PhD

17 Vaccinating Remote Indigenous Communities   105
HOMER TIEN, MD, MSc, FRCSC

Part Four: Stories from Forgotten Places

18 COVID-19 Pandemic and the Fate of Indonesian Children   119
KURNIAWAN TAUFIQ KADAFI, MD, AND RIRIE FACHRINA MALISIE, MD, PhD

19 Caring for Paediatric Patients with COVID-19 During the Pandemic in Peru: Experiences from 2020 and 2021   126
JESÚS DOMÍNGUEZ-ROJAS, MD, AND ALVARO CORONADO-MUÑOZ, MD

20 From the Four Directions: Healing on Navajoland   131
MELISSA BEGAY, MD

Part Five: Learning Under Fire

21 Waiting in the Wings: A Medical Trainee's Pandemic Experience   139
GABRIELLE KARLOVICH, MD

22 Becoming a Psychiatrist During a Pandemic   147
HOUMAN RASHIDIAN, MD, FRCPC, AND SABRINA AGNIHOTRI, MD

23 PANDEMIC RITES: Rites of Passage as an International ICU Fellow and the Journey Back Home   151
ONION GERALD VERGARA UBALDO, MD, MBA, FRCP, FPSCCM

24 Resident Training in COVID-19 Times   160
PAMELA H. ORR, MD, MSc, FRCPC

Part Six: Systems on the Verge of Collapse

25 Anticipation, Dread, and Worry: Preparing for the Arrival of Sick Patients   169
MATYAS HERVIEUX, BSc (Hons), DHS, MA, MD, CCFP(EM)

26 "The War on COVID-19": Reflections from the ICU Front Line   179
PETER G. BRINDLEY, MD, FRCPC, FRCP

27 Seven Days in the ICU   183
LAURA A. HAWRYLUCK, MSc, MD, FRCPC

28 The Pandemic Was a Powerful Teacher: Ramping Down Services   191
FAYEZ QUERESHY, MD, MBA, FRCSC, FACS

29 COVID-19 Seen from a Preventionist Physician's Point of View: Will We Be Able to Draw Lessons for the Future?   197
JEAN RALPH ZAHAR, MD, PhD

30 Treating the Unvaccinated During COVID-19: Did I Sign Up for This?   205
PETER G. BRINDLEY, MD, FRCPC, FRCP

31 Siloed Still ...   208
LAURA A. HAWRYLUCK, MSc, MD, FRCPC

Part Seven: Lessons and Transformations

32 Turning Pain into Progress   219
JODY THOMAS, PhD

33 A Dumpster Full of Flowers   224
INGRID DUFFY, RN, FNP

34 The Same Room   234
HASSAN AL-HABEEB, MD

35 No Visitors   236
REV. KRISTEL CLAYVILLE, PhD

36 History Will Judge Us. And That's OK.   240
    JOE VIPOND, MD, CCFP(EM), FCPC, AND KASHIF PIRZADA, MD,
    CCFP(EM)

Part Eight: Those Left Behind

37 The Other Epidemic: Overdose Crisis   253
    MEAGHAN REABURN, PharmD, BScPhm, RPh

38 Accessing Mental Health Services: An Expanding Public
    Need   257
    TROY RIECK, PhD, C.Psych

39 From the COVID-19 Ashes: A Journey in Life Transformation   263
    DORRETTE RUDDOCK, RN

40 Leading from the Ground: Families Supporting Families and
    Children with Disabilities   266
    TINA TRIGG, PhD

Part Nine: Reconsider/Reflect/Revisit/Return

41 How COVID-19 Made Salient the Need to Reconsider the
    Relationships Between Health Care Providers, Their Family,
    Friends, Co-Workers, and the Public   275
    MATYAS HERVIEUX, BSc (Hons), DHS, MA, MD, CCFP(EM)

42 Science and Truth During and After COVID-19   288
    PETER G. BRINDLEY, MD, FRCPC, FRCP

Afterword: Where Do We Go from Here? A Time to Reflect,
a Time to Heal   293
LAURA A. HAWRYLUCK, MSc, MD, FRCPC

Glossary   295

Contributors   301

Figures and Tables

Figure

4.1 Maslow's Hierarchy of Needs   21

Tables

4.1 Ways to Meet the Maslow Hierarchy Needs of Health Care Workers   26
13.1 Serious Adverse Events Identified in Prone Patient Transport During the First 127 Cases   87

Preface

Nathan D. Nielsen, MD
Associate Professor, Departments of Internal Medicine and Pathology at the University of New Mexico School of Medicine

15 February 2023

As I sit writing the introduction to this collection of essays nearly 3 years since I saw my first case of COVID-19, my mind keeps returning to a quote and a parable. The quote is from the twentieth-century philosopher George Santayana, and reads: "Those who cannot remember the past are condemned to repeat it."* The parable is the ancient Indian story of the blind men and the elephant: a group of blind men who have never encountered an elephant before attempt to describe the creature, but each can only describe a single part, not the totality – for the totality is just too large to be described by a single person.

The quote and parable reflect the ethos behind this collection: while it is indescribably important to remember the events of the pandemic, no one person's recollections are sufficient to tell the whole story. The essays presented here are meant to be a record of the pandemic through the memories of those on the front lines, intended to capture as much of the pandemic experience as possible through an array of viewpoints. We attempted to capture a chorus of voices from across health care, not just those of the seasoned doctors and nurses whose COVID "war stories" dominated the media narrative in much of the world but the lesser heard voices – pharmacists, hospital chaplains, administrators, psychologists, physicians-in-training. Our intention is for this book to be a record of these lesser told stories – a bulwark against the fading of memory as the darkest days of the pandemic fall further and further behind us. For while forgetting can be easy (and sometimes welcome), we believe that it is important to remember how a tiny virus turned our

---

* The quotation comes from George Santayana's work *The Life of Reason or the Phases of Human Progress*, published in five volumes by Charles Scribner's Sons in 1905–06. It is found on page 284 of volume 1, *Introduction and Reason in Common Sense*, published in 1905.

collective worlds upside down – and we should remember, not just as preparatory lessons for possible future pandemics, but as touchstones for conversation (or commiseration) with colleagues, friends, and family, perhaps even as an anchor point for sorting out the confusion that was the past 3 years.

Our hope for the health care professionals who read these pieces is that they hear some of their story in these pages, feel just a little less alone in their "COVID memories," and find comfort in shared experience. For our layperson readers, we hope that these essays are able to provide a better answer to the question, "What was it really like?" than those provided by general media reports or informal verbal accounts from friends or family. In short, this book is our attempt at describing the COVID elephant in its terrible totality.

This collection is divided into nine general thematic sections: "Prices Paid" starts off with a patient's story of life-threatening illness and recounts the effects of the pandemic on the people of health care – personally, educationally, psychologically, and professionally. The pandemic touched every element of the professions, many in ways that will take years to fully understand and heal from. "Scarcity" describes the angst and anxiety of preparing for and dealing with the mass shortages encountered in health care during the pandemic – shortages of drugs, personal protective equipment, hospital beds, and staff.

"Necessity Is the Mother of Invention" includes accounts of the overwhelming upheaval across the medical systems top to bottom and the creative, on-the-fly adaptations that emerged in order to simply keep functioning. "Stories from Forgotten Places" is a collection of pieces from locations that did not receive the global media attention as, say, China, Northern Italy, New York City, or India but were no less devastated, no less disrupted. We include perspectives from South America, Southeast Asia, and from the Native peoples of the United States. "Learning Under Fire" describes the challenges of becoming, and training, health care professionals during the pandemic – disruptions to traditional learning methods and locales, the strain of being tasked with work outside the standard scope, the difficulty of finding one's place in health care systems in chaos.

"Systems on the Verge of Collapse" recounts the strain on medical systems brought about by the pandemic: how systems prepared (or didn't), adapted, and kept themselves from breaking (or didn't), all from an insiders' perspective. "Lessons and Transformations" provides vantage points on the front-line pandemic experience that were all too often overlooked – from a nurse practitioner "air-dropped" into a New York City in lockdown to a pain psychologist, a hospital chaplain, and personal reflections of physicians and nurses who experienced life-changing personal events and loss. "Those Left Behind" gives voice to those with unique struggles during the pandemic – those caring for children with special needs, those struggling with addiction or mental health challenges in times when resources for either were basically non-existent in a chaotic landscape. Our collection ends with "Reconsider/Reflect/Revisit/Return" – a pair of reflections: one on how health care relationships changed as a result of the pandemic, both among health care professionals and between health care workers and the lay public; the other on lessons learned about truth, science, and advocacy through the pandemic years.

I feel it important to state openly that the pieces within these pages were not written by professional authors, not by journalists, not by bloggers, or even Twitter (now X) mavens – these are all authentic voices from the front lines, sharing their experiences, their memories, their pain, and their loss. These essays were not heavily edited for we wanted the authors' true voices to be heard – raw and unpolished on occasion, but undeniably *real*. So, forgive us our literary imperfections (among them the frequent use of the colloquial "COVID" rather than the more scientifically accurate COVID-19 or SARS-CoV-2) and listen to the stories we tell. And let us all never, ever fail to remember our "pandemic past" – for none of us have any desire to repeat it.

PANDEMIC VOICES

PART ONE

Prices Paid

In this opening section of our collection of essays, authors recount the personal losses stemming from the pandemic: personally experiencing severe illness, watching loved ones suffer, caring for patients through various phases of the pandemic, and accounting for the damage to self and psyche that resulted. "My COVID-19 Journey" provides a harrowing account from a survivor of life-threatening and protracted COVID-19 contracted during one of the first waves of the pandemic. "Dania: Riyadh Hospital 2020" is a heart-rending account of helplessly watching a friend and colleague die in front of one's own eyes. "Raging Fire: An ICU Physician's Experience as a COVID-19 Patient" addresses the age-old dilemma: what do you do when you know too much about the illness ravaging your body? "The Person in the Health Care Worker" reviews the psychological and emotional impact of the pandemic on health care workers through a Maslow's hierarchy model and provides a prescription for how health systems could better support the persons operating within them in the future. "COVID-19 on the Front Lines: Mental Health and Resilience" is a critical assessment of the "resilience" concept and a critique of the emergence of a "resilience industry," and illustrates the often half-hearted attempts within the health care industry to foster resilience among their distressed staff. "Trauma and Trepidation: The Emotional and Moral Toll of Dealing with Sick Patients" focuses on the many sources of moral injury that health care workers experienced while on the front lines of the pandemic, treating patients afflicted by the virus and watching them suffer and die, many needlessly, and delves into the long-term impacts of those moral injuries on those still in the health care arena. "Compassion Fatigue: The Palliative Perspective" describes the pathway to compassion fatigue (emotional and physical exhaustion from repeated stress leading to a diminished ability to empathize or feel compassion for others) experienced by the most compassionate practitioners in the health care arena, those practising palliative care, underscoring that the pandemic drained the empathy reserves of even the most empathetic among us.

1 My COVID-19 Journey

Anthony McDermott, MD
COVID-19 Survivor, Ontario, Canada

Submitted 16 October 2022

11 to 18 April 2021

My wife and I met up with my good friend JC at a local park to give our new dogs a chance to play. It was a beautiful day for a 10 kilometre* hike, and afterwards we enjoyed a sandwich and my favourite beer, Guinness. When I woke the next day, Sunday, I was achy and sore. I thought it was from the hike, but by the evening I had developed a cough and fever. On Monday, I was feeling much worse with a high fever and achy all over. I suspected COVID-19. On Tuesday, the day I got tested at Sunnybrook Hospital, my symptoms included excessive diarrhoea that continued all week. By Thursday, I was extremely dehydrated with a very high fever. I couldn't drink much or eat. Terry, my wife, had been taking my vital signs all week. On Friday, we agreed it was time to go to North York General Hospital (NYGH), the closest hospital to our house. Unfortunately, my hospital visit by ambulance was a short one. So many people were being admitted that Emergency had to triage admittance. Since I was severely dehydrated, I was given 1000 ml saline IV and sent home. On Saturday afternoon, things were worse. With a temperature of 106°F† and delirious, I went back to the hospital. With Emergency overflowing with COVID patients, I still was not sick enough to be admitted. The nurse walked with me to see if my oxygen levels would drop, but they did not decrease enough. Apologetically, they sent me home. When we got home, I told Terry I thought I was going to die that night. That evening Terry phoned

---

* 6 miles.
† 41°C.

the COVID helpline at Sunnybrook Hospital and spoke with Dr. Nick Daneman. He had been answering the helpline continuously for over a week. Terry, a registered nurse, phoned him regularly throughout the night, reporting my vital signs and deteriorating symptoms. On Sunday morning at 8 a.m. after the latest set of vital signs, Dr. Daneman found me a bed on Sunnybrook Hospital's COVID unit. With both of us wearing N95 masks and the car windows wide open, Terry drove me to Sunnybrook. Dr. Daneman instructed us to go to a specific entrance where a nurse met me. She wheeled me up to the fifth floor. Before entering the hospital, I turned to Terry, told her I loved her and that I was scared. I still didn't think I was going to make it, but at least now I had a chance.

The doctor who had turned me away from NYGH was genuinely concerned and upset that he had to send me home. He followed up with Terry a few days after I got admitted and was relieved that I was at Sunnybrook. At that time, so many people were contracting COVID. I understand why he couldn't admit me.

19 to 24 April: In the Hospital

The first week in hospital was a blur. My breathing continued to deteriorate. I found I needed to stay on my belly more and more to breathe. The phlegm and blood I was spitting up were increasing as the week went on. By the end of the week, the towel I was spitting into looked like a Jackson Pollock painting. I had oxygen on all the time, and by the weekend it wasn't much help. The dried blood in my nasal passages was constantly blocking my breathing. I needed to take the mask off and blow out all the dried blood. This cycle continued until I was so tired I would fall asleep, and then my laboured breathing would wake me up. My fever would subside for a short time and then spike again. One afternoon, a priest came to see me. He heard my confession and gave me the Sacrament of the Sick. I was extremely grateful that this man risked his own health to console me. Four days later, the doctors spoke to me about my condition. I could read between the lines, and I asked them if I could go on the ventilator. I didn't really know what that meant, but I knew I had to do it. I was exhausted trying to breathe. The doctors and nurses were amazing. They kept me calm as they explained what would happen. They phoned my wife and some of my kids who still live at home so I could speak to them before going on the ventilator. I told everyone I loved them and that I would see them on the other side. Shortly after my call, the doctors said it was time.

Two days after being put on the ventilator at Sunnybrook Hospital, I was transferred to Toronto Western Hospital since Sunnybrook was expecting an influx of COVID patients from across the province who were worse off than me.

25 April to 6 June: On the Ventilator

The last thing I remember was the medical team helping me go on the ventilator. After that, I remember having vivid, often scary dreams, but I don't know whether they occurred while I was in an induced coma or while being weaned off the ventilator.

My bizarre dreams were night terrors that I was convinced were real. Every terror or hallucination had the common theme that I was trapped and couldn't escape. Sometimes I was trapped underground or in water. It's very hard to explain without thinking I am crazy. I was in various types of tunnels. There were different worlds and times all challenging me to escape. I dreamed about best friends being executed in horrible ways, dear people I know being killed. All of it seemed very real. In another dream, I was sitting in an open-air amphitheatre with the sun burning me up. Someone walked towards me and put a bag of ice on my head. In my dream, it felt so good and eased my heat exhaustion. Later, my wife explained that, because I had a very high fever, they needed to cover my entire body in ice to bring my temperature down.

The medical team was in constant communication with Terry. Since she is a registered nurse, they gave her detailed updates, which she appreciated, and involved her in all their decisions. When I had been in the intensive care unit (ICU) for 2 weeks, Terry was allowed to visit, and she helped with my care. I developed many blood clots and secondary infections that needed massive amounts of many different drugs. Terry said it felt like a game of musical antibiotics as the team fought every infection that developed, sometimes trying two different drugs at a time. Eventually, the team was able to insert a tracheostomy. Blood clots that developed around the tracheostomy meant that I needed surgery to stop the bleeding. The hospital phoned Terry at 4:30 a.m. to get her consent. She was shaken but appreciated their decision.

7 to 13 June: Starting to Wake Up

Speaking about this time is the most difficult for me. According to Terry, once the medical team started weaning me off the ventilator, they worried I was not waking up in a timely manner. Terry asked the staff to do an electroencephalogram (EEG) to check for brain activity. I could have told them that it runs in the family. My mother was the same – very sensitive to anesthetic. It's hard for me to put into words these first weeks of coming out of the coma. I thought the staff were trying to kill me by not feeding me or giving me water. I also thought they were moving me from province to province. One day I thought I was in a Calgary hospital, the next in a Brampton one. I kept pulling out my tubes and trying to escape from the bed. I think back on all the burdens I put the nurses through. I cannot thank them enough for their patience with me. I had no concept of how sick I was.

When I started to regain consciousness, I thought I had been hit by a train. I couldn't move very much, and I hurt all over. I couldn't speak and was too weak to lift my limbs. I thought I was paralysed and unable to move. I quickly learned that nothing about my body was working properly, and I was frustrated, scared, and emotional. Everyone was speaking around me and about me, but I couldn't contribute. I couldn't shout out because I couldn't speak. I had no voice. To improve my breathing, they would deep suction me. This procedure was very painful but necessary. I dreaded pushing the button to be suctioned, but the alternative was worse. My mouth was dry, and all I could think about was getting a cold drink of water, which I was not allowed because I would aspirate. My swallowing muscles were not working. My bladder and bowels were no longer under my control. No one was able to tell me when I could eat, drink, go to the bathroom on my own, walk, or go home.

14 to 30 June

The staff were outstanding and very patient with my confusion when I woke up. After a week or so, they moved me to the post-anesthesia care unit (PACU) since I was regarded as stable. I had lost 70 lbs[‡] and had no strength in my body to move on my own. I was extremely depressed, which is not normal for me. Dr. Laura came to see me on her day off. With some of the staff, she put me in a wheelchair, and we spent a good half hour outside in the sun watching the world go by. This small visit really helped turn my despair into hope.

[‡] 32 kg.

I went back into the ICU for another couple of days and then moved to the eighth floor general medicine. My first attempt to sit up on the side of my bed with the help of Jonathan, the physiotherapist, instantly set my brain on fire. At least that's what it felt like. Every new movement – sitting up, standing for the first time, taking a step – always had the same results. My head would overheat, and I would sweat profusely. Someone told me this reaction was my brain coming out of hibernation.

29 July: Rehabilitation and Home

After 6 weeks at Toronto Western Hospital, I was moved to Toronto Rehab Bickle Centre. I needed a wheelchair but was now able to speak. My breathing had improved enough that I was close to getting the tracheostomy out of my throat. I was the first COVID patient for the physiotherapy team on the fifth floor. My dreams and hallucinations had stopped, thank goodness. My coughing had increased to the point where I was spitting blood due to the irritation of the tracheostomy. In a meeting with the doctor, speech and language pathologist, respiratory therapist, and my wife, they decided to remove the tracheostomy. With great patience from the staff, my rehabilitation started to pay off. By the time I left the Bickle, I could move around with the help of a walker. My bodily functions thankfully started to recover. My swallowing would not recover until well into December.

Today, 16 October 2022

I still have swallowing, fatigue, dizziness, gastrointestinal, and bowel issues. I will be feeling fine, but all of a sudden I am completely drained of energy and need to lie down. I sometimes have episodes of brain fog. Without warning, I need to find a bathroom very quickly to avoid an accident. Reports in the media constantly remind me of long-haul COVID effects. It is not very encouraging.

I prefer to acknowledge my current state and make the best of it. I know I am not the same person I was before COVID, but I can't do anything about that. All I can do is focus on the present and not worry about tomorrow. I have a lot to be thankful for. This past Thanksgiving, my sons and I spent time together at Wasaga Beach. I am so grateful to have this chance. In some ways, this illness has made me more aware of how fragile our lives are and shown me that we need to make the most of our lives for others and ourselves. I owe my life to God, my family, friends, strangers who prayed for my life, as well as the medical teams who worked so hard to keep me alive.

Thank you and God bless you all,
Anthony McDermott

Are You 100% Yet?
People ask me are you 100% yet
I used to say more like 90%
But really what does that mean
    Walking slower
    Easily tired
    Getting dizzy for no reason
    Trouble finding the right words
    Not as focused as I used to be
I say I am what I am now! That is my new 100%
I will not ponder on what was or should be
Just today's reality of what is
Tomorrow's reality may be better or worse
That will be my new 100%

2 Dania: Riyadh Hospital 2020

Hassan Al-Habeeb, MD
Critical Care Medicine Consultant and Neuro Critical Care Consultant, Riyadh National Hospital, Riyadh, Saudi Arabia

Submitted 13 February 2023

Dania is a promising young woman who is always smiling, humble, and loved by all the hospital staff. She is a 30-year-old radiologist, jovial to a such a great extent that everyone knows her. She lives to serve, is dedicated to her work, and understands the needs of patients, doctors, and staff. Everyone loves her as a hard-working and collaborative employee, friend, and sister. We met in the hospital in 2008. Since that first meeting, I fulfilled the conditions for a scholarship in Canada. I completed 3 years of specialization there, starting in 2017, and I returned home in the second half of 2020. Many life-changing events happened along the way. I received several professional degrees and certificates, and I travelled a lot. I met people and lost others. I walked away from the Kingdom (of Saudi Arabia) for 3 years, forgetting many things. Memory doesn't store everything – only the things that leave a vivid mark.

When I came back, I was told that a patient in her 30s had coronavirus, was in severe respiratory distress, and had contracted pneumonia because of the virus. Like any patient I deal with, I had to see the file and the medical history. She had entered intensive care before I returned to the hospital from abroad, and she was then transferred to my nursing department at the request of her family. Her family seems to know me. Although I don't recognize them, I think that perhaps we have met before, for the core of my work is to sit with the patient's family. Reassuring families and taking into account their psychological conditions, or at least that of the patient's attendant, I have learned important lessons about how to convey bad news (news about serious illness, disability, or death). I try to convey such news always in the most comforting way possible so it doesn't come down on the family like a strike of lightning.

These meetings are hard to do. So, once again, I sat down with this patient's family. I don't recall anything out of the ordinary in that meeting or anything that affected me more than usual.

Later that day, while I was bringing a cup of coffee from the cafeteria, I heard her sister's voice, and it was so close … almost hers. The sound and timbre of her voice rose from the depths of my memory. It was so deep within that I could never forget that voice. "Doctor." She called my name. Oh my god, she knows me! But the face didn't match. My confusion and embarrassment grew even more. My memory took me back 3 years to before the fellowship in Canada. In 3 seconds, I saw the past right in front of me like a burning film. It must be Dania. I rushed to her, "Dania!" "No," said the voice. "I am her sister."

I closed my eyes and recalled Dania's voice on the phone and the radiology department and its equipment when I used to run down to ask her for help with patients. Oh my god, how torn is my memory? I became shattered, filled with holes like a sieve. I had checked on Dania when I had started a few days ago and read her name. But I couldn't remember anything anymore. I rushed to the file and again found the name, the pathological history, and the situation that had worsened. I sat with Dania's family and shared their pain. She had been more than 2 months in intensive care before and after I arrived at the hospital. I tried to reassure her family, and they told me everything since her illness began. The virus was very exhausting to her respiratory system. Her sister told me that they asked to transfer her to my department because they knew me. I felt embarrassed and afraid that they thought I had ignored her. I was horrified that my memories were only triggered by her sister's voice, so very like her own, a ringing bell in my head warning me of failure to recognize one who had been a close friend.

I passed by and checked on her. She was in her last hours, with a severe pneumonia. It didn't last long in the intensive care. Dania had changed a lot, so much that I didn't and couldn't recognize any of her except her name after reading it for the twentieth time in her medical file. She is a colleague in the department, a friend. One of the nurses came to me, crying intensely, saying, "She passed away, Doctor." It's my duty to stand with her family, to reassure them a bit. Her sickness exhausted them as it did her, as it destroyed her body. The ongoing calls from other friends and colleagues and WhatsApp messages wrecked them.

I hope I was able to communicate the news of her death in as kind and compassionate a way as possible. I can't forgive myself, though, for my failure to recognize her when she came under my care. I ask myself every day how this could ever have happened. Sure, there was that time away. Sure, she had markedly changed from the long illness. Sure, I never expected that Dania would be in my ICU. We, physicians, often think that no one we know or care about will ever become critically ill – much less die and die so young. But still…

The news of her death was devastatingly sad for all the department's staff, doctors, nurses, and administrators. Dania died, but her name is still among us. We pray her mercies.

3 Raging Fire: An ICU Physician's Experience as a COVID-19 Patient

Keith Azevedo, MD
Assistant Professor, Critical Care and Emergency Medicine, Departments of Emergency Medicine and Internal Medicine, University of New Mexico School of Medicine

Submitted 1 July 2022

I remember the taste of earth in my mouth as I began to awake, a faint ringing and a warm sense of calm while dampness slowly dripped across my face and down my neck. This warmth and stillness gradually faded like the slow waves receding during low tide, and I sluggishly realized that I was face down in a gully, dirt in my mouth, with blood seeping down my head and neck. Before I could move, I lay there trying to remember where I was. Then I heard swifts darting by, smelled the sweet scent of ponderosa pine and the burning trace of fallen rock. I was at the base of the 1000-foot* rock climb my wife and I had been working on establishing for the prior 8 months.

This rock climb is approximately a 2-hour hike from our home in the mountains of the Cibola National Forest, where we live off grid, producing all our own electricity via sun. The hike is over relatively austere terrain, gaining 2000 vertical feet† over 3 miles‡ to reach the base of the route, my location on that day. I was alone, working on finishing up the last bit of crack cleaning on the climbing route we were establishing, when I decided to clean up a part of the cliff where someone had left a rope tangled in a tree for the past few years. I had looked at this rope over the seasons and decided today was the day that

---

* 305 metres.
† 610 metres.
‡ 4.8 kilometres.

this obnoxious thing had to come down. While attempting to free the rope from below, a refrigerator-sized boulder dislodged from 50 feet[§] above, hitting my right side, spinning me clockwise, and then a basketball-sized rock, hidden behind the refrigerator, hit the now exposed left side of my head, sending me head down into a rock-filled gully.

Finally understanding my current location and the events leading to my recumbent position, I attempted to get up and make my way to my backpack, a mere 75 feet[¶] away, and reach my phone. Each time I tried to reach my phone, I woke up 10 feet[#] closer. The closer I got to the phone, the easier it was to fight against losing consciousness and the slow fading of that fiery sunset I could see over my home 2000 feet[||] below. I had a distinct, somewhat peaceful, thought – if I die here, it is not a bad place to rest, in my back yard, a beautifully dying fire of a sunset streaking the western sky above.

It was 15 November 2020, a month before the first COVID-19 vaccine was available and 3 months after waking up in that rock-filled gully, and I was getting ready to start day 17 of 21 in a row in the hospital, switching from working in the intensive care unit (ICU) to the Emergency Department. I told my wife that I was not feeling great, but it was probably just the long hours over the last 17 days mixed with continued headaches from the accident. My wife is an emergency medicine physician and asked me to check my temperature. As it would turn out, we did not own a thermometer, and we had to pick one up! The first reading was 101°F.[**] I thought it must be wrong and asked my wife if we could just check it again in an hour as it was likely erroneous – I had to head to work in a few hours anyway and was starting to feel better as I awoke. One hour later, I tried to convince my wife that it was probably the cold water I drank before checking the first reading that resulted in an elevated temperature. But … second reading, 104°F.[††] Shoot, I think the thermometer might be broken.

I tested positive for COVID that evening and quickly became more symptomatic as the days progressed. On the fourth day, I remember feeling particularly well and told my wife I wanted to hike to the base of our route as I had not been there in months. She understandably disagreed, and we came to the compromise of a short walk into the

---

§ 15 metres.
¶ 23 metres.
# 3 metres.
|| 610 metres.
** 38.3°C.
†† 40°C.

mountains, basically to the start of the route. As I walked by myself up the mountain, I felt my legs give out. I would collapse every 15 to 30 minutes, having to rest before moving onward. I was in total denial, as I had felt this similar sense of weakness at altitude on expeditions in the Himalayas and the Andes. After returning home, where my wife asked why my clothes were dirty from lying on the ground, we bought a pulse oximeter and found that my oxygen saturation was in the 70s. I now understood I needed oxygen but made the decision at this point to decline hospitalization if things got worse, resigning myself to die at home if necessary. Though seemingly premature, the previous months I had spent taking care of patients with this disease in ICUs formed my decision to not seek hospitalization.

Several people have asked me for the details of my decision to stay home instead of seeking care at the hospital. I would have to say that, while I am fairly decent about recounting a story or objective events, I am very poor at talking about how these events affected me or the specific reasons behind such a personal decision. In attempting to explain, it feels as though I am somehow complaining or bothering people with mundanity. In most circumstances, I'd rather listen than talk about myself, and therefore the decision to write this essay and describe this decision was not without consternation. All that being said, perhaps similar to a great many of the complex decisions in life, multiple prior experiences informed such a conclusion. These experiences date back to before the conclusion of my undergraduate training. Between my second and third years, I left the United States and worked for the Ministry of Health of Ghana on the Guinea Worm Eradication Project. During that time, I began to learn about the vast inequities that existed in health and education globally, as well as the resultant suffering from these inequities. At one point, I contracted typhoid and malaria at the same time and was told I would need to speak with my family to let them know I would not survive the night. I was 20 years old, and it was the first time I was acutely aware of my imminent, potentially painful, death. Although in considerable pain and exhausted, I remember thinking that my circumstances were immeasurably more hopeful than the majority of the patients I had cared for up to this point, making my current circumstances feel insignificant when viewed in the context of so many others' suffering. After a long recovery, I returned to the States, eventually finishing my undergraduate training, and founded a non-profit organization focused on health care and education. As part of this work, I spent 3 years cycling through twenty countries to understand more clearly the global barriers that restrict access to health care and education. While what I was able to witness and the lessons I learned from that work are outside the scope of this writing, I did experience a similar sense of awe for the vastness of deprivation and for the oftentimes hopelessness, yet honour and dignity that can come with death. Several hundred miles from the airport and 3 days before my return home to start medical school after this 3-year expedition, I was working my way towards the airport in Ulan Bator, Mongolia, when I had a bad accident on my bicycle. I spent several days in a makeshift closet in a local Mongolian clinic as my injuries were too severe for the clinic there to address, and ultimately no one wanted to bear the responsibility for my death. Eventually, I was sent by private vehicle on day 3 or 4 to the capital before being air evacuated to Singapore. I do not remember a great deal of this experience as I was in and out of consciousness for the first week or so, but I do remember feeling what I believed was an inkling of desperation and lack of hope, perhaps similar to so many of the people I had met over the years who were ravaged by illness, ultimately only holding onto the possibility of dying with dignity and honour in the face of futility. I think all of these past experiences, as well as my more recent witnessing of the horrors of months of prolonged patient hospital courses with COVID, too often resulting in undignified death, ultimately shaped my decision to stay home and not seek hospital care. I was certainly hopeful of recovery, but I also understood the likely circuitous path of the route ahead.

Within a week of contracting COVID, I could no longer walk steadily. Night-time was particularly difficult. I would sit at the side of our bed each night, in a tripod position, gasping for air for hours on end, until eventually I would either pass out or fall asleep from exhaustion for a few minutes before awakening again to breathe. This essay is actually the first time I have written or talked in any detail about these days, and I am reminded and amazed at how strongly our bodies yearn for oxygen. It reminded me of the same compulsion for water I experienced while riding my bicycle across the Pamir Mountains of Tajikistan, where water was scarce and I would often wake up totally consumed with the compulsion to obtain even a drop of liquid. Night after night in my home, I would gasp away with oxygen saturations in the 60s, often thinking of that calm, warm, western dying light at the base of our route; but I would continue to breathe, taking one breath after another, oftentimes raging a bit to remember that dying sun.

Those months and weeks from today's vantage point now have a bit of cloudiness, seemingly blending together in memories of laughter and sorrow. I remember wanting to take a shower one day and then feeling the familiar warm sensation of water pouring down my back and neck as I woke up on the shower floor. No more showers for a while, I thought, as my wife with her tireless patience reminded me. We had a particularly long stretch of sunless days one week and did not have enough power to run my oxygen concentrator, so we decided to run an extension cord from our camper van's homemade battery supply to provide power. Hours later, our plans were dashed with only 2 hours of battery available from our camper, leaving us to sit in darkness while packing up to access power at a nearby hotel. These mixed memories of tempered joy and worry paved a way for my wife and I to remember these times with less apprehension.

Today, it is now 19 months since I was diagnosed with my first COVID infection. I have been off oxygen for almost 4 weeks now, which is the longest consecutive stretch I've experienced thus far. My wife and I finally finished our rock-climbing route, Rage Against the Dying Fire. My sense of smell and taste are a bit of a distant memory, which is quite insignificant when viewed in light of so many deaths. I am solidly aware of the paltriness of my illness, after seeing entire generations die in our ICUs. Looking back now from a personal vantage point of relative recovery at my decision to possibly die at home, I more clearly understand the ramifications of this decision. I regret the embarrassing and often anguishing times my wife had to witness as I would struggle to be human – unable to eat, breathe, or wash myself, the often-mundane parts of life that embody such an integral part of our humanity. This struggle, along with the ever-tortuous course of recovery and relapse, left me at times feeling helpless and hopeless. And yet, knowing too well the "hospital alternative," if I had to make the decision again, I would likely choose the same.

I believe many of us who worked clinically during the pandemic have perhaps at times felt a similar sense of helplessness – feeling like an ineffectual bystander, watching our patients die day after day. I think we honour the patients whose dignity and lives we struggled to preserve by remembering their stories and by utilizing what we have learned about humility, honour, selflessness, pain, resiliency, dignity, and courage to better care for our current and future patients, families, and friends. With our perhaps less distant return to a new normal, it can be easy to be softly lulled to complacency and forget these difficult lessons. But, as I start to find myself losing focus, thoughtlessly complaining about the mundane, I often remember the stories of so many patients I have cared for, and I try to continue to rage against that dying fire.

4 The Person in the Health Care Worker

Rima Styra, MD, MEd, FRCPC
Professor, Department of Psychiatry, University of Toronto

Submitted 22 October 2022

Health care workers are devoted individuals who want to help others and during COVID-19 frequently took on risks in the care of their patients. They had spent years learning their profession and were highly motivated to use their skills to better the health and quality of life of their patients, whom they saw suffering with COVID-19. It is easy to forget that the caring individual who comes to our aid is also an individual with their own personal life. No one was immune to the stress of the pandemic, and even though health care workers care for others, they are individuals – persons not only defined by their work but individuals with feelings, aspirations, and relationships. Health care workers were not immune to the stresses that we all faced during this major global challenge.

Media and social networks have highlighted the stress and subsequent distress that health care workers facing COVID-19 were experiencing throughout the world. The scenes of patients infected with COVID-19 were prominent across the screens of everyone's home, resonating deeply with those who were on the front lines. As most of the population went into quarantine within the safety of their homes, health care workers went to work to face this new threat. We remember during the early days of quarantine driving to get to the hospital, a city usually crowded with cars, now deserted and quiet. We wondered how many of the other drivers were "just like us," heading in to care for our patients and to support each other.

Work done during previous outbreaks of novel emerging infections outlined the distress in both health care workers and the general public. Recent outbreaks of SARS (severe acute respiratory syndrome), MERS (Middle East respiratory syndrome), and Ebola virus were traumatizing events for many health care workers.[1] It was quite common for health care workers to experience symptoms of anxiety, depression, and post-traumatic stress disorder as a result of these outbreaks. COVID-19 is similar in its psychological effects on health care workers,[2-4] although the severity and magnitude of this worldwide pandemic, with massive numbers of the public and health care workers becoming infected and dying around the world, far exceeded previous events. The distress may have been further exacerbated by the ongoing reporting of increasing numbers of infections and loss of life by the media, leading to further vicarious traumatization and a change in health care workers' world view of safety and health care.

Emotional support and social support are often effective in mitigating the distress of traumatic events. Some health care workers delayed retirement or their search for career advancement to stay in their current jobs at the bedside. However, as the surges of patients continue with new emerging variants, we have seen that health care workers, many of whom had stayed throughout the pandemic, are now leaving the health care field or opting for less stressful positions. While some migration of health care workers out of stressful roles into administrative positions or out of health care is normal, what is happening now is not. This exodus is massive and is causing a crisis in manpower in the health care system worldwide, which affects patient care as well as workload for the remaining staff, thus further negatively impacting the workplace environment and satisfaction. How did we get to the point where this exodus is happening? Is it just the effects of a pandemic, or is the exodus unmasking other problems? At times throughout their history and evolution, health care systems have been accused of depersonalizing patients. Has the pandemic unmasked the dehumanization of its workers? Health care workers were intensely aware that each of them had a story to tell of their experiences: the fatigue, declined vacation time, inequitable remuneration, redeployments, and the stress of long shifts with little time to address basic needs. But who was to listen and make the changes? Many of us who worked at our hospital started to notice that our colleagues were voting with their feet. As numbers of staff dwindled, so did spirits among those who remained, and they started to reflect on their own personal journey.

Abraham Maslow was an American psychologist who developed a hierarchy of needs to explain human motivation. His theory suggested that people have a number of basic needs that must be met before they can move up the hierarchy to pursue more social, emotional, and self-actualizing needs. Maslow's hierarchy of needs can help us to better understand some of the consequences of the COVID-19 pandemic. The key concept of Maslow's hierarchy is that everyone has basic needs that need to be addressed first in order to move to achieving psychological satisfaction and self-fulfilment in life. Maslow's hierarchy of needs

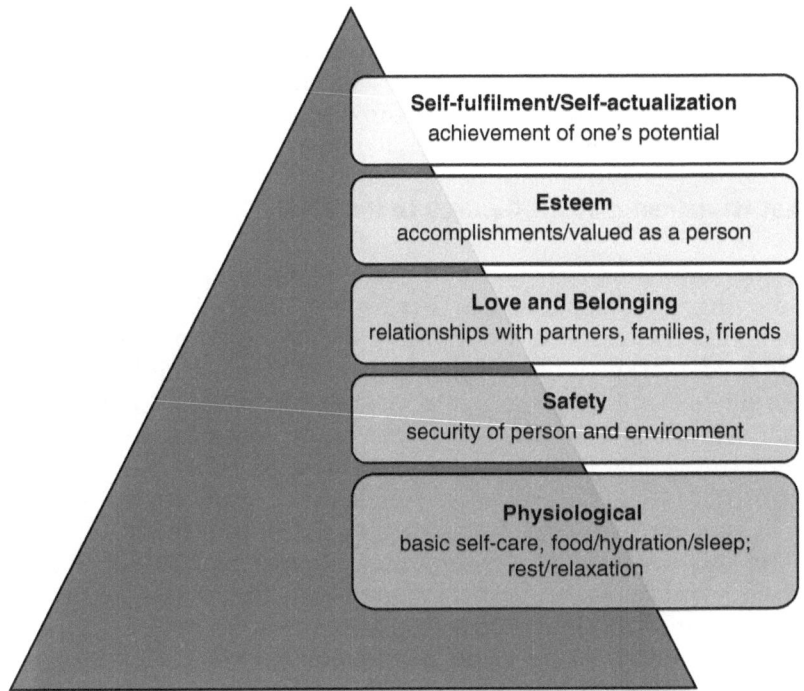

Figure 4.1. Maslow's Hierarchy of Needs

is a well-established theory that outlines these needs and also ranks them according to their perceived importance.[5,6] It is portrayed as a pyramid, with the most essential needs forming the base and the least essential constituting the peak of the pyramid (Figure 4.1). Maslow's theory suggests that lower basic needs have to be fulfilled before advancing to higher levels of functioning. If basic needs are not met, or are limited at various stages, this situation can result in both mental and physical health issues.

The hierarchy consists of a progression of needs:

Physiological – food, water, sleep
Safety – security of body, of resources, of employment, of the family, of health
Belonging – friendship, family, romantic relationships
Esteem – self-esteem, achievement, confidence, respect by others
Self-actualization – morality, creativity, spontaneity, problem solving

Maslow's model provides a framework to understand the basic needs of health care professionals as well as career development plans, goals, and the effect of experiences on their self-esteem and self-actualization. It empowers individuals with the knowledge needed to identify their interests, skills, strengths, and overall values.

What Happened during COVID-19 to the Person in the Professional?

Feeling safe and nourished and cared for as an individual is vital to moving on to achieving higher needs. The COVID-19 pandemic threatened this sense of basic safety for health care workers. They were tired, worked long shifts, often missed meals, couldn't get away from the bedside long enough to meet their physiological needs (for example, bathroom breaks), and were unable to get adequate rest and sleep. The pandemic threatened their sense of safety because of the risk of infection, concerns regarding personal protective equipment (PPE), and often doubts as to whether they could manage to work within this very stressful environment. The availability of PPE was a major worldwide stress. It was suggested that masks be used for longer wear without any scientific evidence to substantiate the use being promoted and no clear information provided to address the anxiety of risk with this practice. The emotional anguish was there with no clear and, seemingly at times, no honest acknowledgement by those in leadership roles that no answers existed because the answers could not be known. The impact of seeing nightly reports of worldwide COVID-19 fatalities and personally witnessing the number of colleagues becoming ill was indicative to health care workers of the infectivity and of their lack of knowledge about adequately protecting themselves.

Family and friendships play a major role in one's sense of belonging and being loved. Everyone treasures the time they spend with their loved ones. Health care workers are no different in this aspect. They may in fact rely even more on these bonds in view of their exposure as professionals to challenging and traumatic situations, even in usual times. Such circles of care entail bidirectional relationships of giving and taking but also of protection. The fear as a family member of bringing additional risk of falling ill and harming their loved ones by exposing them to COVID-19 because of their work as a health care professional and/or causing their family additional worry and fear because they were working with COVID-19 patients was very real. Health care workers who could not discuss their perception of the risk and distress they experienced with their loved ones, often due to a perceived or actual need to not distress family members or those who felt alienated, were found to be more anxious.[7] Colleagues were often a common source of support, and yet with restrictions in gathering and overall fatigue, it was difficult to have the interactions that lead to dialogue, comfort, and camaraderie. Not fully sharing information can lead to an uncomfortable sense of apprehension and stress, which impacts overall functioning. Without the support of family and friends, who are the basic framework of support, striving towards higher levels such as self-esteem, confidence, and self-actualization can be difficult and possibly not attainable.

Self-esteem for the work being done was highlighted early on by society, but health care workers continued to have doubts and concerns as to the appropriate care of patients with COVID-19. They often agonized over decisions made and experienced moral distress when faced with limited resources. The sense of overwhelming distress was sadly manifested by the loss of life of some health care workers who took their own lives. Health care workers looked towards organizational support, which they anticipated would be there for them in the same way as they were there for their organization. But often they expressed disappointment about the lack of reciprocity.

Work carried out early in the pandemic at the University of Stanford identified that health care workers were asking for several things: to be heard, to be protected, to be prepared, to be supported, and to be cared for by their organizations.[8] Unfortunately, many of these needs were not fulfilled in the early days of the pandemic, resulting in severe stress, isolation, disenchantment, lack of trust, self-doubt, and anxiety about the future. There was a need for transparency, honesty, and addressing controversies openly. People were often reassured when it was admitted that the evidence for such reassurance was lacking, might be oversimplified, or was based on assumptions that may in time be proven false. As the pandemic progressed, many of the earlier challenges were addressed; however, many of the feelings of health care workers continued to be impacted by the experience of the early days of the pandemic, which had affected overall trust. As time went on, organizations got better at searching for supplies, strengthening supply chains, and obtaining timely access to vaccines for staff and their families. Organizations started to address high patient volumes and the triage of surgical services to assist those in areas that had particularly experienced distress. There is a necessity to identify the needs of the individual – to be happy, supported, healthy, and able to reach goals outside of the hospital setting within their community and their family.

Consequences

In a poll of 1000 health care workers conducted in September 2021, 18 per cent had left their jobs, and 19 per cent had considered leaving their health care position.[9] The system continues to require a large number of health care workers who are being lost to the system during a time when we are seeing COVID-19 surges and still face pent-up need for surgeries and care. The newspapers and media are filled with stories of resignations and units being closed, of patients being turned away or not receiving timely surgical treatments because of human health resource issues. Numerous teams are understaffed, emergency departments are in crisis, and patients are suffering.

Even before COVID-19, health care workers were suffering from exhaustion and burnout. Burnout is exhaustion brought on by prolonged or repeated stress, often in an occupational environment, which results in emotional, cognitive, and physical symptoms frequently leading to a low sense of personal accomplishment at work. Burnout is not an individual mental health diagnosis but is considered an occupational syndrome. It is a distinct workplace phenomenon that primarily calls for systems-oriented organizational-level solutions in a system that was previously already struggling, now impacted by the pandemic. A lack of success and stress in one's professional life can lead to increased dissatisfaction at home, as well as broken relationships, and can precipitate depression and suicide.

As highlighted, one of the most important aspects in a person's life, be they a health care worker or not, is reaching the level of self-actualization. Between COVID-19 surges, health care workers started to review their goals and their purpose – what was important to them in their life. Health care workers had the chance to breathe and to think about who they are as a person, what motivates them, and what they want to achieve in the long term. What became apparent was that many who had been in the health care system felt they could no longer achieve these higher levels of self-actualization within the system. This realization has led to a crisis in health care. It would be important for organizations to consider each health care worker as a person impacted by numerous personal variables and professional self-esteem. The U.S. Surgeon General's advisory report on health care worker burnout has identified the importance of the workplace culture.[10] The culture must be one that addresses the needs of the worker and builds a culture of safety in the work environment in order to be a path towards decreasing burnout and moral distress.

Maslow's hierarchy of needs can only be successfully achieved when both the individual professional and the organization work together to address these needs. Possible interventions for the hierarchical needs[11] include examples such as physiological aspects required for the individual to focus on time management to meet basic self-care needs, whereas the organization could promote an effective workflow strategy; safety would be dependent on the individual utilizing rapid antigen testing, with the organization ensuring a secure PPE supply and access to testing. Respect for the individual needs to be acknowledged by including staff in decision-making and by appreciation expressed by leadership for the work of the health care workers during difficult times. Self-esteem is the key to positive mental health and well-being, and is a conduit to handling adversity and developing coping skills when faced with stressful events.

Individual health care workers need to feel empowered to recognize signs of distress in themselves as well as in their colleagues and to utilize resources that are available, such as family and friends, as well as professional resources when required. The health care system needs to provide space for health care workers to prioritize some time for themselves, to acknowledge the valuable work that they do, and to focus on the caring and positive aspects of their work – the reasons why they chose this work and why they are still there. Health care workers, like everyone, are people first and health care workers second. They care deeply about their patients but need to stay healthy so they can continue their work.

Where Do We Go from Here?

The changes needed to ensure that we retain an engaged and healthy workforce for the future are extensive and encompass numerous areas. As the news and personal experiences of health care workers has shown, health care workers are opting to leave the profession by retiring early, moving to part-time positions, and seeking out other careers where they can utilize their knowledge and experience.

Table 4.1 offers some suggestions to consider, based on Maslow's hierarchy.

The pandemic has made us aware of the need to address the system so that health care workers can thrive and excel in their work and their lives. As individuals, they have a personal requirement to strive to achieve life satisfaction, whereas organizations have an obligation to ensure that the work environment adds to the perception of self-worth of the individual.

Table 4.1. Ways to Meet the Maslow Hierarchy Needs of Health Care Workers

Needs	Tools to help meet the needs
Physiological	Time to meet basic self-care needs Understanding the need for relaxation, vacation Provision of respite centres Attention to staffing numbers and patient load Review of work-life balance by the individual and the organization
Safety	Devising safety plans grounded in scientific knowledge as it exists and that evolve as the science changes (includes PPE, work environment, cleaning procedures, etc.) Communicating the evolving understanding of risk to health care workers and their families Considering what measures can be taken by the organization to maintain the health of their staff and to decrease the risk of infecting their own families/friends Obtaining feedback from front-line staff regarding effectiveness of safety planning, challenges in rollout, gaps that haven't been addressed, and impact on workflow
Belonging	Valuing the contributions of all health care workers Listening to concerns of staff and suggestions Acknowledging the important role health care workers play and recognizing their training and experience Providing support for mental health stress that is easily accessible
Esteem	Including health care workers in decision-making, which acknowledges the valuable contribution of each individual staff member Providing opportunities equally to promote advancement and projects Appreciating the work that staff provide every day and expressing thanks on behalf of the organization
Self-actualization	Facilitating health care workers' abilities to use their expertise in improving the delivery of clinical care through the optimization of available resources Recognizing, valuing, and engaging health care workers' individual skill sets in ways that allow them to contribute to the organization's response and achieve their professional goals such as improving quality of clinical care, improving patient safety, improving communication with patients and families and the public, community outreach, devising and participating in research

REFERENCES

1. Kisely S, Warren N, McMahon L, Dalais C, Henry I, Siskind D. Occurrence, prevention, and management of the psychological effects of emerging virus outbreaks on healthcare workers: rapid review and meta-analysis. *BMJ*. 2020;369:m1642. https://doi.org/10.1136/bmj.m1642. Medline: 32371466.
2. Lai J, Ma S, Wang Y, et al. Factors associated with mental health outcomes among health care workers exposed to coronavirus disease 2019. *JAMA Netw Open*. 2020;3(3):e203976. https://doi.org/10.1001/jamanetworkopen.2020.3976. Medline: 32202646.
3. Styra R, Hawryluck L, McGeer A, et al. Surviving SARS and living through COVID-19: healthcare worker mental health outcomes and insights for coping. *PLoS One*. 2021;16(11):e0258893. https://doi.org/10.1371/journal.pone.0258893. PMID: 34758047.
4. Rossi R, Socci V, Pacitti F, et al. Mental health outcomes among frontline and second-line health care workers during the coronavirus disease 2019 (COVID-19) pandemic in Italy. *JAMA Netw Open*. 2020;3(5):e2010185. https://doi.org/10.1001/jamanetworkopen.2020.10185. PMID: 32463467.
5. Maslow AH. *Motivation and Personality*. Harper and Row; 1954.
6. Kolko-Rivera ME. Rediscovering the later version of Maslow's hierarchy of needs: self-transcendence and opportunities for theory, research, and unification. *Rev Gen Psychol*. 2006;10(4):302–17. https://doi.org/10.1037/1089-2680.10.4.302
7. Styra R, Hawryluck L, McGeer A, et al. Support for psychological distress in health care workers: thinking about now and beyond the COVID-19 pandemic. *Health Promot Chronic Dis Prev Can*. 2022;42(10):421–30. https://doi.org/10.24095/hpcdp.42.10.01. PMID: 35766916.
8. Shanafelt T, Ripp J, Trockel M. Understanding and addressing sources of anxiety among health care professionals during the COVID-19 pandemic. *JAMA*. 2020;323(21):2133–4. https://doi.org/10.1001/jama.2020.5893. PMID: 32259193.
9. Galvin G. Nearly 1 in 5 healthcare workers have quit their jobs since COVID-19 hit US. *Morning Consult*, 4 October 2021. https://morningconsult.com/2021/10/04/health-care-workers-series-part-2-workforce/
10. Office of the Surgeon General. *Addressing Health Worker Burnout: The U.S. Surgeon General's Advisory on Building a Thriving Health Workforce*. US Department of Health and Human Services; 2022. https://www.hhs.gov/sites/default/files/health-worker-wellbeing-advisory.pdf. PMID: 37792980.
11. Hawryluck L, Styra R. ICU mental health in the ongoing pandemic: how will we be okay? *ICU Management and Practice*. 2021;21(2):78–82. https://healthmanagement.org/c/icu/issuearticle/icu-mental-health-in-the-ongoing-pandemic-how-will-we-be-okay

5 COVID-19 on the Front Lines: Mental Health and Resilience

Peter G. Brindley, MD, FRCPC, FRCP
Professor of Critical Care Medicine, Adjunct Professor of Anesthesiology, Adjunct Professor, John Dossetor Health Ethics Centre, University of Alberta, Edmonton

Submitted 5 July 2022

Health care workers performed superbly during the COVID-19 pandemic, but our collective mental health likely took a beating. What's more, I suspect the effects could be every bit as long lasting as the putative physical symptoms of long COVID. By year 2, as COVID continued its march through the Greek alphabet, the cumulative effort became obvious, and staff were harder and harder to find. Furthermore, those who turned up were quicker to anger and more openly voicing their desire to quit.

Even when we did not have an especially crushing week, it felt exhausting. Some of us took to a debrief or "emotional pat down" before we returned to the "real world." These check-ins confirmed we were all tired – fair enough. What was more concerning was an unfamiliar sense of despondency and listlessness. Perhaps it was because, after 2 years of a pandemic, even an average week adds to the toll. Perhaps it was a combination of so much unnecessary death but more institutionalized deaths with families more excluded than ever before. Perhaps this despondency was simply what it feels like being a half-century old and a quarter-century at work. Perhaps it's because health care is a peculiar job that reliably includes sadness and sleep deprivation.

This chapter is adapted from Peter G. Brindley's editorial, "Wellness and Resilience: Beyond Buzzwords and BS," published in the *Canadian Journal of Emergency Nursing*, 2022;45(3):E1–E2. Used with permission.

Perhaps, perhaps, but the bigger point is that these gnawing frustrations require more than a coffee card and an occasional weekend off. They also appear to be widespread and commonly discussed around the proverbial watercoolers (ironically, the literal watercoolers have been removed because of COVID). Regardless, it's not just the staff, and it's not just the patients, and it's not just the families: for once, we really were all in this together.

Personal well-being matters before, during, and after pandemics, but we have plenty of work to do on this portfolio if we wish to attract the next generation of workers. It is not only a matter of looking after ourselves so that we can look after our patients. After all, it is well recognized that fatigued, burned out, and otherwise frazzled health care workers make more mistakes and cost the system more. In short, to do well you must be well. Ergo, a physician lacking resiliency could be a danger to patient care. If so, then physician heal thyself and do so STAT.

Fortunately, during COVID, there were no shortage of articles, committees, and workshops telling us how to grow our resilience. Unfortunately, who had (or has) the blinking time? We have been told that resiliency is a muscle, so get out there and train. We are told that mindfulness starts with peace and quiet, so pretzel into that lotus position now. We know we need to exercise, ought to meditate, and need to rebuild the dam before the next storm. However, when exactly are we supposed to find the time, and how much of our hard-slogged money ought we to spend?

As summarized in the 2019 book *McMindfulness: How Mindfulness Became the New Capitalist Spirituality*, Well-being (with a capital W) has now become an industry with products to shift. It also has its high priests and lowly sinners. It has also morphed into a moral requirement during off hours rather than a non-judgmental aid. No more eating ice cream in your underwear or drooling on the couch while snoozing to Netflix. No dear Doctor, get out there and seize some wellness – you owe it to your patients. Come on, be better!

Often things are best defined by what they are not. If so, then it's worth knowing that antonyms of resilience include fragility and weakness. However well intentioned, it felt like not engaging in this resilience culture (or is it a cult) comes with a faint odour of failure. It might also fuel a vicious cycle ("Oh no, now I also suck at meditation"). For a profession already driven by insecurity and the imposter syndrome, we didn't need these further admonishments. I suspect that some also ended up in an exhausting catch-22. In other words, we were working on resiliency during time when we should really be working at nothing at all. The point is, as a profession we needed to learn that we don't always have to "do"; sometimes we need to take time just to "be."

The resiliency industry also distracted us from awkward but necessary questions. For example, why does this job require so much (insert your own expletive) resilience in the first place? Have we actually set ourselves up for longevity and success, or merely undertaken a 30-year endurance test? Why does our lack of resiliency feel like a personal failing akin to the 65 per cent we got in chemistry? To be fair, many areas of medicine have recognized our collective pathology and made amends. Unfortunately, however, this recognition tends to be in places where there is a glut of staff and trainees to share and shoulder the load. For others, we lean in ever harder, keep ever quieter, and leave the building with little left for our long-suffering spouses and bewildered kids.

Medicine is a challenging and, at times, wonderful career, no ifs, ands, or buts. Moreover, many other jobs are similarly challenging but without our job security or societal prestige. As such, it is important not to moan. Regardless, one of the issues peculiar to health care is that, to be truly empathetic, we often take a small dose of the patient's poison ourselves. In other words, we need to let it in to understand it. Neuroscientists would explain this idea by talking about mirror neurons. In simple terms, these neurons re-create a small copy of the sadness within ourselves as the first part of fashioning a response. Resilience is desperately needed for these situations and so that we can truly care for patients, not merely process them through.

Resilience shouldn't be a buzzword or a product to buy. It should also not be a crafty technique to enable you to survive crushing work hours and chase almighty bucks. For too long we have avoided frank discussions about our work environment and what drives us to work the way we do. We may have helped many patients, but we have no doubt harmed some too. We have also harmed ourselves and modelled dysfunctional behaviour from one generation to the next. In other words, before, during, and after COVID, we are both victims and perpetrators, and everybody and nobody is to blame. It would be a very fitting legacy from COVID that we commit to doing better so that we can finally feel better.

6 Trauma and Trepidation: The Emotional and Moral Toll of Dealing with Sick Patients

Matyas Hervieux, BSc (Hons), DHS, MA, MD, CCFP(EM)
Department of Emergency Medicine, University Health Network, Toronto

Submitted 18 October 2022

The period before the onset of COVID-19 and the arrival of actual COVID patients in our emergency departments was extremely stressful because we knew we were not adequately prepared. We did not have the right personal protective equipment (PPE); we did not have appropriate isolation procedures or decontamination procedures; we did not have a way to protect ourselves from our colleagues in cramped working conditions, lunchrooms, washrooms, and shared spaces. We had no way to protect ourselves, let alone our patients in waiting rooms or adjoining clinical areas, from COVID.

We also had been severely beaten down and demoralized by our public institutions – governmental agencies and public health – and the institutions we worked for – hospitals, nursing homes, ambulatory care centres – which we had expected to help prepare us for COVID patients and protect us from COVID once these patients arrived. When the realization hit us that these institutions had neither prioritized our safety nor listened to our voices as we shared our knowledge and expectations about how to respond to COVID, the result was that, even before COVID patients arrived through our doors, many of us were feeling the betrayal, anger, and disillusionment that accompanies institutional trauma (trauma that results from institutional acts of omission or commission that can worsen the effect of a traumatic experience or cause trauma as a result of violating the dignity or safety of a worker).

Once COVID patients began to flood our Emergency Department doors, the fallout from institutional trauma – caused by unsafe workplaces; variable, confusing, and illogical PPE policies; and a lack of consultation with front-line teams – was intensified. Obviously, not all patients who presented with COVID were gravely ill; many had moderate flu-like symptoms. But the uncertainty and the potential for severe outcomes, mechanical ventilation, and death magnified the terror patients felt. For clinicians, we similarly felt frightened as we hoped that our protocols and limited resources would be sufficient to protect us. Without vaccinations, we were all vulnerable to the full effect of this virus.

When patients began to present in respiratory distress, the reality and scariness of the situation intensified. It was clear that many of these patients, given their comorbidities, would not survive. Many were elderly with families who lived in different cities (or out of country) and trying to provide information and expectations to their family members over the phone was problematic. The "no visitor" policies at most institutions also meant that health care providers became surrogate family members for patients who would otherwise have been isolated and alone when they were seriously ill and as they were dying. Though no visitor policies were made public, we became the gatekeepers who had to tell family members that they were not permitted to see their sick loved ones, even though such a visit may have been their last chance to see their loved one and say goodbye.

In addition to the personal pain associated with refusing these visits, this gatekeeper role inverted the normal advocacy role we play for our patients and put providers in opposition to family members and patients. The impact of the desperation and hostility that family members and patients expressed towards us was intensified by our having to act against our own individual cultural and personal expectations about access to loved ones when they are dying. Many providers struggled with denying families these opportunities.

Yet, we were even put at odds with many patients who had minor symptoms. Many patients simply did not have enough sick days to be off work for 2 weeks or simply could not afford to miss work: they were living paycheck to paycheck. Yet, we had to be the gatekeepers who would tell a patient who felt well enough to work that they could not; patients who disregarded instructions would be reported to public health.

Similarly, many patients with flu-like symptoms arrived at the hospital expecting admission, either in hopes of being monitored in the event they deteriorated or in hopes of being in a safe place where they would not have to worry about infecting their families. Many were angry to be told that their oxygen saturations were too high to qualify them for admission. The instructions to return to the Emergency Department if they were feeling even worse and could not breathe aroused frustration and anger from many patients. Those patients who were caring for sick family members or who lived with elderly parents or partners were in a particularly hard situation: they were not allowed to stay in hospital and had no choice but to go home and potentially infect their loved ones. Many who lived alone were frightened to be alone. Again, as the gatekeepers for admission, emergency physicians were seen as insensitive and mercenary, and many patients outwardly expressed their frustration. Sadly, patients and their families simply were too angry to understand how difficult it was for us, at times, to send them home.

In addition, many of us felt the wrath of family members who became enraged when their loved ones – who presented to hospital with a non-COVID illness – died in hospital from COVID contracted due to a hospital exposure. In addition to dealing with the loss of our patients and their families' anger, we also had to deal with our feelings of failure and anger at inappropriate hospital and public health policies that caused many of these avoidable deaths.

The entire situation was made even more difficult because of patients and family members who were "COVID deniers." These patients and family members would become aggressive and verbally abusive when they were told that they had COVID or that their loved ones were likely to die of COVID. Many became threatening and accusatory, suggesting that we were not looking hard enough to find the real cause of their or their loved one's illness and angry that we were refusing to provide antibiotics. They were angry that their entire family needed to be isolated and would threaten to send, or did send, their children to school, even though their families were COVID-positive. This hostility had two effects: our workplace became even more unsafe, and it further intensified our disillusionment. Now, we were not only disillusioned by our policymakers and administration but also by members of our own community. Our efforts seemed disrespected on many fronts.

There was also the reality of how exposure to COVID patients negatively affected our own lives. The likelihood of infecting our loved ones before we had symptoms of COVID was real. We all had to establish our own "disinfection" routines before going home: many of us changed our clothing in garages or front porches, and we established elaborate routines to prevent contaminating our homes. Since most hospitals were already short staffed, there was also particular onus on us to not get COVID from our families, so when family members were sick, we either slept in garages, porches, or hotels (which in themselves were a risk).

Many of us were mandated, when outbreaks occurred in our institutions, to live in hotels. Others were redeployed or lived with the threat of redeployment, which meant that many clinicians were being asked to practise outside of their usual scope of knowledge and skill – for example, psychiatrists working as emergency or intensive care unit (ICU) nurses! This practice caused a lot of anxiety and stress for providers and patients alike. It was also, perhaps, especially difficult for hospital shift workers to have children at home since working from home was not an option, and hospitals were unable (or unwilling) to work around childcare needs.

Another serious issue that came to the forefront when COVID patients started to arrive with serious illness was the potential for moral injury among health care providers and the consequence to health care providers' mental health as a result of this exposure. Moral injury is defined as a strong cognitive and emotional response to events and situations that violate a person's moral or ethical code and can arise from actions or, when actions are required, the lack of action of a person themselves or of others. In medicine, moral injury can be experienced when the standard of care is breached, when its quality is poor, when health care workers perceive they are being asked to act against their professional ethical code, and when their personal safety is knowingly placed at risk and/or compromised. Moral injuries can result in loss of trust, changes in perception of self and others, and feelings of guilt, shame, and decreased self-worth. These changes may in turn lead to social withdrawal and self-destructive behaviours such as alcohol, sleeping pills, substance misuse, and even depression, suicide, and post-traumatic stress disorders (PTSDs).

Indeed, even before these patients arrived, our pre-pandemic planning made it clear that both seasoned and new front-line workers would likely experience moral injury. Part of our ongoing pandemic "training" was constant reminders and triage guidelines/instructions about the potential need for ethical triaging and resource allocation, especially for ventilators and end-of-life care. These conversations, for many physicians, caused extreme moral distress: there is no appropriate training that can prepare a provider (intensivist, emergentologist, hospitalist, family physician, respirologist, and so on) to deal with the idea of having to "play God" and decide who lives and who dies.

Even for those workers without decision-making powers (nurses, respiratory therapists, registered practical nurses, and the like), these conversations were traumatic because they could not advocate for their patients or advocate for their patients with the expectation that their advocacy would be heeded. We also had to try to brace ourselves for the frustration and hostility we anticipated receiving from family members when informed of our decision to palliate instead of trying to resuscitate their loved ones. Combined, the realities of our health care system meant that, even before we were confronted with our first COVID patients, we were all facing terrible situations in which we would be forced to make decisions that prioritized resource allocation and survivability over our own emotional and moral inclinations.

When patients started to arrive, the reality of the severity of some patients' illness made this type of decision-making more difficult. In some instances, we were expected to have these conversations as a provider who had just met a patient in distress. Providers were expected to assess comorbidities and, on the spot, determine which patients were less likely to benefit from care and should therefore be denied a ventilator or other life support that they needed. We were, similarly, expected to immediately determine which patients would not receive life support should their condition worsen to the point of requiring it. Worse yet, given the nature of hospital restrictions, physicians would have to have these conversations, as mentioned, with families who were not allowed to visit or who had not even seen the condition of their family members who were in hospital. The limitations of phone calls or video calls to have these types of visits became quickly apparent.

The reality is that there is simply no training on how to refuse resources to a patient that would have likely been tried in other circumstances. Given the extremely high risk of moral injury in these scenarios, it is disappointing that triage guidelines were presented in a matter-of-fact manner by those providing the instruction – often in the form of Command Table/Ministry memos/directives, hospital info bulletins, or via clinician/non-clinical administrators, detailing how the triage plans would be operationalized – who in almost all cases would not themselves be having to make these types of decisions. Plans for operationalization were very inconsistent in approach, with wide variability over who would be making actual triage decisions; most placed the responsibility on the front-line physicians. Even before formal triage was needed, it was equally disappointing to have some critical care consults act in equally inconsiderate and dismissive ways as we tried to advocate for our patients whom we believed required critical care but were being denied.

In short, while there was acknowledgment that making these types of decisions would be difficult, there was no systemic support offered to mitigate the distress of front-line workers who were being asked to make these decisions nor any way to ensure consistency in patient assessments so that access to resources could be determined free from bias. This point regarding bias in clinical decision-making should not be overlooked; clinical decision-making has always been plagued by intentional and unintentional biases: ageism, nepotism, cronyism, systemic racism, sexism, classism, gender inequity, homophobia, and the like, despite efforts to make decision-making more objective. Unfortunately, health care workers are people and at baseline are subject to the same influences as everyone else in society, no matter their efforts to be unbiased. For many front-line workers, it quickly became clear that bias among clinicians influenced who received admission and potentially life-saving treatments and who did not. The antagonistic nature of this situation, whether bias informed the refusal for critical care or not, further demoralized front-line workers and caused deepening tensions among providers who had previously worked collaboratively as one team.

Moral distress was especially challenging for those who work in smaller communities. As they had only a few ventilators, if the health care system became overwhelmed and/or if people came to hospital so severely ill that they couldn't be transported to a larger centre, the likelihood of triaging ventilators for friends, family members, or other known community members would be a real-life possibility. Within rural areas, it was also clear that administrators and specialist physicians, who for the most part are often not originally from these communities, did not understand the lifelong and multigenerational connections that front-line staff (family and emergency physicians and nurses) have with the patients they see. There seemed to be a lack of empathy for the type of moral injury we were being asked to endure: we were not being asked to ethically triage "patients"; we were being instructed to "unethically" triage friends, family, co-workers, and neighbours. We were being asked to determine whether people we cared about lived or died by the use of some administrative algorithm.

Such a request to triage in tight-knit communities and the effect it would have on rural front-line workers seemed to be completely unappreciated by clinicians and policymakers at governmental tables. For many, it laid bare the very real differences in practice between larger cities and smaller communities – differences in what it means to be human and even humane as a health care worker. Future discussions should engage smaller community front-line workers in the development, implications, and implementation of any triage guidelines and discuss how steps will be taken to ensure smaller communities with fewer resources do not bear most of the burden of any limits placed on accessing resources. Moreover, supporting those tasked with making such decisions before, during, and after any period of triage must be discussed, and plans must be devised in any future planning.

The lack of understanding of the moral impact that front-line workers would endure as a result of poor policy and pandemic preparation seems to have been completely lost on our policymakers. The suggestion that guidelines or other clinical decision-making tools would allow providers to "objectively" triage our community members is simply part of an illusion perpetrated by decision-makers to deny the "subjective" harm front-line workers were being asked to experience. This type of administrative denial compounds moral injury with institutional trauma and only deepens the harm caused to front-line workers.

This problem is not a new phenomenon: in fact, soldiers, peacekeepers, police officers, and paramedics are faced with this type of dilemma on a regular basis. The fallout from a lack of appropriate policy in these fields is well documented: suicides, PTSD, substance abuse, and so on. While there has never been "objective" decision-making in medicine, the pandemic laid bare the truly "subjective" cost of clinical decision-making. But, for many of us, the suggestion that we "subjectively" somehow "ethically" triage those we know (or do not know) laid bare the inhumanity of the demands made of us by our decision-makers.

The result was that experienced staff left, and junior nurses and new hires were then asked to cope without the experience, skills, and guidance of senior nursing staff. Nurses who remained in emergency departments were often overwhelmed and stressed by their workloads and patient acuity even before the arrival of significant numbers of COVID-positive patients. As the pandemic progressed, the attrition in emergency departments inevitability increased under the strain of such a high-risk environment. A vicious cycle began and continues.

The manner in which public health measures were implemented half-heartedly and inconsistently within our communities, provinces, and country, in combination with inconsistent and non-responsive policies and procedures being implemented within our health care institutions (hospitals, ambulatory care clinics, nursing homes, and so on), sent a clear message to front-line workers that our policymakers were not committed to protecting front-line workers' health and safety, nor were they committed to protecting the large and ever-increasing number of patients we were treating. As the human consequences of these poor policies materialized, we came to fully appreciate the ramifications of having policymakers who were not committed to mitigating the effects of the pandemic to the fullest possible extent.

Clearly, there has been much talk about burnout among front-line workers during the pandemic. The assumption has been that, as the pandemic dragged on, the combination of fatigue, stress, and staffing shortages with the increased acuity of our COVID and non-COVID patients has contributed to this burnout. There has also been the suggestion that a lack of "normalcy" in our everyday lives and the isolation we all experienced during the pandemic has contributed to a deterioration of front-line workers' mental health.

But I believe that much of this "burnout" originates from moral injury and institutional trauma inflicted upon front-line workers: poor pre-pandemic planning left front-line staff feeling vulnerable and unsupported early on and throughout the pandemic, which resulted in continued psychological trauma and distress. I believe that this trauma and distress are the core reasons so many made the decision to leave their clinical practice. Sadly, the anxiety created from apparent mismanagement across all levels of government and public health/health care administration has created an unnecessary tension between front-line workers and these decision-makers. This tension will be unlikely to ever fully dissipate unless decision-makers are held accountable for the harm they have inflicted and policy changed to ensure that this type of trauma is eliminated, as much as possible, from our workplaces.

7 Compassion Fatigue: The Palliative Perspective

Sonia Malhotra, MD, MS, FAAP, FAAHPM
Associate Professor, Internal Medicine and Pediatrics, Tulane University School of Medicine, New Orleans

Submitted 20 September 2022

The Blur of Life

I don't know where the past two and a half years went. I remember the blur of early morning awakenings, leaving my home at 4:30 a.m. to make sure I made it to work by 5 a.m. so I could start rounds in the medical intensive care unit (MICU) and trauma ICU (TICU). Exactly 9 days after Mardi Gras, our first COVID-19 patient came in. New Orleans was one of the first cities to surge with this unknown virus. We had boards all over the ICUs to indicate which patients were followed by our service line, the palliative medicine team. As the first surge of the COVID-19 pandemic progressed, more "P's" with a circle showed up on the boards to indicate more and more patients being followed by my team. My team expanded with borrowed members from other areas of the hospital that had been shut down. We quickly developed protocols and algorithms for symptom management, end-of-life care, goals of care conversations, medical updates, video visits, and documentation. As the medical director of the service line, I had to think about the safety of my own team members, and I changed us to a 7-day-per-week service (from 5 days per week) and staggered my members coming in to work versus working from home. Our trainees all worked from home. But at 9 a.m. each day, we gathered in person, socially distanced from each other or on the phone, to talk about our growing patient list. At one point, I remember our list (which usually was approximately twenty-five to thirty patients) climbing to ninety patients. I wasn't sure how we would manage such a high volume and do this work on a daily basis.

Keeping the Candle Burning

In the world of palliative medicine, we have proven ourselves as physicians and teams that care for ANY patient living with a serious illness, with a special focus on symptom management, communication around goals of care, and emotional support. But in those first few months of the pandemic, the amount of death and dying we saw was tremendous – and heartbreaking. Even for a group like ours that was used to death and dying, it was a lot of death to manage in such a short period of time. Some people helped us through and asked us how we were doing. Others asked us to keep pushing through and caring for others, especially for our ICU teams, to make sure they were OK. And through it, we felt like we were lighting candles daily to keep a flame going for our patients, families, colleagues, and ourselves to keep pushing through day by day. We lifted each other up, checking in on one another, and communicating as frequently as we possibly could. We worked together, rounding alongside our ICUs and meeting daily with our hospitalist colleagues to ensure protocols were being followed and families were being given updates. During that first surge, local organizations brought in food, and kids sent cards. Our hospital and medical student organizations secured personal protective equipment (PPE) for us. We all had to find ways to care for each other, and no deed was too small to lift each other up.

Functioning Like a Brake Pad

I remember the daily struggles of managing life. From my start at 5 a.m., I would make it home by 12 p.m. so my husband could get to his full-time medical director job. I would then continue the tasks of virtually schooling three children. I was particular about returning home, taking my shoes off outside, and going straight upstairs to change my clothes and shower for fear of transmitting an unknown infection to my family. While my youngest napped, I made as many phone calls as I possibly could to families. The operators knew me well. Each time I called them for an outside line, they asked, "Doc, you OK?" Oftentimes, the conversations with families were short medical updates. Sometimes, they were long and full of complex emotions. I often felt like a shock absorber to the varied responses I got. With visitor restrictions in full effect, there was no way for families to see their loved ones. Although we had put together several methods of communication, such as a weekly televideo visit so families could see their loved ones and a daily text messaging service for medical updates, it was not enough. I didn't blame the families – it wouldn't have been enough for me either.

Brakes on a car are designed with pads that serve as shock absorbers. Over time, the pads wear thin, and then there is no absorption of the shock that the brakes place on stopping the car. I often felt my brake pads were wearing thin. There were so many things out of my control, and while I was absorbing this shock, I didn't have a replacement set of brake pads. In that time, all I could do was look at my children. Their lives changed with the closure of schools, the inability to do activities with other kids, and having to utilize screens to interact with others. My husband and I live far from our families, and we served as the core for our kids. Anytime I felt low or that I couldn't absorb any more, I looked at my kids, and they filled me up. When I imagined their lives changing so drastically, I was pushed to create some semblance of normalcy for them and myself. I knew I couldn't change much for the families I spoke to. However, I could serve as that normalcy from the hospital, the familiar voice that called them each day and spoke to them.

The New Normal

Walking saved me from feeling low. For the first 6 to 9 months of the pandemic, I walked with my family on the weekends. Despite the frequent phone calls from the hospital and text messages from my colleagues organizing who would be calling which families (since we were all pitching in to cover 7 days per week), we took our kids and walked for 5 miles.* Our youngest was in his stroller, and our older children took their scooters. It felt nice to see people getting out to see the sun and feel the air. It felt refreshing to feel something outside of the hospital's closed-off rooms, the IV poles that cluttered the hallways, and the constant beeping noises. Despite the sweltering southern heat that drenched our clothes and tanned our skin, and sunscreen that left a film, we walked and walked and walked. To this day we walk – not the same 5 miles† but we have incorporated walking as a weekly practice. And I remember each one of my colleagues and I speaking about the practices we adopted to keep us going. Some of us had weekly video calls with our families and friends; others walked or ran; and those who had

---

* 8 kilometres.
† 8 kilometres.

family or friends nearby held outdoor gatherings to feel some form of connection. We built any connection we could to the real world that felt so far away when we stepped foot in the doors of the hospital. To this day, despite multiple COVID-19 surges, many of us keep those weekly practices. It feels like an engrained response to what could happen again at any point in time with any new disease that comes through.

The Devil

Compassion fatigue (CF) is emotional and physical exhaustion from repeated stress leading to a diminished ability to empathize or feel compassion for others, often described as the negative cost of caring.

Professionals in health care who are regularly exposed to the traumatic experiences of the people they serve have a combination of secondary traumatic stress (STS) and cumulative burnout (CB), and are at high risk for compassion fatigue. CF can lead to symptoms of exhaustion, anger, irritability, inability to feel empathy, and an overall decreased satisfaction with work, often leading to absenteeism and impaired decisional abilities. Other terms that have been used to describe CF include vicarious traumatization (VT). However, compassion fatigue is the result of CB and STS that is not mediated by compassion satisfaction, a method to mitigate and transform negative aspects of a job towards the positive.

The Devil. That is what I was called by a family member during the second surge when I asked her to wear gloves and an N95 mask while she went in to say her goodbye to her dying father. She was unvaccinated, as was her father, who had contracted COVID-19, likely from a large gathering. Once 2021 rolled around and we had access to vaccines, much of health care became a political war ground. Many people proudly announced their unwillingness to "receive the jab." We saw patient after patient come in with severe COVID-19 who had access to a vaccine – and yet chose not to receive it. A few patients still stick with me, including the home nurse who was seeing patients with COVID-19 and was not vaccinated. That patient died, leaving two children behind, including one who was graduating from high school. Though we live in a global world, it was tough to imagine that, in our country, people were willing to be unvaccinated, while in other countries that lacked access to the vaccine, people were pleading to receive supplies of it to protect their own.

When I think about compassion fatigue, I don't think about the first surge of the pandemic, even with as much uncertainty and disruption of routines that occurred. CF certainly felt more pervasive during subsequent pandemic surges. Once we identified how to better treat the COVID-19 virus, once restrictions started lifting, once families had an ability to come in and see their loved ones, it felt like the anger towards us health care clinicians worsened. The food and kind cards thanking us for the work we were doing stopped. Our families, who spent months socially isolated from others, didn't hold back from blaming us for their loved ones getting the virus.

There was not enough compassion satisfaction for many of us taking care of patients who refused to listen to public health guidance. It was sad, frustrating, and challenging all at once to see patient after patient who refused to get the vaccine. These patients were very sick and died in large numbers. Many of my colleagues felt the effects of cumulative burnout. Not only were they caring for people who didn't want to listen to medical guidance, but they were also being yelled at, sometimes spit on, and for a few, followed when leaving the hospital. In a profession where we learn from day 1 to be compassionate towards those whom we serve, our own safety was threatened. It was hard to be compassionate when we ourselves were experiencing a heightened sense of mistrust, anger, and even danger aimed at our lives.

Many people working in health care left altogether. The constant harassment and fear of losing your life at the hands of patients and families were too much. Since then, the workforce has not recovered. Systems have been scrambling to find people to work. In some states where violence against health care workers has occurred (such as mine), laws were put into place to protect nurses, physicians, and other health care workers.

There is a body of research studying compassion fatigue and methods to mitigate it, and yet one thing is clear: *we haven't figured it out*. Simply, if we had better answers for it, we wouldn't be losing so many health care workers. And yet, when I think back to my experiences with COVID-19, I am reminded that, the more we checked in on one another, the more we acknowledged each other and our daily contributions, which led us all to feel more comfortable during a time of high uncertainty. I am reminded that, when I reframed what I could into something more controllable, I felt more at ease with the uncertainty of work every day. When I felt gratitude for what I could do with my children and at work, I felt like I was making some form of impact. When our health care systems allowed us to be fluid and flexible with staffing, we lost fewer people from health care altogether. Most importantly, when I felt that my workplace was doing the right thing by securing PPE, supporting structures to support health care workers, and communicating with us, I felt I was an important part of the mission that we all were a part of.

As patients and families, how do we help clinicians fight compassion fatigue? As health care systems and fellow clinicians, how do we help our own fight compassion fatigue? I don't pretend to have the answers, and yet I remember that, each and every day during the COVID-19 surges, I reminded myself to do the things that kept me going. I needed my colleagues to check in on me, to validate that it was OK to not be OK. I needed fluidity and flexibility to be a doctor and to take care of my children. Empathy and sustainable structures helped make the unbearable somewhat bearable.

I listened to "Hymn for the Weekend" each and every day as I drove into work. My "Hymn for the Weekend" became my daily hymn that helped me keep my feet on the ground.

PART TWO

Scarcity

The pandemic gave rise to stresses on the health care system not seen in generations, often resulting in a lack of the fundamental elements of patient care: staff, space, equipment, and medications. This section, "Scarcity," is a collection of accounts of the efforts to prevent, deal with, or simply adapt to these various shortages. "The Last Bed: Triage and Triage Avoidance" describes the moral, ethical, and philosophical challenges underpinning the concept of "triage" and the struggles with allocating the last of finite resources, knowing the effects on those who are excluded. "PPE During COVID-19: Scarcity, Science, Logistics, and Paper Bags" is an account of the sometimes mad scramble within a large hospital to obtain the proper protective equipment for its staff, and how creative solutions and the stretching of material to previously inconceivable extremes became necessary. "OMG, We Are Running Out of Propofol!" provides the pharmacists' perspective to the baffling and seemingly unending drug shortages during the pandemic – the perspective of those tasked with breaking the news to physicians that bedrock drugs were simply not available and with providing workarounds, alternatives, and rationing plans.

8 The Last Bed: Triage and Triage Avoidance

James Downar, MDCM, MHSc, FRCPC
Head and Professor, Division of Palliative Care, and Clinical Research Chair in Palliative and End-of-Life Care, Faculty of Medicine, University of Ottawa; Adjunct Professor, Queensland University of Technology School of Law; Staff Physician, Department of Critical Care, The Ottawa Hospital; Investigator, Bruyère Research Institute

Bojan N. Paunovic, MD, FRCPC
Provincial Medical Specialty Lead, Adult Critical Care, Shared Health Manitoba; Medical Specialty Lead, Adult Critical Care, Winnipeg Regional Health Authority (WRHA); Section Head, Adult Critical Care, and Assistant Professor, Department of Internal Medicine, University of Manitoba; Site Critical Care Lead, Health Sciences Centre, Winnipeg; Past President, Canadian Critical Care Society

Submitted 10 August 2022

Philosophers, ethicists, politicians, and economists have long struggled with the question of how to fairly allocate a limited resource, whether food, water, fuel, or other necessity. In moments of crisis, resource allocation ethics take on an additional sense of importance as people are faced with the prospect of needing a resource and being told that it simply is not available. Critical care bed allocation is probably the most extreme health care–related example of a high-stakes crisis resource allocation problem, so clinicians, ethicists, and other key stakeholders had tried to prepare for this scenario through the development of protocols, which were then subject to discussion, revision, and testing in simulations for decades before the COVID-19 pandemic struck. However, despite all the time and energy spent preparing for this scenario, it is fair to say that nobody was truly prepared to deal with this possibility when it happened.

The scene in early 2020 was chilling. Reports from China suggested that we were facing a highly infectious virus with a relatively high probability of progression to critical illness that lasted longer than most other viral illnesses and had a higher overall mortality. China's acute care capacity had been rapidly overwhelmed, and they were building hospitals as quickly as possible. Northern Italy was next, and their critical care capacity was also overwhelmed in a matter of weeks. Stories emerged of heartbreaking decisions being made at the bedside: refusing to give a ventilator to someone because of their age or comorbidity, or taking a ventilator from one person to give to another who was more likely to survive. (Note: these stories emerged in the media and were reported online, but we cannot independently confirm to what extent these decisions occurred.) Northern Italy has one of the highest standards of critical care in the world, with intensive care unit (ICU) capacity similar to that seen in North America and elsewhere in Europe. If Italy was overwhelmed, what chance did any of us have?

It was at this point that many jurisdictions started looking in earnest at their own ICU bed allocation plans and making them public whenever possible. This analysis led to two types of problems: (1) the realization that there was no plan; or (2) the realization that the plan itself was problematic. One of the most notable problems with existing plans was that they had been developed with an influenza pandemic in mind and were therefore heavily based on acute illness severity indicators that were found to be unreliable prognosticators for COVID and many other conditions.

But regardless of whether jurisdictions had a plan, needed a plan, or needed to update their plan, another substantial issue emerged. As people became aware of the potential for an overwhelming surge in demand for critical care, they started to react negatively to the contingency plans being developed. It must be noted that any resource allocation framework is going to be value-laden and controversial. As such, there is no single way to balance principles such as consequentialism (for example, trying to maximize lives saved) and non-discrimination (for example, limiting disproportionate effects of prioritization on different races, age groups, socio-economic groups, and so on). For that matter, people may reasonably disagree on what the most appropriate (or realistic) goal will be. If it is to improve overall survival, how is that to be defined? Does it refer to surviving the acute illness, surviving to ICU discharge, or surviving to a future time point? If the issue of "equity" is raised, there may be disagreement on whether equity means that some demographic groups should be prioritized over others in order to compensate for inequities in social determinants of health or perhaps for historical injustices. Everyone hopes to make the system fairer; the problem is that there is no unanimous view on what fairness looks like.

Questions at this level are interesting from an intellectual standpoint, but in a crisis, we are often forced to choose answers that reflect what options we have available to us. If we consider prognosis, we need to use the prognostic tools that we have rather than the ones we wish we had. If there is no means to objectively determine who belongs to a given demographic group in a matter of minutes (for example, race, education) or how to objectively balance competing forms of inequity (for example, gender vs sexual orientation vs poverty), then we may not be able to realistically incorporate these considerations into a time-sensitive prioritization system no matter how socially conscious or well-intended we might be.

But much of the discussion around prioritization did not centre on such practical or even value-laden considerations but rather on more basic issues. Some people were concerned that we did not have enough resources in the first place and suggested that the shortage was an indication of failure at the governmental level. Such criticisms are problematic: first, this critique is retrospective and does not offer a solution to the crisis; and second, critical care capacity depends on the availability of multiple contributors – space, supplies, and most importantly, qualified staff. That said, an approach that would have historically maintained substantial excess ICU capacity as a contingency for an unprecedented event would have been very costly and come at the expense of other important priorities that affect health outcomes.

However, early in the pandemic more discussion was inappropriately focused on the availability of ventilators and how this equipment should be rationalized – so much so that some so-called experts suggested more than one patient could be managed on the same equipment to mitigate potential triage. This example highlights the disconnect within both the medical and bioethics communities since this concern initially failed to recognize that, even if ventilator availability was unlimited, the appropriate provision of critical care is more dependent on appropriately trained staff than on pieces of equipment. As such, a neglected area of discussion in both areas was consideration of models of care delivery that could be adjusted to accommodate increased numbers of patients but minimally affect care.

Others were upset at the idea of any prioritization scheme, particularly one that would favour those more likely to survive. They argued that this concept was morally wrong, that it valued some lives over others, or even that it was a violation of human rights. Again, these criticisms are highly problematic because (among other things) they fail to consider the alternatives to the plan presented or the consequences of having no plan at all. The core injustice of a pandemic – that people who want critical care and who could be saved by critical care would not receive it – is the result of the pandemic itself rather than an attempt to mitigate the effects of the pandemic. When confronted by an overwhelming demand for critical care, there are literally only three options: (1) first come, first served; (2) purely random allocation; or (3) some form of prioritization. In all cases, people are denied critical care, including some who might have benefited from it. It is hard to argue that "first come, first served" is any fairer than a prioritization scheme. It is equally hard to argue for random allocation if it would result in more deaths overall. From a fairness perspective, if you feel that all lives are equally valuable, you should try to save as many as possible. If you choose a plan that results in fewer lives saved, you are effectively implying that some of those lives are more valuable than others. People may disagree with a given prioritization plan, but to critique that plan on the basis of human rights, they would have to present an alternative plan that would not violate human rights (or, at least, violate them to a lesser degree).

We also have to recognize the important role of the front-line health care providers and how they feel about the allocation system. In normal times, health care providers generally assign ICU beds on a first-come, first-served basis, with some degree of prioritization for particularly ill patients. From the experience in Italy, where there was no explicit prioritization scheme, clinicians began to prioritize beds based on an arbitrary, subjective assessment of mortality risk. They did not make these decisions because of an inherent character flaw but because the training and ethos of health care is to use resources to potentially save a life rather than to treat someone who is almost certain to die regardless. For that reason, health care providers would probably struggle or refuse to implement a plan that did not prioritize somewhat on the basis of mortality risk. Anecdotally, a frequent comment from front-line ICU providers pointed out the moral distress they felt at the idea of *not* using an approach that would save the most lives.

In the end, no jurisdiction has formally acknowledged using a prioritization scheme for ICU admission at any point. There are two possible explanations: either every jurisdiction had adequate ICU beds available for the entirety of the pandemic, or informal triage decisions were made without being acknowledged or approved. We will likely never know the extent to which informal triage may have taken place, but we may be able to estimate it based on retrospective data of those admitted and not admitted to the ICU.

The other key reflection point is the degree to which resources were shifted from other health care services to prioritize a "surge" in critical care in order to avoid a formal triage scenario. This "macro-triage," in which critical care was prioritized over organ transplantation, urgent surgery, or cancer care, likely affected large numbers of people and led to substantial morbidity and mortality. But we must be careful not to criticize the decision to reallocate services because we do not know the counterfactual – how much morbidity and mortality might have occurred if we had implemented a triage plan at some point. Ultimately, macro-triage decisions had to be made at a time when the magnitude of the surge was unclear. With the benefit of retrospective data, we may be able to estimate some of the short-term effects of these decisions, which may be helpful for informing future pandemic decisions.

But even before our retrospective data becomes available, there are some clear lessons that we can draw from an ethical standpoint. The bioethics community, which is positioned to discuss controversial topics and frame difficult decisions and to bridge the fields of philosophy, law, and health care, often struggled during the pandemic. Resource allocation is a core aspect of bioethical training and discourse, and yet many bioethicists refused to engage in practical discussions of ICU bed allocation frameworks. Others suggested that triage frameworks should only apply to those who consent to be part of them, which would of course convert any framework into a first-come, first-served approach. Some insisted that any prioritization scheme was a violation of the basic principles of human rights without providing any reference to support such a claim. Although the bioethics community has had decades to deliberate these issues, we still await viable alternatives to the prioritization plans that were discussed in the early parts of the pandemic. Resource allocation is about balancing priorities to achieve the best compromise and, ideally, the least harm. In that sense, people can only criticize the shortcomings or potential harms of a plan if they are able to present an alternative option with fewer shortcomings or potential harms.

However, perhaps the most justified critique is one of implementation. Even if a prioritization process was widely accepted, how could it be consistently and appropriately applied? The resources required to review, decide, and act on these types of decisions, even when well laid out, are considerable. Often these resources will need to draw from the very teams that are required to deliver care at a time when staffing would already be stretched. Navigating this issue requires pragmatic discussions that are not hindered by the above-mentioned concerns.

Many aspects of the pandemic have been unpleasant or even regrettable, and the knowledge and experience we have acquired has come at a significant cost. To assume that resources can be infinitely reallocated to prevent the need for allocation decisions would be neglectful. Hopefully, our experience with triage discussions and ICU bed allocation planning will catalyse ethical and legal discussions at a higher level to inform future decisions.

9 PPE During COVID-19: Scarcity, Science, Logistics, and Paper Bags

Steve A. McLaughlin, MD
Chief Medical Officer and Hospital Regents' Professor, University of New Mexico School of Medicine

Erik Kraai, MD
Associate Professor, Division of Pulmonary, Critical Care and Sleep Medicine, University of New Mexico School of Medicine

PPE Committee of the University of New Mexico School of Medicine

Submitted 26 August 2022

In March 2020, I saw my first case of SARS-CoV-2. That is what we called the virus back then. Apparently, it is the official name, although we were soon using the informal "COVID-19," "coronavirus," the "rona," and then eventually just "delta" and "omicron." The case I saw was one of the first ten cases in New Mexico. He was sick, struggling to breathe, and wearing a high-flow face mask with a procedure mask over the top. I saw him briefly, and I wore a procedure mask since he was in an isolation room and we weren't doing any high-risk aerosol generating procedures (AGPs). It's kind of shocking when I think back on that first patient and how much the world has changed and how much personal protective equipment (PPE) has changed. Out of an abundance of caution, and because we were cancelling all non-essential meetings, I worked from home for a bit after that case, and I isolated from my family. During that first week and while isolating, I did an interview with a national news outlet about COVID and talked about the way it felt to be on the front lines of the pandemic. It was like standing in the sand at the edge of the ocean and seeing the water recede (the Emergency Department [ED] was mostly empty in those days), knowing that there was a tsunami out there coming but we were not yet able to see it and that, knowing our line of work, we wouldn't be able to run for higher ground. Well, the news outlet mistakenly thought I *had* COVID, which is what was said to the entire country.

Oops. I got scores of texts from people I hadn't seen in years offering to send food and expressing concern for my life. Our hospital was also closely following the events taking place in New York City, and we worked around the clock to prepare for the patients that we expected to soon come into our ED needing our care and fighting to breathe. At the same time, our institution was quickly fit testing the front-line clinical staff to make sure everyone would have a properly fit N95 mask to use in high-risk situations. There were thousands of us needing to be tested and trained. What became apparent by the end of March 2020 was that we were burning through our PPE supplies, especially our N95 masks. We were using them at a rate that was going to exhaust our supplies in the first weeks of the pandemic, well before the peak of the first surge, which several staff who were later part of our PPE Committee pointed out:

> Early on in the pandemic was such a surreal experience. Being in New Mexico meant that we had the opportunity to see what was happening in other cities before we got hit with the pandemic. First Wuhan, China, then it spread throughout Europe, to New York and Seattle before finally taking over the rest of the world, including us. It was always the same stories: overwhelmed hospitals, not enough beds, ventilators, medical staff, and PPE. We certainly felt the calm before the storm: as the world shut down, hospital admissions for other things dramatically decreased, bringing down the census in our ICUs, normally at 100% capacity, down to about 50%. This, however, was short lived. First a couple COVID patients, then a few more, and soon our ICU was 100% full of COVID patients.

> During the early days of the pandemic, our supply chain team and I felt good about where we were, given that we had supplies set aside in a pandemic supply warehouse. We learned within the first week that our 45 days of normal supply was not going to be enough to support our hospital through COVID-19. Our inventories started to deplete almost immediately as staff were consuming the supplies at a rate that was not anticipated. When it became apparent that supply orders were not going to be filled, especially PPE supplies, a real sense of worry and concern set in as this was new territory for all of us. All the standard supply chain best practices and principles were no longer working, and the team had to pivot immediately into uncharted waters and develop its own processes

to overcome the strains brought on by the pandemic but also needed assistance to understand what was needed to ensure clinician and patient safety were considered during this time. That assistance came in the form of the PPE Committee.

On 29 March 2020, our institution created the PPE Committee as part of our Emergency Operations structure. The team included nurses, physicians from a variety of specialties, infection prevention professionals, residents, and logistics and supply experts. I think the entire group would agree that we were about to embark on a journey that, although difficult, would be one of the most powerful and positive experiences of our careers. We met every single day starting at 4:00 p.m., including weekends. Three days later, on 1 April, we released our first set of conclusions and our guiding principles:

Based on our work to date, we have the following conclusions:
1 Despite a strong logistics effort, two key kinds of PPE (N95 masks and eye protection) will be in critical short supply or completely gone within 2 weeks.
2 Available evidence suggests that simple (procedure) masks can help reduce the spread of COVID-19 within the workplace.
3 The staff and providers are highly concerned about their personal safety at work.
4 Existing PPE guidance on both supply and procedures is inconsistent, lacks unit-level specificity, and has not been communicated effectively to ensure confidence and compliance of providers and staff.
5 In most situations, droplet and contact precautions with eye protection are adequate to prevent transmission of COVID-19 to health care workers, meaning that, in the vast majority of instances, N95 masks are unnecessary.

Guiding principles:
- Keep health care personnel and patients as safe as possible.
- Be good stewards of our PPE through thoughtful use, cleaning, and reuse.
- Evolve our behaviours to both increase safety and reduce anxiety.
- Consolidate care (people/locations) to increase safety and reduce PPE use.
- Operate in a coordinated fashion internally and with our partners.

We also made this statement at the end of the official report: *"Finally, the committee requests urgent consideration of these recommendations. We have only 2–3 days to act if we are going to make an impact."* We were about 10 days away from running out of N95 masks.

> I remember walking in and watching a colleague of ours grab a whole box of masks because "who knows what's going on out at our community hospital" and being caught in this precarious place of knowing that behaviour wasn't sustainable but understanding where it came from. We locked down masks that day.

> Even as an ICU doc, I was certainly not immune to the anxieties and fears. I remember one of the first times I saw the green/yellow/red chart and heard that we had less than 10 days of N-95s on hand. It scared the heck out of me and made me feel helpless. I was also frustrated that many of my partners were angry and didn't believe me that we were doing everything we could to keep them safe. Again, being on the PPE Committee helped me with many of my own worries and concerns, allowing me to feel like I was "doing something" and also feel certain that the hospital was indeed doing everything it could to provide everyone with the best protection possible.

The institution acted quickly, and that week we had the logistics team take direct physical control of all N95 masks and eye protection. We limited N95 use to specific high-risk areas and used procedure masks in other areas. We generated specific PPE guidance for every single unit, area, and job description at the institution. Our guiding principles were essential. As we worked on supply, there were other aspects that became equally important, including the communication plan and transparency.

> I was pregnant early in the pandemic and so little was known about what impact COVID had on fetuses and pregnant women, so I was isolated from taking care of patients suspected of having COVID. My family was terrified when I would go into the hospital, and yet here I was on this committee helping to make protocols for how so many front-line people would be protected from this unknown entity. I remember feeling like a fraud – since I wasn't seeing the patients myself, I just felt like I really wasn't actually helping. And so it became really important to me that our committee drive forward efforts for transparency around supply and that we speak to our front line and answer people's questions. That we be specifically accountable for our decisions. There were times that accountability meant hard questions got asked, and I remember leaving a meeting with a particular group of staff and realizing how close they were with patients, how much anxiety they were feeling with that contact and with

our proposed PPE strategy. I remember meeting with our team afterwards and us asking hard questions of our own strategy. I think our committee's push for accountability and transparency made us better and taught me a lot about leadership. No one person on that committee had all the right answers all the time, but I think as a group we pushed forward, we listened, and we created something that was so needed at that time in our hospital. For me, it gave me a sense of purpose within that period of time that didn't replace the guilt I had but at least helped me through.

Because of the very real concern of running out of N95s, there was a big push to reuse masks and to save them for future cleaning and sterilization. Hospital units were purchasing Tupperware and paper bags so that their staff could preserve masks between duty periods. We had a whole team working on plans to sterilize masks for reuse, and we were reviewing every piece of literature that addressed the maximum number of duty periods for which a single mask could be used. Finally, we developed hospital-wide *daily* PPE reports and a communication plan to share with the entire workforce.

> PPE is a term most nurses and doctors use in our everyday work vocabulary but was not something we were accustomed to hearing outside of that setting. But here we were, seeing headlines talking about the shortage of PPE worldwide. Being a nurse in the COVID ICU, this made me feel increasingly nervous. It did not take long before rationing of the N95 masks began to take place, with ever-changing rules on when you could obtain a mask. I specifically remember a week where use of N95s had tightened so much that you were not given one if your patient was on a ventilator, the logic being that the virus should be maintained in a "closed circuit" inside the ventilator. While this logically made sense, the uneasy feeling of walking into these rooms without an N95 certainly put me on edge while spending 20 to 40+ minutes in the room. I was also hyper-aware of making sure the connections on the ventilator did not accidently get knocked loose, which can happen when patients are moving around. Thankfully, we quickly realized we could at least spare N95s for these situations as long as people used them for an extended amount of time. Joining the PPE Committee some weeks after this experience helped me feel empowered to advocate for my fellow ICU staff but was also incredibly humbling to see just how extensive this PPE problem was and all that everyone in the committee was doing to help mitigate this problem.

There was a deep disbelief that, here in the United States, we could truly be out of something that we needed. This experience was now common at the grocery store but was still hard for people to believe regarding medical supplies. Here is a communication from my daily email to our department from those first few months.

> Hello Team: With the announcement of the "stay at home" order this week, it seems that the good people of the world have gone to the stores and stocked up on all matter of items to get them through this next wave. I do understand that impulse. There is a bit of a stockpile/prep mentality in my family. For example, my parents have a gas-powered generator in suburban Seattle. Just in case. It is pretty funny that the toilet paper is cleaned out. Shelves empty. I can laugh at that. We have plenty of smooth rocks as a backup. But seriously, I have not been able to find half and half for the coffee. We are down to about 2 days' worth with no more to be found. Online ordering from Whole Foods, Target, and even the gas station mini-mart is out. I'm not kidding – this is troubling. We can get through almost anything but that is predicated on rolling out of bed, pulling two shots of espresso, adding cream, and preparing to face the day. I am freaking out … Plenty of broccoli though. Anyone have a cow? I am willing to work out a trade. Text me.

During the time when we were rationing N95 use, we had daily emails from staff members and providers telling us to just order more masks on Amazon or that they had seen masks for sale from a number of online vendors. There was so much anger and disbelief. The assumption was often that the hospital was just too cheap or not trying hard enough. The reality was that the country was simply out of masks at *any* price. That was an experience that most of us had never had in our professional or personal lives, so it was easier to blame someone than to embrace the reality that we were in a global pandemic and there just were not enough masks. That anger and frustration evolved over time from initially being focused on wanting PPE that we could not provide to ultimately not wanting to use the PPE that we were recommending.

> One of the things that struck me early on was the degree of anger that came from so much of the staff in the medical ICU. Many were furious that we were not providing them with adequate protection. I remember quite clearly the morning that I was crossing the street to get to the hospital from the parking structure, and there were a number of staff members out on the sidewalk with picket signs demanding PPE. As I got closer, I recognized several of our ICU nurses among the protesters, and we had an awkward exchange of glances as I realized I was likely one of the targets of their protest. I was tremendously thankful to have been asked to

be on the PPE Committee and was hoping I would be able to address their fears and concerns ... Those fears and anxieties shifted over time, so much so that eventually the committee was trying to convince many of those same people that they needed to wear their PPE! The decrease in fear and anxiety could be directly seen in the level of concern about having "enough" PPE.

One of the really tough decisions we had to make was addressing the requests from individuals to bring their own PPE from home. Examples included full elastomeric respirator sets, modified scuba masks, and other non-approved masks and face shields. Because of the work of the PPE Committee and the incredible efforts of every single person in our institution, we always had just enough masks to provide a reasonable level of protection. We ultimately decided that personal PPE would not be allowed as long as we had a supply of N95s and procedure masks. Our decision was heavily influenced by a desire to be equitable for the entire workforce. We wanted the entire team to be *equally* protected. We felt that this decision increased unit cohesion and morale, and was ethically the right decision. Simply, we felt we needed to avoid the situation where someone with money could buy their way into a higher level of protection.

In May 2020, we started getting regular shipments of N95s – initially not enough to allow the single use of masks but enough to expand the availability of masks to situations where the risk of exposure was only moderate. By that summer, we were balancing expansion of PPE use with the incoming supply. It was a fascinating logistics exercise. I was very proud that, from May 2020 forward, we were consistently able to increase PPE availability and never had to take a step back into rationing.

> And finally, after months of scrambling and restricting and fighting, we had enough stock to last for a meaningful amount of time. Essentially, watching the predicted curves of use and available stock go from a sharp decline with a scary number of days to empty. Then, as our logistics team worked its magic, we slowly began levelling and eventually climbing. When I once again disposed of a mask after just 9 hours of use, it was a big day for me.

The winter of 2020 was an awful time for COVID in New Mexico. Case numbers peaked in the middle of November, and our ICUs were full of people dying despite our best possible care. We did have enough PPE at that time, but the fear of dying was still ever present for the medical teams. You saw death from COVID every day and wondered if it was going to happen to you next.

That December was both the low point and the high point of the pandemic for me. On 13 December, my father-in-law died from COVID. Four days later, at 5:20 p.m., I received my first COVID vaccine. It was hard to reconcile those two events in a single week – such sadness and yet also such hope for a better future.

Everything changed after the health care team was vaccinated that spring. The PPE Committee had to change its focus to *encouraging* PPE use since many people no longer felt they needed to be as careful. We spent a lot of effort trying to encourage safe behaviours at work, such as not eating in groups, to prevent spread. The fear of dying started to fade, and we became more focused on preventing illness in the workforce so that we could maintain safe staffing levels.

On 12 March 2021, the PPE Committee met and determined that it had completed its mandate. We had plenty of masks, face shields, and other equipment. All of the protocols for PPE use were in place. That week we moved to a "ready reserve" status. The committee stopped regular meetings yet remained available for questions. We thanked each other, provided small gifts to recognize the countless hours from a team of more than twenty people, and then basically went back to our regular roles at work.

> I had a meeting just recently with our infection prevention team about hand hygiene. We were reminiscing about the PPE Committee and how, despite meeting as often as 6 days a week and sometimes at the end of very long days, we always looked forward to that meeting and connecting with all the members. Although we were addressing PPE, I think we were also providing each other with support and encouragement, which I very much needed and appreciated.

> I learned so much by being a member of the PPE Committee team. I was able to translate what the needs of the institution were into a cohesive plan that the supply chain team could adhere to in its efforts to source all the different types of available medical supplies. We had to reconfigure supply usage from what the established norm was into usable and science-driven modifications that allowed us to carry out a very difficult mission. I was especially impressed when I saw how our staff accepted these recommendations and the new ways of carrying out their patient care tasks, which were huge in being able to calm fears and anxiety among many of the staff. It was an experience in true teamwork, and I am better at my job and as a person for having gone through such a difficult time.

What we experienced as a team managing PPE for a hospital with over 7000 employees and hundreds of patients was both intense and scary, and yet ultimately surmountable, just like COVID. Our institution had the foresight and courage to take the steps and build the structure necessary to address PPE shortages. We felt fortunate to be on the PPE Committee as it gave us each a sense of purpose and a place to find support during the toughest days. We did our work well, although certainly not perfectly. We made tough decisions based on science and with integrity.

And then it ended. Just like that we went back to our regular work, although to this day we are still not fully aware of how profoundly we have been changed by this journey.

10 OMG, We Are Running Out of Propofol!

Scott Roach, PharmD, MBA
Director of Pharmacy Operations, University of New Mexico Hospital, Albuquerque

Preeyaporn Sarangarm, PharmD, BCPS, BCCCP
ED/ICU Pharmacy Supervisor, University of New Mexico Hospital, Albuquerque

Submitted 12 August 2022

I was working a shift in the Emergency Department (ED) as an ED pharmacist when I first heard of the national normal saline flush shortage. I reached out to the Director of Pharmacy Operations Scott Roach and very eloquently asked, "Are you serious?" I never would have thought that something so simple, a 10 mL syringe filled with normal saline, could be the cause of so much angst. As we dealt with nursing units hoarding flushes in cubbies and nurses grabbing and pocketing handfuls of flushes "just in case," we realized that normal saline flushes were the new toilet paper. How did we get here? How did these medication shortages become so dire?

Drug shortages are a consistent, unrelenting (not to mention frustrating) problem for pharmacy departments. The causes of medication shortages are complex. A hurricane hits Puerto Rico? Be prepared for a dialysis fluid shortage. Manufacturers in China are closed due to COVID-19 lockdown? Expect shortages of IV contrast. The US Food and Drug Administration (FDA) does a facility inspection? That could mean delays in everything from medication tablets to emergency medications used in a cardiac arrest. Therefore, the question is not whether there will be medication shortages but rather how manageable. To a certain extent, we colloquially grade them from "We've got this if we are creative" to "This is getting bad" to "OMG, we have to tell providers they can't use first-line therapy" (sometimes with some choice words thrown in). Pre-pandemic, the responses from providers could be harsh. But at this point, we hospital pharmacists have seen the entire spectrum of reactions to medication shortages: Acceptance – "OK, what are the alternatives?" Disbelief – "Well, X hospital has this, why don't you?" Scepticism – "Are you sure that you can't get this because I just used it?" Fear – "Are you trying to hurt our patients?" And a personal favorite that evokes an equal mixture of head banging and deep breaths: Anger – "My patient needs this, why can't you just make this happen?" Sometimes, depending on how bad a day it is, this demand can sound an awful lot like Veruca Salt from *Charlie and the Chocolate Factory*: "But Daddy, I want it now!"

Pharmacy departments go out of their way to solve these shortages on their own to avoid all of the above. And sometimes it is *stressful*. There are so few "easy button" solutions. It feels like everyone has the same grand plan to address the newest shortage, from using secondary expensive compounding pharmacies to panic buying everything that is available. Every decision ends up inevitably putting a huge burden on our staff or is incredibly costly or, worse yet, sometimes both. The impact on our IV room technicians are especially keen. It may mean anything from tasking our IV technicians to make huge batches of fentanyl or norepinephrine infusions or using twenty tiny vials to make a single infusion. The steely look that our lead IV technician supervisor gives us when this happens alone makes it worth seeing if there are *any* other alternatives before we go down that path. In reality, although feasible in the short term, in the longer term these compounding processes for our IV room and staff are not sustainable.

All of what we described above is just how we manage shortages for *some* IV products. In the background, our pharmacy technicians are shuffling medications around the hospital wards multiple times a day, trying to make sure providers have the medications they need close at hand. We are also purchasing extremely marked-up alternatives because often they are the only options available, which is frustrating in itself, watching capitalism at its finest. By the time we contact providers to inform them of medication shortages, we are usually down to our last bit of supply and have exhausted all of our normal tricks. Like a seesaw, juggling the communication cascade that results from the efforts to ensure all stakeholders are informed is a difficult path. We desperately try to avoid the Chicken Little phenomenon – "Here comes pharmacy with another shortage. The last five shortages never impacted us, so why should we stress now?" – when the reality is that we are begging for an immediate change in practice to get through a shortage. Or sometimes, even worse, we feel the chagrin after realizing we accidently left out a certain medical service from the email about a shortage. We, of course, only discover the omission because of the (appropriately) irate provider who needed that very specific medication at a critical moment. What is even more deflating is knowing an apology doesn't correct the inconvenience this omission might have caused the team and the patient. But this discomfort doesn't even compare to the gut-churning feeling when we have to let folks know that we are out of something with no alternatives. Nobody wants to be the person who can only provide a defeated shrug of the shoulders when no answer exists to the question, "So what do we do now?" These shortage situations have a mysterious way of popping up out of the blue, and sometimes we only have hours to decide what to do to optimize a nonexistent inventory, feeling like the sand in the hourglass is rapidly funnelling to a point where an immediate decision has to be made, with an associated, gnawing feeling as we wonder, "Did we do the right thing?"

The pandemic added a completely new level of complexity to managing medication shortages. We are based in New Mexico, a more rural and less wealthy state, so it was difficult to guess how COVID-specific shortages would affect us based on the early pandemic experience elsewhere. In early 2020, the pandemic was still so intangible that, for our first pharmacy administration meeting to discuss how to handle the potential drug shortages, we all piled into a single conference room. Looking back, it was probably not ideal to have twenty-five key pharmacy personnel unmasked in a room designed to accommodate ten! Basing our decisions on what we had heard from areas like New York, we stocked up on medications and (for better or worse) began what also leads to drug shortages: panic buying. Although we did not "hoard" per se, we did make our best guesses on what we would need, from pain medications to cough suppressants to paralytics, and bought what we could. And then we waited. And waited. As medications piled up in the pharmacy conference room and in spare refrigerators throughout the hospital, we began to think that we did not need all of the extra supply and even began to return some of it. But then the pandemic hit – and our ICUs felt the force of the first wave of COVID.

Despite all of our preparations, in so many ways we were still unprepared. Because of how little everyone at that point knew about potential COVID treatments and just how long critically ill COVID patients would be hospitalized, it was apparent that, despite the best-laid plans, *everything* would need to be continually assessed and reassessed.

As the weeks passed, we really began to feel the shortages. It started out small: reduced deliveries of certain medications, new medications appearing on the shortage list almost daily, and end dates for known shortages extending far beyond the original projected duration. Then came the shortage that shall forever live in infamy: propofol.

We managed this shortage the same way that we do all shortages. The problem was, at this point, no shortage was "normal." It was *not* normal to have a message sent from the Governor to see how our supply of X medication was. Nor was it normal to tell providers that first- and second-line, and possibly third-line options were affected. Managing the panic had become part of the new "normal." Dealing with the rumours of supposed shortages (some real and some not) and the inevitable reactive whiplash of "We need to fix this now" was part of the new normal (and headache inducing). Therefore, while we were exuding an air of calm in response to the external panic of "OMG, we are running out of propofol," internally we were fretful. First, we tried to obtain the medication directly from the manufacturer. It turned out that everyone was feeling the propofol shortage – so that was unsuccessful. (Though we did order *any* sedative we could get from our normal distributor.) Pre-pandemic, propofol (the backbone sedative for our ICUs and operating rooms [ORs]) was available in the ICU medication "vending" machines on override, meaning that nurses could pull the medication before an order was placed in anticipation of its need. We removed this option to minimize waste – but funnily enough (which really was not funny at all), everyone found creative workarounds. The ICUs developed algorithms to minimize the use of sedatives with a particular eye towards propofol use, but changing prescribing culture that quickly was like using a toy hammer to break down a steel wall. Our pharmacists tried to intervene as much as they could to discontinue infusions and limit new starts, but with limited success and, frankly, a lot of frustration (see the Chicken Little phenomenon above). At this point too, the change was so stark to clinical practice (although still very much appropriate care) that there was almost a sense of guilt from staff – "Were we really doing the right thing for our patients?" A new low moment was when the propofol shortage became so dire that our pharmacy purchaser had to report on a *daily basis* how many intubated COVID patients we had to one of the propofol manufacturers just so we could obtain our allocation. That sparked a true moment of alarm that we would not be able to "creatively" solve this shortage as we had done in the past.

Our fears were not unfounded; eventually the amount that we were able to procure just was not enough. We pharmacists are proud of our ability to adapt, and this solution was one of our more "out of the box" moments. Normally, we use 100 mL vials of propofol to run continuous "drips" and 20 mL vials for short-term sedation, such as for procedures. The question then became, could we "pool" the smaller propofol vials to make larger volumes to run for drips? While this idea may sound simple, developing this process was stressful and slightly anxiety provoking. Propofol is tricky. Since the medication has a lipid (fat) base, it is prone to problems with sterility after manipulation, which means that it is not as simple as drawing up a whole bunch of smaller vials and putting the contents into a bigger bag. Expiration became a huge issue since we could only give this "pooled" propofol a 12-hour shelf life. Although I heard many a time, "This is COVID – the normal rules are out the window," there were so many ifs and so many questions as to whether this solution was the right path. Can we justify this plan? Is it the safest option? If we pursue this process, how can we make enough medication to ensure the ICUs and ORs have enough medication and at the same time minimize waste of this now precious resource? At this point in the pandemic, we had already put incredible pressure on our IV pharmacy room technicians. Our IV room had become like a mini manufacturing plant, adapting quickly to make batches of many more medications than usual to help cover other medication shortages. Adding a labor-intensive medication like propofol to that list was a big request. (You can only imagine the look from our IV supervisor.) And yet, eventually, despite all of our best efforts and creative solutions, we had to tell the providers the very unpleasant news: we were nearly out of propofol.

The reaction we received was a bit unexpected and almost anticlimactic, given the feeling of impending doom experienced while composing that "Don't shoot the messenger" email. Rather than the usual grumbling over yet another medication shortage, the responses from providers to nursing were universally more positive than negative. ICU leadership checked in often on what should be done to help ameliorate the shortage, and nurses closely followed new sedation algorithms and tried to limit medication-related waste. All of these efforts led to changes in ICU pain control and sedation practices that had been long overdue. Eventually, the propofol shortage eased, and we "moved on" to other medication shortages.

We all now dread Tuesdays – the day of our weekly medication shortage meeting. As the pandemic continues, the shortages have become the worst our Pharmacy Department has ever seen. Pre-pandemic, on a good week, we had half a page of shortages to keep an eye on. That list is now three to four pages. And it's not just medications now; it's also the syringes to make the medications or specialized cassettes to hold epidurals.

But at the same time, all is not doom and gloom. In some ways, COVID helped unite us. As we bring up new medication shortages to providers, they may sass our department for always being the bearer of bad news, but they are more willing than ever to help solve the problem and have a better first-hand understanding of the struggles with medication shortages. We are fortunate to work in such a collaborative environment where everyone comes together to tackle the worst situations. Perhaps, in part, it is because we have all been impacted by shortages of once readily available household goods, or we have watched the news, where there were close to 100 container ships waiting to unload in the Long Beach and Los Angeles ports, and thought to ourselves, "I wonder if our medications, toilet paper, or <insert your delayed package here> was on one of those container ships."

At this point in the pandemic, we have heard it all and tend to be less surprised by the latest shortage. Regardless, each shortage requires a pause, a deep breath, and the need to move forward to ensure we can continue to provide optimal patient care. We all look forward to the day when medication shortages no longer dictate the therapies we choose. Until then, we can only hope that manufacturing processes will better adapt to COVID realities and become better able to handle the increases in patient numbers and the backlog of medication shortages created by the pandemic.

Thinking back on the saline flush syringe shortage, I still remember laughing on the inside when we heard that nurses had sometimes used these syringes as impromptu squirt guns and that we needed to ensure they were being used properly and not wasted. Although outwardly quasi serious, on the inside, I felt some joy, knowing there were folks still finding ways to decompress, even in the middle of yet another (stressful) COVID surge. It's interesting that something so simple as a syringe of salt water could, on one hand, create shortage-inspired angst but, on the other, also serve as a reminder that we can still take a moment to pause and have some fun! Yet, whether it's a saline flush or something more critical like propofol, we will continue to be ever ready for the next drug shortage on the horizon. Although some say the only certainty is that nothing is certain, shortages are eternal.

PART THREE

Necessity Is the Mother of Invention

This section, "Necessity Is the Mother of Invention," carries on the theme of the Scarcity section – the needed adaptations and creative solutions required by the unique, unprecedented challenges presented by the COVID-19 pandemic. "Anchored in Family: Starting a Business in Health Care Innovation During COVID-19" describes the challenges of trying to launch a business within the health care sphere during the pandemic, with the particular challenges posed by pandemic restrictions piled on top of the standard challenges of starting a business. "A Voice from the Operating Room to the Intensive Care Unit: An Anesthesiologist, Redeployed" provides an account of what it was like to be a "fish out of water" during the pandemic, tasked with clinical work outside of the sphere of one's training and prior experience. "How COVID-19 Changed the Way We Transported Patients Between Ontario's Hospitals: Prone Patient Transports" recounts the adaptations required for inter-hospital transfers of the sickest COVID patients – those whose oxygen levels were so low they had to be kept prone ("belly down"), even while being transported by air. "Transporting Patients: Kilometres to Go to Find a Home" continues in a similar vein, this time exploring not only the logistic challenges posed by transporting COVID patients but also the very indications and appropriateness for doing so. "When the Going Gets Tough, the Tough Get Going: A 'Hybrid Model' of Paediatric and Adult Critical Care During the COVID-19 Surge" describes the peculiar challenge of adapting facilities built for the care of children to the care of the overwhelming flood of COVID-affected adults and the successes that came from pushing past traditional barriers and delineations. "Lessons Learned from COVID-19: Personal Perspectives from a Low- and Middle-Income Country" provides a different viewpoint from those thus far presented and certainly a far cry from the accounts provided by the global media – in this case, an account of the lessons learned facing the additional challenges posed by a raging pandemic to a South African health care system that, even on the best of days, literally struggles to keep the lights on. The section concludes with "Vaccinating Remote Indigenous Communities," a description of the logistic and political challenges faced in the delivery of essential life-saving vaccines to some of the most remote territories on the planet.

11 Anchored in Family: Starting a Business in Health Care Innovation During COVID-19

Sabrina Fiorellino, JD
Chief Executive Officer, Fero International Inc.

Submitted 9 February 2023

This article is dedicated to every member of the Fero family. Thank you for your teamwork, relentless pursuit of greatness, and belief in our moto – that there are no limits.

On 11 March 2020, the World Health Organization declared that the COVID-19 outbreak was a global pandemic. Just a few weeks earlier, my family was vacationing in Mexico. Everyone was there – except me, as usual, because I was working. I was working even though I was in the process of exiting from my existing business in 2020, making the beginning of 2020 particularly busy for me. But exiting a business during COVID and then trying to figure out what to do next is not for the faint of heart.

The truth is, I've never done anything that was easy. Almost every business I've built or every career I've had was in a difficult field and required me to work an endless number of hours to succeed. I am a lawyer by background, specializing in mergers and acquisitions, but I am a true entrepreneur at heart, having bought or built, grown, and successfully exited local and international businesses. Most endeavours I chose were male dominated, which was always fine by me as I was used to it. But what I wasn't used to or prepared for (and I would come to realize) was how hard it is for female entrepreneurs to raise money and how very much harder it is during an economic slowdown, which gives you a hint about what I chose to do after my exit.

I knew well before I actually left my previous business that I was leaving, and so I began the normal process of thinking about what's next. I knew I had no intention of practising law again (although I will always be grateful for how much knowledge I gained in my practice and how much it helps me in my daily business dealings), and I knew that I wanted to work for myself, but I had no idea what I would do. For quite a long time, the thoughts around what to do next didn't take up too much space because I was so busy with my exit, but the idea for my current company came from a life event that was the single most devastating event I had ever faced in my life – the death of my grandfather, who was not just my family member but my best friend.

Growing up, I lived in a house with four generations. There is an old saying that "it takes a village to raise a child," and that was certainly the case in my family. My mom was a single mom who worked to provide for us, leaving my other family members to watch us when necessary. In my opinion, we were lucky, and we were loved by everyone at home, but my grandfather went above and beyond everyone else. He drove me to every sporting event I had before I got my licence (and taught me to drive my first car, which was manual); he stayed up late with me when I had assignments to do just to keep me company; and when I eventually moved out of the family home and went back to visit him, he insisted on cooking me one of his famous meals, even though I insisted that I would cook for him. But then he got sick, and not just a little sick – he was really sick. And it wasn't just him who was sick. You see, my family was small – actually very small. By the time I was an adult, my only close and immediate family members were my mom (who was an only child), my grandparents, and my brother (I was so happy to eventually include my sister-in-law and nephew in our tiny family).

My grandfather was diagnosed with Sjogren's syndrome in the same year my mom was diagnosed with stage four sarcoidosis. Both were autoimmune conditions, and in both my mom and my grandfather, the conditions were quite severe. My grandmother also suffered from rheumatoid arthritis, which was also quite harsh, and I have (currently, well managed) ulcerative colitis and some other autoimmune conditions. My brother, an anesthesiologist, and my sister-in-law, a nurse, spent their entire careers in health care, and I couldn't be more grateful that they were around when things went south.

First my mom. By the time she was diagnosed, her condition was already quite severe and continued to progress quickly, which resulted in her carrying around an oxygen tank to breathe. As her condition progressed, her mobility decreased, and her hospitalizations became frequent. She had a number of pneumothoraces (lung collapses), complex infections, and a pleurodesis on both lungs (a process that sticks your lung to your chest wall permanently), all requiring prolonged hospitalizations. Eventually she was too sick to leave the hospital; she went into respiratory arrest, was placed on life support (extracorporeal membrane oxygenation, ECMO), and had a double lung transplant (we are so happy to have her with us). Her story is a miracle and one to write in more detail another day.

Next comes my grandfather. Similar to my mom, his condition also required him to carry oxygen off and on (not as significant as my mom). My grandfather was in and out of hospital, often crashing, being near the brink of death, and eventually recovering. During every single hospital admission he had, I stayed in the hospital with him – until COVID hit. His hospitalization during COVID was very sadly his last and most heartbreaking. My grandfather was admitted in the normal course for a "crash" that did not seem out of the ordinary for him. What was different this time was that I couldn't stay with him or even visit. I was more concerned than usual, however, because he was taken by ambulance to a hospital that wasn't the regular hospital he and my mom went to. The hospital where he landed happened to be the same hospital where my mom waited in the intensive care unit (ICU) for 15 hours on high-flow oxygen with her lung collapsed because none of the staff knew how to turn the chest tube machine on. My brother and sister-in-law had to show up after their shifts and literally turn on the machine to reinflate her lung. When I found out that he was at that same hospital, I panicked, and I asked my brother to regularly communicate with my grandfather's care staff to make sure he was OK. The care staff regularly reported to my brother that my grandfather was fine, but when my brother accessed his medical charts, he requested to visit my grandfather because the verbal reports he was getting differed vastly from the charts. I want to be clear here: In general, I love the Canadian health care system, and I know it's one of the best in the world. These particular experiences do not in any way reflect the care that I and my family have received at any other hospital.

Somehow, my brother managed to get us into the hospital for a visit with my grandfather. When I arrived, I couldn't believe my eyes. A man who had raised me, lived in the same house as me for the majority of my life, and was my best friend didn't even recognize me (even though he was fine a few weeks earlier). We quickly discovered that he hadn't been fed, his teeth hadn't been brushed, and he hadn't even been tended to for at least 3 days. All the memories of my mom suffering for 15 hours came crashing back, and my worst fears came over me like a wave of debilitating sadness. I FaceTimed my mom immediately and told her that she had to say goodbye to my grandfather because

I knew instinctively that he wasn't going to make his normal miracle recovery this time. My brother and I fed him, gave him water, and he significantly improved before we left, but I knew it wasn't enough.

My brother, working at a teaching hospital where my mom had her lung transplant, and I, sitting on a board of a community hospital where a close friend experienced excellent care, were appalled at the experiences we were having at this hospital. But because of COVID, there was nothing we could do because there were no inter-hospital transfers during that period. So my grandfather, an extremely sociable person who loved to be around people, died alone, 3 days after our last visit with him.

To make matters worse, we had a funeral for a man who was one of the most social people I know with only eight people. An injustice to his legacy. This tiny funeral also meant that I had to be a pallbearer and give his eulogy. I barely managed to get the words out, but to give you an idea of the type of man he was, here is part of what I said:

> Upon his death, hundreds of phone calls for condolences came in to honour the memory of my grandfather. Almost consistently, people recollected about his warmth, compassion, sense of humour, and flamboyant story telling. His stories were legendary. He once described that he had read almost every law textbook and medical textbook while me and my brother were going through school. He wasn't sure if he would be able to pass the medical boards but was sure that he knew more than any lawyer in Toronto … Above all else, he was a dedicated family man. He worked endlessly and selflessly to provide for his family and ensure they could live a better life. He essentially did everything for each member of his family. He helped to feed, wash, clothe, and care for them, over and over again for days and years. He was a father to both me and my brother, even though we were his grandchildren. He would take us to sporting events and trips, help with homework, and sneak us sweets and candies when no one was looking. He was always there to offer advice and encouragement in a non-judgmental way. He taught everyone so much about resilience, even when no one understood that was the lesson they were learning. When friends and family began to have babies and began to comprehend the heroic labour it takes to keep a child alive, the constant exhausting tending of a being who can do nothing and demands everything, it is at that time that we truly realized that my grandfather had done all of these things for each of us before any of us could remember. Each member of the family was fed, washed, clothed, taught to speak, and given a thousand other things, over and over again, hourly, daily, for years. Every one of us whom he touched believed "he gave us everything."

I think the fact that he died alone and we weren't able to celebrate his life at his funeral are two of the things that still haunt me the most to this day and ultimately were the inspiration for my business.

My grandfather's death elicited feelings in me of both anger and sadness to a degree that I had never felt before. My immediate thought after the numbness started to wear off was that the health care system was in trouble during COVID, and I was single-handedly going to fix it (a bit too ambitious but I was determined to do something).

In the news, there were several stories covering companies that were producing new innovative medical infrastructure solutions, and I wanted to be part of that innovation. I knew that I wasn't able to help with increased staffing, but I could find someone to align myself with to build space. I started speaking about the idea to friends and family, and I got introductions to several manufacturers – some better than others. One in particular, whom we spent quite a lot of time trying to work with, eventually told me that we could form a company together but my contribution was worth between 5 and 10 per cent, and probably even less. As you can imagine, I abandoned that ship before it left the harbour.

Eventually, I started to expand my team, and we worked hard at finding a manufacturer that could build our vision. By sheer chance, on 14 April 2020, I saw an article (I still read the news – but mainly on my phone!) about a manufacturer in southwestern Ontario that was turning shipping containers into mobile triage units. I immediately decided to call the company's owner the next day, and by the following Monday, we had decided he was going to build what we wanted: a modular, pressurized medical unit that would assist with acute care, up to and including intensive care and operating room care.

From a medical infrastructure perspective, I had limited knowledge about what was required. I knew we could hire professional engineers to ensure the infrastructure met codes (that part was easy), but we needed specialized expertise related to workflow. I reached out to a world-renowned doctor working at the University Health Network (UHN) for help. He was kind enough to introduce me to Dr. Laura A. Hawryluck, who is an intensivist at Toronto Western Hospital, the critical care response team lead, and a professor of critical care medicine at the University of Toronto. Without Dr. Laura's help, our company wouldn't exist. Dr. Laura was instrumental in assisting in an endless number of ways. And our manufacturer did not disappoint either, delivering a high-quality, beautifully built, volumetric health care unit.

With Dr. Laura's help, we also connected with the senior team at the UHN as well as with the UHN's health care human factors (HHF) team, who eventually conducted a week-long assessment of our health infrastructure after it was built and assembled. The work culminated in a written report from the HHF to the Ontario government about our health infrastructure, both outlining the HHF's assessment of the infrastructure as well as the benefits of its use. From there we were off to the races. We had an incredible amount of earned media coverage and many sales inquiries.

Taking a step back, it's really, really hard to be an entrepreneur. When you are starting a small company, society, investors, banks, and so on dismiss you. When you scale your business, you can be lumped with others that some people suggest have an unfair advantage in life and don't necessarily care about those who work for them. Here is what I want to share about my experience of being an entrepreneur: I have created several companies from scratch, created lots of jobs, and positively contributed to the economy my entire life, but I've done so at great personal expense. For most of my life, I've worked 7 days a week, often more than 16-hour days (even on the weekends). I've lost friends, missed family events and vacations, and still don't have a family of my own. I've been insulted, laughed at, and even recently called a liar (a story for another day), all of which I didn't deserve, and never received an apology for any of the mistreatment over the years. I've often put my entire life savings into new businesses (through unsecured loans, not knowing if I would ever get the money back), signed personal guarantees for bank debts (secured against my personal property), and went without a paycheck for months or years on end – all to ensure the company would be successful. And most of all, I've done everything in my power to ensure my businesses would be successful so that my employees and subcontractors and their families would be OK. AND I wouldn't trade any of it for the world. (As an aside, in all of my businesses, I knew all of my employees by name; I knew their families, kids, birthdays, and so on, and I personally called each one of them or even visited them on milestone events.) I don't want a pat on the back for any of these things because I believe that is how business leaders should run their businesses. I really care about my businesses and the people who make them possible.

As a result of the endless hours I work, many people tell me that I need more work-life balance. But no matter how hard you try, when your business is in startup state, it requires your full time and attention; no matter how hard you try, your personal life is often not your own. You can't simply hire more people to help because there is not enough money available. So you do as much as you can to get the business to a point where it's possible to hire – where the business is in a steady state and it's much more manageable. But again, it's a personal choice that I go into with open eyes, and I love *almost* every minute of it.

I've already said it's hard to be an entrepreneur, but from experience, none of my previous new businesses compared to being an entrepreneur during COVID. Government support (at the municipal, provincial, and federal levels) for start-ups during COVID was non-existent. I want to be very clear here: This point is absolutely not a criticism of government but simply a fact. I would not have wanted to be a government official during COVID. Officials had to deal with health crises, long-term care crises, school crises, global supply chain issues, a new war in Europe, and eventually an economic crisis. These are all extremely complex issues, and taken together, there is no one solution to dealing with all of them, especially all at once.

Government supports were plentiful for existing businesses – businesses that existed prior to COVID and had to shut down during the pandemic. There was also infinite money for companies that could retool to provide COVID-related supplies. But for a startup, there was nothing, just crickets. While other businesses shrunk, our business grew; while other businesses laid off people, our business hired. And still nothing.

Our team worked remotely from home for over 2 years. There were days, sometimes weeks, when I didn't leave the house other than to walk around the block. It was isolating and unmotivating, but I knew I had to continue. We had to hire virtually, never being able to meet people in person, and we had to raise capital from investors virtually for the first time in history, a time when investors could simply shut off their cameras, ignore what you were saying, and much more easily say no to your ask.

It's exceedingly difficult for female entrepreneurs to raise money – the well-documented statistics around this issue speak for themselves. Women-led startups received under 3 per cent of venture capital funding in 2020, and this percentage went down during COVID after years of going up. Our business is majority female owned and led. I can't tell you how many people we pitched our business to before we were successful at raising money. We saw so many of our male counterparts pitch, receive enormous amounts of money, and fail. But with no investor money, we continued to move forward and succeed.

On top of these statistics working against us, we were pitching during one of the worst economies to raise money to date. But eventually, we got our growth money! Similar to Dr. Laura, our business would not exist if it weren't for our initial major investor. In our joint press release, Joe Mancinelli, chair of LiUNA Pension Fund of Central and Eastern Canada, stated:

> On behalf of the LiUNA Pension Fund of Central and Eastern Canada, we are proud to support strong female entrepreneurship and invest in

female-led companies that will continue to have an impact across Canada and the potential for positive growth on a global scale ... Female-led companies only received 2 per cent of venture capital funding in 2021 – the lowest since 2016.

Our investor believed in us and supported us against all odds, and we will always be grateful for the major investment that gave us our real start.

Today, it continues to be exceedingly difficult to raise money and grow, but we continue to move forward in spite of the odds. For me, my investors are like my colleagues – I feel an absolute need to protect their money (similar to protecting my employees' jobs). I love my life and my career no matter how challenging it is – in fact, I love overcoming the challenges. But above all else, I'm serious about protecting my investors and my employees, and I would do that no matter what!

Currently, we are a growing company. Our mission has always been to bring state-of-the art, sustainable, and cost-effective infrastructure to the most vulnerable populations around the world. More specifically, we design and manufacture rapidly deployable, volumetric modular infrastructure solutions for hospitals, long-term care, remote communities, laboratories, mining, and the military. We can also deliver infrastructure where natural disasters, war, or other similar events occur. We are now organically receiving inquiries on our website from internationally recognized organizations, and we continue to fabricate, hire, and grow. We even get inquiries from various government agencies in the United States who want to give us money to move our operations south (very tempting!).

As we continue to expand, our plan is to grow both organically and through acquisition, explore new frontiers where our infrastructure can impact (such as food shortages), continue to raise money to grow our team, and eventually expand globally, becoming, in our Chief Financial Officer's words, "a great Canadian growth story."

When markets improve and our company is in a steady state, our ambition is to list our company on a Canadian stock exchange. When we do, we will be the first female CEO/CFO to take their manufacturing business public in Canadian history. Look out for us.

12 A Voice from the Operating Room to the Intensive Care Unit: An Anesthesiologist, Redeployed

Gianni R. Lorello, BSc, MD, MSc (Med Ed), CIP, FRCPC
Associate Professor, Department of Anesthesiology and Pain Medicine, University of Toronto

Submitted 16 June 2022

I remember the start of the pandemic as if it were yesterday, working during the March break with uncertainty infused throughout the medical system and in society at large. The uncertainty not only resided in the COVID-19 pandemic; uncertainties of what the future held for our patients, our colleagues, and ourselves also lingered. One certainty that remained was fear: fear of the virus, fear of the availability of personal protective equipment (PPE), and fear of death. I recall having profoundly emotional discussions with my mother, discussions that no mother would ever fathom having with her child, discussions around my very own goals of care, and frantically finding a lawyer to create a living will. I can still hear my mother's voice cracking, telling me that a "mother dies before her kids," only realizing afterward that she was trying to comfort herself as the stark reality of death flashed by her eyes.

I attended numerous virtual meetings where contingency plans were being created. One such plan was redeploying health care providers to the intensive care unit (ICU). The idea of being redeployed simultaneously worried and excited me; perhaps it would be one of the only occasions since residency that I would be offered the opportunity to provide my expertise as an anesthesiologist within an ICU setting. Although the ICU was a foreign environment, the opportunity to engage in and enact the moral, ethical, and social responsibility that I took upon entering medicine excited me, as well as being surrounded by intensivists, nurses, trainees, respiratory therapists, and spiritual care providers, among many more, for whom I have utmost respect.

As I continue to reflect on my redeployment experience, I turn to the lasting detrimental effects of words being thrown around in health care and in social media, words that are activated differently by each individual and thus carry different meanings for different people. I focus on the disjuncture between policies that socially organize our daily work and lived experiences as a front-line worker. I took solace in speaking with trusted colleagues and in knowing that they too had very similar internal reactions. Although the discourses on the following terms could be separate chapters and books by themselves, an overview is provided.

Upskilling. "Upskilling" became a newly popularized term by leadership among nearly all organizations worldwide. As words have profound lasting effects, I started analysing the term "upskilling." Although I remain cognizant of the numerous discourses around upskilling, one underlying narrative is that I, a physician, an anesthesiologist, do not have the skills required to take care of critically ill patients, despite caring for some of the sickest patients within the operating room environment, dealing with acute physiological changes, blood loss, intra-operative emergencies, and so on. The simplistic nature of such a term can be activated into, and create a reality of, a perception of intellectual rivalry rather than celebrating complementary skills for the common goal of patient care in a time of crisis. It appeared to me that there was a sense of professional and social stratification. As I was concurrently in my second year of a PhD program studying critical social theory, at that time I could not help but see this situation through Gieryn's boundary work[1] – division between knowledge, fields, and people – where delineations for the people living these demarcations have profound effects. For me, the issue was not a protection of critical care specialty but rather a sharing of relational expertise; it was not diluting anyone's expertise but rather realizing that it would be impossible to take care of the number of patients that would potentially overwhelm the health care system, in particular the ICU, without resulting in otherwise preventable deaths and without becoming burned out. Furthermore, as an anesthesiologist, I brought a unique skill set to the ICU: the ability to intubate and place a critically ill person on life support safely, effectively, and in a manner that reduced the risk to other health care team members as much as possible. As anesthesiologists, we extended these services and expertise across all areas of the hospital, creating intubation teams in collaboration with operating room nurses, attending all Code Blue calls and any calls where sick patients required assessment for intubation. Why was this stratification through "upskilling" therefore even required? Everyone within the hospital complex played a vital role in caring for patients, from environmental services, to spiritual care, to social workers, to nursing staff, to respiratory therapists, to physicians, and to many other key people who actively contribute to patient care.

When redeploying people, organizations need not think about "upskilling"; rather, they need to conceptualize redeployment by looking at who can participate in sharing their professional knowledge and skills to ensure that the team workload is reduced and not increased through a need for a greater amount of refreshment of knowledge and skills among those joining any team in need. An approach that consistently seeks to provide real help quickly helps ensure team morale is not further diminished.

I luckily was redeployed to an ICU that welcomed me with open arms. The relationships that I already had further materialized into friendships; these friends and colleagues became my family, family with whom I connected frequently. No amount of medical training prepared us for the emotional work that ensued. Organizations are frequently charged with anticipating emerging and changing needs in an iterative fashion while enabling resilience. However, the term "upskilling" implies that one and one's specialty is obsolete; rather than building resilience, it diminishes morale and self-worth. In the event of future pandemics, particular attention must be paid to the impact that words have because words matter and have lasting effects on people.

Hero. As the pandemic progressed, health care professionals were being called "heroes." I remember thinking to myself, "But how can I be a hero?" I am extensively trained to help people who are very sick. I was privileged to be employed when many people were laid off work. I was fortunate to be able to socialize at work with other people. I was lucky to be able to take care of people, people who became sick because they were forced to work to provide for themselves, their families, and their friends. Many of these people did not have the luxury to physically distance ("social distancing") from their families and loved ones, or appropriate PPE, or safe work environments.[2-4] I was not a hero but rather fortunate to perform a job that I am so privileged to be able to perform.

As I further analysed the term "hero," I started to think about how "heroism" is conceptualized positively and how unchallenged assumptions of heroism can backfire and hurt the individuals involved, producing a negative effect. One underlying narrative of heroism is that of resilience, the ability to always be there when needed, to continue despite everything falling apart, and to rescue everyone in need, as well as the inability to fail and burn out. As humans, we are all prone to burnout, and we all perform immense emotional and physical work caring for patients, especially during a pandemic. Another discourse is that around normalization of exposure-prone risk.[5] An epistemic shift in the conceptualization of a hero from one of infallibility to one that rehumanizes health care providers is one way of reclaiming the term "hero," since any and all health care providers are susceptible to burnout and mental health issues. If we reclaim the term "hero," can it be said that being a hero is doing what one can under extraordinary circumstances to help others, yet knowing that there will be more to do?

We are all in this together. Signs emerged with the phrase "we are all in this together," trying to depict how societies were uniting during the pandemic. However, the pandemic proved to have the complete opposite effect, and pre-existing inequities were further exacerbated and widened, disproportionately affecting some people more than others, especially people already socially marginalized. The loss of small businesses and their ability to employ others, which had been created through years of hard work, the inability to lose income and consequently having to work, the inability to physically distance in the workplace, and the miscommunication, among many other reasons, disproportionately affected socially marginalized people, further widening the social gradient. Although inequities have always existed, the pandemic has worsened the social divides that we are experiencing today.

Further social divides and inequities impacted the health care system as well: redeployment of trainees and missing electives that may have impacted future career opportunities; training time extensions due to a lack of exposure; cancelled surgeries from elective procedures impacting quality of life to cancer surgeries; and redeploying people to areas outside of what they signed up for at the start of the pandemic. These lived experiences are not synonymous with "we are all in this together" as they have potentially very real negative consequences on individual lives.

As an anesthesiologist, I am honoured and privileged to have been able to work with some of the most supportive staff who welcomed me with open arms in the ICU. Navigating a new environment is a big feat at the best of times, and entangling the stress and fear of the pandemic further compounded my lived experiences as an anesthesiologist in an unknown environment. Many nights were spent with patients, family members, and nursing staff, engaging in emotional dialogue. I was not "upskilled"; rather my knowledge and skills were shared with my ICU colleagues, and some were refreshed from my previous time during my training years. I am not a "hero," and we were not "all in this together"; rather, I was fortunate, privileged, and honoured to be able to engage in my calling as an anesthesiologist, extending my care and compassion into the ICU and across the hospital. Despite continuing to live and work in a pandemic, reflecting on the earlier days of the pandemic and being redeployed to the ICU reinforces my original motivations for entering medicine. I would without a doubt in my mind be one of the first to be redeployed to the ICU should my services be required again.

Words have immense power with the potential to motivate but also to deflate people and their actions. The words within our environment shape and impact us. I encourage everyone to think and rethink about all the potential discourses around words and phrases. This thinking and rethinking of words before they become popularized may help mitigate the profound effects that words have on people; although the use of certain words may be well intentioned, the negative effects of words linger. The cautious and deliberate use of thoughtful and positive communication is a key to positive cultural change. This voice from the operating room to the ICU reinforces how words matter and how words have lasting effects. I want each and every one to think – how are you using words?

REFERENCES

1. Gieryn TF. Boundary-work and the demarcation of science from non-science: strains and interests in professional ideologies of scientists. *Am Sociol Rev.* 1983;48(6):781–95. https://doi.org/10.2307/2095325
2. Wright L, Steptoe A, Fancourt D. Are we all in this together? longitudinal assessment of cumulative adversities by socioeconomic position in the first 3 weeks of lockdown in the UK. *J Epidemiol Community Health.* 2020;74:683–8. https://doi.org/10.1136/jech-2020-214475. PMID: 32503892.
3. Wang Z, Tang K. Combating COVID-19: health equity matters. *Nat Med.* 2020;26(4):458. https://doi.org/10.1038/s41591-020-0823-6. Medline: 32284617.
4. Ahmed F, Ahmed N, Pissarides C, Stiglitz J. Why inequality could spread COVID-19. *Lancet Public Health.* 2020;5(5):e240. https://doi.org/10.1016/S2468-2667(20)30085-2. Medline: 32247329.
5. Mohammed S, Peter E, Killackey T, Maciver J. The "nurse as hero" discourse in the COVID-19 pandemic: a poststructural discourse analysis. *Int J Nurs Stud.* 2021;117:article 103887. https://doi.org/10.1016/j.ijnurstu.2021.103887. Medline: 33556905.

13 How COVID-19 Changed the Way We Transported Patients Between Ontario's Hospitals: Prone Patient Transports

Andy Pan, MD, FRCPC (EM CCM), DRCPSC (PTM)
Faculty of Medicine, University of Ottawa

Michael Peddle, MD, FRCPC, DRCPSC
Associate Medical Officer, Operations, Education, and OCC; Transport Medicine Physician; Associate Professor, Schulich School of Medicine and Dentistry, Division of Emergency Medicine, Western University, London, Ontario

Russell MacDonald, MD, MPH, FCFP, FRCPC, DRCPSC
ORNGE, Ontario Air Ambulance; Toronto Paramedic Services; Faculty of Medicine, University of Toronto

Submitted 18 November 2022

In response to the COVID-19 pandemic, the critical care community dusted off the old policies and procedures to cope with the severity of respiratory illness due to the SARS-CoV-2 virus. They included revisiting the use of prone ventilation (turning and treating patients on life support so that they lie in bed on their stomachs instead of lying on their back [supine position] in the usual way). This procedure was once a common intervention to increase the amount of lung tissue available to help a person struggling to breathe; it had fallen out of favour due to lack of clear evidence that it made any difference until only recently, due to the PROSEVA trial.[1] The PROSEVA trial is one of those trials that revolutionized the care of some of the sickest patients in the intensive care unit (ICU). Large and international in scope, the trial showed improved outcomes in patients with the most severe respiratory failure. It does have risks, including the loss of the patient's airway (because the endotracheal tube, the tube that connects them to the ventilator, falls out), the loss of IV access, and the loss of other tubes such as feeding tubes, as well as the risk that it doesn't work and the patient worsens acutely and is difficult or impossible to restabilize. However, many critical care practitioners were still not comfortable with prone ventilation, and its use remained limited as a result. Moreover, prone positioning in bed was not used in patients who were very sick but had not yet reached a point of needing life support. The practice of prone ventilation in the transport medicine environment was even less well known or accepted, with only a handful of organizations globally having formal protocols on how to transport a patient in the prone position.

Once the pandemic renewed interest in prone ventilation, and seemingly early evidence, even anecdotal in nature, suggested that it was helpful, transport medicine systems began to develop and refine ways to transport these patients between hospitals as local resources became depleted and it was clear people needed to be moved to where resources remained in order to avoid the initiation of triage plans. Once patients were stabilized in the prone position, returning them to a supine position risked destabilizing them and made any consideration of an attempt to move them to another centre simply impossible. This need to explore transporting people in a prone position became an increasing necessity as time passed due to increased demands for critical care beds and the availability of staff to care for these patients. The emergence of extracorporeal membrane oxygenation (ECMO), an artificial heart-lung machine used to take over lung and potentially heart function, as a potential treatment modality for some of those who could not be stabilized even on a ventilator also prompted the need to move the very sickest of critically ill patients to centres capable of providing ECMO.

Prior to the start of the pandemic, the health care system had already developed the capacity to identify patients who were starting to decline and transport them to quaternary care centres early in their disease course for consideration of specialized treatments that they couldn't receive in their present location and for advanced therapies such as ECMO. When dealing with people struggling with severe lung illnesses – those who deteriorated quickly and could not be safely transported – specialized retrieval teams were readily available to place the patient on ECMO at the referring hospital and transport them safely to quaternary care. However, the pandemic quickly outstripped these ECMO retrieval resources and ECMO hospital resources themselves. Critical care teams had to widely introduce the use of prone ventilation and inhaled pulmonary vasodilators, with the hopes that some patients would improve and the growing demand for ECMO could be curtailed.

This rapid adoption of less commonly needed and therefore less commonly used techniques to improve oxygenation and ventilation created a problem for transport medicine services. Patients remained in critical care beds of local and regional hospitals much longer as these techniques were tried. By the time it became clear that these methods were failing and the patients would not survive unless they were moved to a quaternary centre, they were sicker and increasingly unstable. Moving critically ill patients and keeping them alive during such moves can be challenging at the best of times – even if for some the needed move is within the hospital in which they are being cared for. Moving these patients safely from one hospital to another prior to the pandemic required specialized teams and careful planning before and during any planned transport. Moving so many of them over great distances with unprecedented severity of illness had never been done. And transport medicine services faced the same challenges as other parts of the health care system, from personal protective equipment (PPE) availability, to staffing, to equipment including ambulances, helicopters, and fixed-wing aircraft.

Recognizing that the need to maintain prone ventilation during transport would be crucial for people to survive, a working group of paramedic educators, transport physicians, and front-line paramedics worked through the barriers and created an education and implementation plan to rapidly roll out protocols and procedures to safely transport prone mechanically ventilated patients.

Overcoming the initial pre-pandemic hesitation and resistance to this mode of transport remained a challenge. Recognition of the system need and the clinical benefits in maintaining prone ventilation during transport was instrumental in breaking down the fears of this "novel" intervention. Critical care paramedics are a specialized group of practitioners who are knowledgeable and highly skilled at managing critically ill patients in the transport environment. They are able to identify risks in transport and know how to implement solutions to mitigate these risks.

The first barrier to dispel was the notion that prone patient transport was a difficult procedure. Practically speaking, proning a patient doesn't require new skills or training, just caution and manpower. Part of the training included developing an understanding of how a patient is proned, emphasizing how to do it safely, and engaging everyone involved in patient care: the transporting crew, the sending hospital staff, and the transport medicine physician (TMP), who provided direct medical control and assumed medical care of the patient during transport. The TMP would typically identify patients who may benefit from prone positioning when the request for transport was first received and discuss with sending hospital staff to ensure the patient was stabilized in the prone position prior to the paramedics' arrival at the sending hospital.

The second barrier was the limitations and risks in caring for a patient in the prone position. The main concern was how to manage a patient who decompensates while in the prone position during transport. It takes at least four people to safely prone and un-prone a patient in a hospital setting. In the back of a moving vehicle, whether on the road or in flight, there may be only one or two paramedics available. Paramedics expressed their concerns about not being able to perform time-sensitive interventions, such as manipulating or reinserting an advanced airway (if the endotracheal tube, the tube placed in the patient's windpipe to connect them to the ventilator, fell out), managing intravenous lines and arterial lines, or performing resuscitation including CPR should the need arise. This barrier was managed by acknowledging its presence, careful pre-transport planning, and a shared care decision between the hospital staff and the patient's substitute decision-makers about the benefits and risks of transport.

The third barrier was the paramedics' stress associated with knowing that there were limited interventions should something go wrong in transport. Managing these situations can be difficult on an already stretched health care provider. Initially, the protocol included a "no CPR" statement in the prone position and "no attempt to un-prone" during transport for crew safety. These protocols were put in place over concerns that a paramedic crew might attempt to un-prone a patient in the event of a cardiac arrest, resulting in physical harm to the providers and the patient. Recognizing that these patients were already in extremis, the expert consensus agreement was that there was a degree of futility in CPR for this patient population. While this approach was meant to address some of the concerns, it had an unintended paradoxical effect on the stress placed on the paramedic crew. For some, it amplified the feeling of helplessness, knowing there could be an intervention but that they could not carry through with it. To address this issue, the protocol evolved to include additional training on the performance of CPR while the patient remained in the prone position should the need arise.

The "see one, do one, teach one" approach in medicine worked well with the rapidly developed and implemented process of prone patient transport. The initial unease was dissipated as crews were able to practise on mannequins, go through the physical process on how to move a prone patient from bed to stretcher and back, and practise these psychomotor skills repeatedly. As the number of prone patient transports grew, the procedure for doing so quickly became second nature to these highly skilled paramedics.

The formal training package had two components: a self-directed online training module and a live session with an educator. The online module comprised a review of operational guidelines and medical directives, review of images on how to secure patient positioning in our assets, and videos on how to prone and transfer a prone patient from bed to stretcher and to load the patient into an aircraft. There was also a live Q&A webinar session as well as a knowledge quiz. This module was followed by a hands-on session at base with a mannequin and aircraft. Given the rapid evolution of the pandemic, the training was developed with the first cohort of paramedics completing the training within 2 weeks.

Being mindful that this procedure is still a novel intervention, transports were closely monitored and reviewed by base hospital staff and the medical director. We published the outcomes of our first 127 patients that we transported in the prone position during the early phases of the COVID-19 pandemic. Of these patients, 117 were transported by land, 7 by rotary-wing, and 3 by fixed-wing aircraft. Over half (52.8 per cent) were vasopressor dependent (required adrenaline-like medications to support their blood pressure), and the mean PaO_2/FiO_2 ratio was 86.7 pre-transport. This ratio is used in critical care medicine to identify severity of illness. Values below 150 are very severe lung injury. The mean transport duration was 50 minutes, with a range of 14 minutes to 176 minutes. Table 13.1 summarizes the serious adverse events identified.

These serious adverse events (SAEs) do not necessarily mean that prone transport was the cause, but it was important to monitor the SAEs to ensure patients could be moved in this position as safely as possible. The SAEs were most in keeping with the severity of illness in this patient population. There were no accidental tube or line dislodgements, which was one of the principal concerns about moving patients while prone. Our review concluded that patients can be safely transported prone by specially trained critical care paramedic crews.

As the pandemic evolved, we were no longer simply moving prone patients to quaternary care centres for ECMO consideration. Critical care beds became so limited at some hospitals that lateral movement of patients from one hospital's ICU to another hospital's ICU was needed to preserve the bed capacity across hospitals. A number of mechanically ventilated patients who were prone were moved for these reasons.

Table 13.1. Serious Adverse Events Identified in Prone Patient Transport During the First 127 Cases

Serious adverse events	No.
Number of patients experiencing a serious adverse event	18
SpO2 <88 on 2 consecutive readings >2 minutes apart or requiring ventilator settings change	15
Hypotension requiring treatment (sBP <80 or MAP <60)	3
New requirement for vasopressors	1

COVID-19 has had an enduring impact on our health care system. Despite its challenges, critical care paramedic crews and the critical care transport service rose to the challenge, implementing a rapidly developed program to meet an unprecedented patient care need in a safe, effective manner.

REFERENCE

1. Guerin C, Reigner J, Richard J-C, et al. Prone positioning in severe acute respiratory distress syndrome. *NEJM*. 2013;368(23):2159–68. https://doi.org/10.1056/NEJMoa1214103. PMID: 23688302.

14 Transporting Patients: Kilometres to Go to Find a Home

Bojan N. Paunovic, MD, FRCPC
Provincial Medical Specialty Lead, Adult Critical Care, Shared Health Manitoba; Medical Specialty Lead, Adult Critical Care, Winnipeg Regional Health Authority (WRHA); Section Head, Adult Critical Care, and Assistant Professor, Department of Internal Medicine, University of Manitoba; Site Critical Care Lead, Health Sciences Centre, Winnipeg; Past President, Canadian Critical Care Society

Submitted 27 July 2022

The transport of critically ill patients is by no means a COVID-19–generated phenomenon. It has been a frequent occurrence in many jurisdictions for decades. Robust transport teams were specifically designed to transport patients, often over significant distances, in order to receive specialized care that was not available in their home areas. Transport of critically ill patients has been especially used in Canada in order to ensure that rural and northern and Indigenous populations have access to higher levels of services. Transport also regularly occurs between provinces for access to care such as organ transplantation.

However, the need to transport critically ill patients between provinces and between jurisdictions within provinces purely due to a lack of capacity was a novel insult to health care systems that was brought on by COVID-19 surges. On the surface, this need may seem to some to be simply an issue of logistics – transport is transport, regardless of the reason. However, for those who were charged with coordinating and implementing this effort, it was immediately apparent that these transports created a complex interplay of reactions similar to the stages related to grief: denial, anger, bargaining, depression, and acceptance.

The concept that surges could result in the need for mass patient transportation was initially denied, not necessarily due to lacking the acceptance of the possibility but due to counting on the ability of the system to quickly expand capacity and the effectiveness of public health restrictions to limit cases. Unfortunately, when it became apparent that case numbers were rising and that capacity was not doing so at the same pace, it seemed that government denial led to delays of, or inadequate, restrictions. This issue quickly became the focus of anger, especially by health care workers who felt the pressure and were "living the numbers" in real time. Bargaining occurred, not as a sequential stage but in the background, as discussions were undertaken at various levels to manage the imbalance between needs and resources. Efforts to move health care staff between areas of the country were undertaken, but this measure was not successful on a large scale. Triage documents were developed to guide decision-making in which patients, who would otherwise have been offered critical support, would not be given that support if their predicted outcomes were poor. To some, these triage documents were the necessary tool to ensure appropriate care would be delivered to the most appropriate patient. However, for many, denying care due to lack of local resource when another jurisdiction had the capacity to do so was an untenable concept. Although debatable, the likely main driver to accepting the task of transporting multiple critically ill patients was to avoid implementing triage on a scale never before experienced by the critical care community.

However, even though it may have "felt better" to transport instead of triage, the task still took a heavy toll. Needing to perform this task when it felt that it could have been avoided engendered a tired helpless feeling, especially as media reports at the time emphasized how it was a result of a "failure in the system." This feeling was compounded by the environment that COVID-19 forced us to work in. Visitor restrictions prevented connecting more personally with families to inform and comfort them as transport was arranged. Personal preventive equipment (PPE) prevented unit and transport personnel from developing team bonds. Decisions regarding the "who, when, and where" of transport were remotely communicated, giving rise to a feeling of depersonalization of medical care. Although grateful that care was not denied to patients, the stress of trying to ensure the most appropriate patients were safely transferred rippled through health care teams as there was a sense of abandonment of our duties. Health care teams are a proud group; they take their responsibilities to heart, and it was very difficult to accept that our patients were being sent out – not to a place that had more expertise but simply to a place that had more staff.

Accepting this reality was difficult but greatly facilitated by the empathy expressed by the health care teams receiving the transferred COVID-19 patients. While Canada is an immense country, the critical care community is small, and interactions between these teams during the transports allowed more connections to develop that likely would not have otherwise. While it is correct to say that the utmost professional conduct was experienced, that is too sterile a term to convey the true comfort those interactions delivered. Also easing the acceptance of transport were the messages of thanks conveyed by numerous families, grateful that extra efforts were made to ensure their loved ones received the care they deserved, even if it did have to occur at a facility remote to them.

As we continue to work through new phases of the COVID-19 pandemic, we have yet to fully decompress and debrief over many aspects, including the role and/or necessity of transport. No medical decision is without consequence, and each decision is weighed between risks and benefits. The decision to transport is no different. The goal to ensure patients get to a place where they can receive care is weighed against the risks inherent in any movement of a critically ill patient, be it within the hospital or across the county. We need to continue to ensure that these transports are facilitated by experienced personal and that decisions for transport are transparent and equitable. It is only by recognizing and supporting these needs that transport can be seen as an ongoing viable option if we were to experience other capacity emergencies in the future.

15 When the Going Gets Tough, the Tough Get Going: A "Hybrid Model" of Paediatric and Adult Critical Care During the COVID-19 Surge

Akash Deep, MD, FRCPCH
Director, Paediatric Intensive Care Unit, King's College Hospital NHS Foundation Trust, London, UK

Philip Knight, MD, MBChB, MRCPH
Consultant, Paediatric Intensive Care Unit, King's College Hospital NHS Foundation Trust, London, UK

Louis Skevington-Postles, BSc, MSc
Team Lead Paediatric Physiotherapist, Paediatric Intensive Care Unit, King's College Hospital NHS Foundation Trust, London, UK

Submitted 7 May 2022

I was amazed by the nurses and staff on the children's unit. They were courteous, kind, and professional. I put my survival and increased recovery down to them.

– A patient in their late 70s, our longest stay adult patient on the paediatric intensive care unit during the pandemic

On 11 March 2020, the World Health Organization officially declared the novel coronavirus disease a pandemic, putting unprecedented demand on global adult critical care services. The scale of the demand was confirmed by the terrible experiences of our Spanish and Italian colleagues as it became clear that the United Kingdom and the United States would imminently face the same challenges.

The number of adult intensive care unit (ICU) beds per 100,000 population varies greatly between different countries. The United Kingdom has 6.6 adult ICU beds per 100,000 population, which is low compared to Germany, for example, with 29.9 per 100,000. With the United Kingdom lying at the lower end of capacity, the question was very evident: will adult critical care be able to cope with the unprecedented surge?

The help from paediatric services to adults could come in three different forms:

1 *Relocate human resources.* Relocation means sending doctors, nurses, and allied health professions to adult critical care. It will inadvertently lead to decreased paediatric intensive care unit (PICU) capacity and could increase the risk of staff burnout.
2 *Repurpose the PICU completely to care for adults.* Repurposing the PICU means that paediatric critical care specific to that unit will not be able to be carried out in that PICU.
3 *Create a hybrid model.* A hybrid model can be created by accommodating adults in the PICU while maintaining PICU activity. It can be done in one of two ways, either by opening additional beds to accommodate adults while keeping PICU beds intact or by managing a mix of adult and paediatric patients on the same unit, in the same space, and with the same staff. This option has the benefit of maintaining PICU services in that region.

In roughly the same 6-week period between March and May 2020, the COVID-19 pandemic led to a "super surge" of critically ill adult patients in the United Kingdom and the United States. Our hospitals were faced with the challenge of supporting our adult colleagues while also caring for critically ill children. While many PICUs across the globe converted their units to provide care exclusively for adults, a few PICUs expanded services to care for both paediatric and adult patients, forming a "hybrid model." This hybrid model required drastic adaptation to manage two very different patient cohorts in the same space and by the same staff. We describe our experience of providing a hybrid model at King's College Hospital (KCH) in London.

Children are generally cared for in two types of hospitals, either a stand-alone hospital for children or within an established adult hospital like KCH, London. As a PICU team, we wanted to help our adult colleagues but needed to ensure that the critical care offered to children did not suffer. There were urgent meetings at the local, network, and national levels to establish how this capacity could be expanded. As result, our national database, Paediatric Intensive Care Audit Network (PICANet), performed bed modelling, looking at regional occupancy of paediatric intensive care beds across the country from November 2018 to June 2019. Modelling showed that, during March and April, capacity was 25 per cent less than in the busy winter months; therefore, PICUs could likely afford to help their adult colleagues. Following this investigation, the UK paediatric and adult intensive care societies released a joint statement that PICUs would care for critically ill adults while providing uncompromised high-quality paediatric critical care. The UK National Health Service (NHS) decided to increase capacity and centralize paediatric critical care. In London, it was done in stand-alone children's hospitals such as Great Ormond Street Hospital for Children and the Evelina London Children's Hospital. This decision increased capacity at the stand-alone hospitals and was used to decompress other PICUs that had ceased paediatric services completely in order to convert to adult units. Out of the twenty-four PICUs across the United Kingdom, seven were tasked with taking adults. Some completely repurposed their PICUs to adult units by replacing all paediatric emergency equipment with adult equipment and using existing adult protocols, while retaining some PICU staff where appropriate. Some units took only COVID adults, while others took just non-COVID adults or a combination of the two. Success was dependent on the timely mapping of the challenges unique to each hospital and appropriate communication between paediatric and adult colleagues. We at KCH, due to the nature of our specialty work, adopted a hybrid model to support specialty adult and paediatric critical care services on the same unit. As KCH is one of the busiest adult critical care centres in London, all non-specialist critical care paediatric patients were transferred to other stand-alone children's hospitals. As a designated paediatric neuroscience centre, trauma centre, and supra-regional centre for liver transplant, KCH PICU allocated 25 per cent of their beds to maintain these specialty services. Incredibly, that number of beds was enough to provide this paediatric specialist care. But had we had cross-infection with COVID on the unit and not had reduced numbers of trauma and local general paediatric cases requiring PICU, the number of beds could have become overwhelmed with little patient turnover.

Before committing to the huge task of caring for adults on a PICU, one needs to ask these questions: Can I provide care outside my usual scope of practice and comfort zone? What support systems will be in place so that patients do not get care that is even 1 per cent less than the expected standard of care? Are we ready for potentially important ethical considerations that might arise? For example, how do we triage between patients of similar prognosis such as a 7-month-old with severe viral-induced respiratory failure versus a 70-year-old with COVID-pneumonia-induced respiratory failure? Fortunately, we did not have to make such decisions as we were able to accommodate all our emergency paediatric specialist care, but our position in offering assistance to adult critical care was always that our paediatric population should not suffer because of it. This position would have been taken into consideration when prioritizing our final specialist beds if faced with such tough decisions. Last but not least, what is the impact of all these unprecedented actions on the emotional well-being and private life of health care professionals, including their spouse, children, and family?

As the number of PICUs across various countries were getting ready to take care of adults, there was a rapid influx of guidelines. The theme within many published guidelines was that the principles of managing adult critical care would be the same as paediatric intensive care, the so called "bigger children," but the key for us was to understand and prepare for the differences that we, as paediatricians, might not be used to, anticipate adult-specific complications, and optimize care in the setting of the novel COVID phenotypes.

Identification of adult patients for admission to the PICU was determined by a tactical lead from the adult team, who would discuss individual patients for admission with the paediatric critical care lead. Initial triaging intentions to care for patients similar to paediatric age and diagnosis were abandoned as the demand for assistance increased. As each clinical area converted to caring for adult COVID patients, our PICU remained one of two remaining non-COVID critical care areas within the whole hospital, supporting specialist adult and paediatric services.

During those 6 extraordinary weeks of the first wave, we admitted twenty-three adult patients with a median age of 53 years while simultaneously caring for twenty-five critically ill children, the smallest weighing 2 kilograms.* We performed a record ten liver transplants, one multivisceral transplant, and facilitated two paediatric organ donations while continuing to support emergency neurosurgery. During the second surge, the number of adult and paediatric patients treated on the PICU was even higher. The second surge was busier with even sicker adults admitted to the PICU, but the experience from the first wave helped prepare the team. This model proved to be a successful response to a surge in adult critical care patients while maintaining a high level of specialist paediatric critical care. Below we share some specific challenges and strategies in six key areas during this unique time.

Leadership and Communication Strategy

We employed an established emergency structure, led by a tactical leader who disseminated updates to the clinical team. The tactical leader

---

* 4.4 lbs.

would address all operational issues, including staffing, bed availability, equipment, and consumables, and particularly, as our understanding of the disease phenotypes evolved, disseminate agreed management strategies as quickly as possible. Technology was used to maximize effective communication while minimizing unnecessary in-person meetings and exposure to the virus. Regular updates were provided from local leadership via email, teleconferencing, live streaming, and frequent multidisciplinary meetings with clearly identified leadership roles, which allowed for early identification and resolution of issues. This structure was vital in balancing the rapid influx of critically unwell patients with the progressive preparation and staffing of new escalation areas to receive them, ensuring that staff were utilized and rested as efficiently as possible.

Educational Challenges

When I woke up, I didn't know where I was. I couldn't talk. I couldn't write. It was like a nightmare, and I was terrified ... They nursed me back to reality.
– A patient in intensive care follow-up recalls their delirium

The potential gaps in knowledge with age-appropriate equipment, medication dosages, and adult-based policies were identified early in the hospital's response to COVID and mitigated through education and protocol sharing. We were able to utilize a unique pool of providers who were dual trained in adult and paediatric medicine, as well as adult ICU trainees who had rotated previously in the PICU. We had the valuable resource of unit-based nurse educators who provided just-in-time education and coaching of all bedside nursing staff and PICU providers. An oversight system was established to ensure that an advisory adult critical care attending physician was always assigned to be available for urgent consultations as required and to review the daily management plans. This cross-pollination of adult and paediatric staff allowed us to work as one big critical care team.

Team Factors

In our experience, keeping the PICU team together in a familiar environment while caring for adult patients mitigated certain patient safety risk factors but also gave resilience to the team in an emotionally and physically challenging period of time. However, some doctors and nurses willingly worked in COVID units so that vulnerable staff could be redeployed to non-COVID areas or shielded. Therefore, additional staff were recruited as part of a "return to PICU" model whereby ex-PICU nurses were recalled to shadow rosters, and the core team supported nurses with previous ICU experience or non–critical care nurses on the PICU. Senior non–critical care staff were utilized in a tier of senior staff members dedicated to updating families on a regular basis to allow clinical staff to focus on direct clinical care. Other differences in caring for the two groups of patients by the same staff posed unique challenges and included differences in visitation needs, end-of-life care, and organ donation. In this context, additional psychological support was provided by our psychology team, and the well-being hubs set up were invaluable.

Challenges for the Therapy Teams

I loved this [being brought outside] and loved the freshness on my face.
– A very sick adult patient who required two long-stay ICU admissions, one on the PICU, recalled being brought outside by the therapy teams and nurses; she had not been outside for 2 months

Adapting to a hybrid model of critical care during the pandemic presented a variety of challenges requiring bespoke solutions from the paediatric physiotherapy, occupational therapy, and speech and language therapy teams. Once the decision had been made to care for both adults and children on KCH's PICU, planning began to ensure that the therapy teams could deliver the high standards of care required to ensure best possible outcomes for both adults and children admitted. Initial steps included establishing staff training records and competencies for therapists across both paediatric and adult critical care; examples of adult-specific competencies included the safe use of speaking valves with invasive mechanical ventilation and delirium screening in adults. In order to ensure the provision of safe and effective care to both paediatric and adult patients, it was decided the paediatric therapy specialties should remain working across the paediatric critical care unit and paediatric units where possible, avoiding redeployment to environments caring solely for adult patients.

Working collaboratively with our adult therapy teams, we established local training sessions to ensure therapy staff were upskilled and had the knowledge to work safely and competently across the critical care units within KCH. Improved accessibility and social distancing guidance meant that training sessions were delivered virtually wherever possible and then supplemented with bedside teaching in smaller groups as appropriate. Examples of training sessions included adult-specific oedema management for occupational therapists and ventilation strategies in adult critical care for physiotherapists. As a paediatric therapy team, we were also communicating and contributing to training sessions at both regional and national levels, sharing our experiences of managing both adult and paediatric patients simultaneously, as well as sharing the initial experiences of caring for paediatric patients admitted with COVID. Reflecting on his experiences, Alex, a paediatric physiotherapist, remarked: "Incredible teamwork was the only way we all got through it, sharing experience and knowledge."

Upskilling of staff also facilitated redeployment of therapy staff from other specialties such as outpatient settings, helping to ensure adequate levels of staffing were maintained across the critical care units. Ensuring equitable provision of therapy services across all of the intensive care units at KCH was an immediate effort. Staff rosters were reconfigured to ensure a full 7-day therapy service was provided in line with all paediatric and adult critical care guidelines. Reconfiguring the rosters facilitated the delivery of therapy interventions such as rehabilitation, complex ventilator weaning, and discharge planning throughout the week, while also ensuring that staff remained supported and were not asked to work in isolation on weekends as part of a minimal staffing structure. Annual leave was also cancelled to support a 7-day roster, and adult therapy colleagues were utilized as required for their experience and skills in adult critical care.

Supporting therapy staff well-being was another challenge faced when repurposing into a hybrid model of paediatric and adult critical care. There was a heightened awareness of the emotional impact of asking staff to work in unfamiliar environments or areas of specialty outside of their own. Additionally, many of the activities or strategies normally utilized by staff to help maintain resilience and well-being were restricted due to government lockdown measures. The therapy team identified "well-being champions" who were responsible for arranging and signposting staff members towards well-being activities including mental health resources, and regular team and one-to-one debrief sessions supported staff and disseminated information.

Paediatric therapists voiced their thoughts and feelings about their experiences, commenting that the hybrid model was "emotionally and mentally draining as well as physical." But some also spoke about the well-being measures taken: "I feel as though the multidisciplinary team as a whole worked hard to keep up positivity throughout both waves."

Strict visiting restrictions throughout both waves of the pandemic created the unique challenge of establishing methods of communication with the families and loved ones of both our paediatric and adult patients on the critical care unit. Paediatric therapists are used to working very closely with parents throughout their child's admission and found it very challenging to work with patients, particularly young adults, in the absence of family members. To ensure our therapy care continued to be holistic and patient centred, it was crucial to facilitate discussion with family members to help build rapport, provide updates regarding therapy progress, communicate discharge plans, and gather key information allowing meaningful goals to be set. As a therapy team, we identified family liaison roles within the team and utilized technology to facilitate communication virtually. Therapy sessions, including rehabilitation and goal-setting sessions, were often completed with family members virtually. Regular timetabled family communication sessions, as well as adapting the intensive care environment with personal items provided by family members, were also key in helping prevent and manage delirium.

Families and patients alike appreciated the measures put in place to ensure patient-centred care and the efforts made to facilitate communication. Feedback from a patient in their 40s, who was admitted to the PICU at KCH during the pandemic, was recorded in a follow-up clinic:

> She said she is full of energy; she has no bad memories of ICU, only good ones. She said she loved you all and is very grateful for all the care. She will visit you all very soon when all this madness is over.

The family of a gentleman in his 80s admitted to the PICU after sustaining a brain injury were also appreciative:

> The family are all excited for his return, and we wanted to pass on our thanks to all the staff who looked after him while he was at King's College Hospital.

Through both waves of the pandemic, the paediatric therapy team continuously adapted their approach to caring for adult and paediatric patients on a hybrid model of intensive care. During the second wave of the pandemic, through experiential learning, less support was required from our adult colleagues due to the increased confidence and skill sets of our paediatric therapists in the care of adults. There were also smoother, more reliable processes established for the discharge and transfer of patients to and from the paediatric critical care unit, as well as for the procurement of equipment crucial to patient rehabilitation. The paediatric therapy teams have shown they can be effective as part of a hybrid model, which remains a responsive and flexible response to repeated adult surges. Reflecting on the team's experiences, the paediatric therapy clinical lead said:

> I am so incredibly proud of the team. They took it all in their stride. Whether they were being redeployed, treating outside their comfort zones, having feelings of doubt or uselessness, they all dug deep and did whatever was asked of them.

Equipment, Supply, and Pharmacy Challenges

As resources became progressively scarcer, we worked very closely with procurement to adjust stock lists and medications to ensure that they were in line with adult requirements. A major challenge throughout the world was the availability of ventilators. Ventilators that could be used to ventilate adults were freed up where children under 30 kgs[†] could be ventilated with high-frequency ventilators or with neonatal or portable ventilators. Each decision was carefully risk assessed to reduce the impact on the paediatric service. The high demand for renal replacement therapy (RRT) led to a shortage of machines and consumables requiring diversion of paediatric equipment. Careful calculation of our predicted needs to provide support for lifesaving paediatric liver transplants was required shift by shift. We also owe a debt of gratitude to the support received from industry contacts and friends.

Emotional Challenges: Supporting ICU Staff

The hybrid model has the unique challenge of responding to the very different physical, medical, and emotional needs of two different patient groups. For example, visitation policies in paediatric versus adult patients were very different. Adult patient visitation was limited to pre-terminal visits, and for parents of paediatric patients, alternation of caregivers for respite was prohibited. Conversations regarding end-of-life care and advanced care directives, including facilitating organ donations, challenging at baseline, often occurred on the phone or over video conferencing. A major focus was placed on the mental health and well-being of providers. Mental health teams set up well-being hubs that provided much-needed psychological support. Recognizing and acting upon the need to manage staff welfare was critical to optimize our ability to care for patients in these most challenging of times.

Conclusion

The advantage of a dynamic hybrid model was that it remained responsive to the rapidly changing demand for critical care beds, providing increased capacity for adult patients at the right time while providing ongoing specialist paediatric services. This flexible modelling also means our units have been upskilled to care for adult patients, a valuable resource for future surges with unpredictable demands. Using a

---

† 66 lbs.

hybrid model, we were able to maintain large numbers of transplants as well as high-level trauma and neurosurgical emergency services during the COVID surge. However, with a strong probability of future surges of various aetiologies occurring in the context of a winter surge for children, with high numbers of paediatric patients, additional consideration should be taken in the planning of specialist services and the available critical care capacity. With this cooperative model, the collective critical care family is better poised to successfully navigate global crises such as COVID through enhanced communication and teamwork. Our adult ICU colleagues have already been ready and willing to assist us in return. We have utilized adult nursing staff on our unit and, on the rare occasion, admitted older children to the adult liver ICU when we have exceeded capacity, but with our support and input. On a regional level, we have prepared just-in-time teaching resources for adult intensivists in preparation for our paediatric respiratory surges, and we have adult ICU fellows rotate through our paediatric unit. If future surges take place that predominantly affect children, these proactive steps will facilitate our adult ICU friends in assisting us.

This hybrid model was nationally and internationally acknowledged as a unique model. Our national society reported this model in a podcast for the members and included an interview with a 78-year-old patient, who had spent several weeks on the PICU, and his partner, who had supported him during this time. We also presented this model in the COVID-19 weekly collaborative hosted by Harvard Medical School. In addition, we collaborated with Columbia University, New York, to publish our respective hybrid models in which the New York team had adults with COVID on their unit as opposed to KCH, where we treated non-COVID adults.

Therefore, partial repurposing your PICU to accommodate adults makes sense when there is a surplus of PICU resources, especially in the summer months. Would we do it again? The answer is yes, without a shadow of a doubt. There will be many challenges on the way for the medical, nursing, and allied health professionals. Looking after your team, focusing on resilience, and allowing room for personal emotions and reflections are absolutely key to success. We extend a heartfelt thanks to the medical and nursing adult ICU colleagues. We never felt pressurized to do anything, we were always consulted, and whenever we asked for help, it was provided.

16 Lessons Learned from COVID-19: Personal Perspectives from a Low- and Middle-Income Country

Mervyn Mer, MBBCh, Dip PEC (SA), FCP (SA), Pulmonology Subspecialty, Cert Critical Care (SA), M Med (Int Med), FRCP (London), FCCP, PhD
Department of Medicine, Divisions of Critical Care and Pulmonology, Charlotte Maxeke Johannesburg Academic Hospital and Faculty of Health Sciences, University of the Witwatersrand, Johannesburg, South Africa

Submitted 13 February 2022

The past two and a half years have been both taxing and tantalizing, eerie and enthusing, intrusive and illuminating, demanding and distinctive, as well as being rewarding and a time that has required reflection. Multiple lessons have been learned from the challenge of the COVID-19 pandemic. Ten simple but important elements emanating from the intensive care unit (ICU) experience in a low- and middle-income country (LMIC) in Africa, where several limitations exist, are shared here. They have universal applicability.

1. Preparation Is Pivotal

We had the gift of some time to prepare as efficiently as we could relative to many other regions. Preparation began shortly after we became aware of the situation that was unfolding in China. Recognizing the potential implications, we got a representative team of relevant role players early on to engage, and after our first meeting, we had already devised a working protocol that was later refined and widely adopted. This protocol allowed us to address and overcome several of the challenges faced, often in the setting of very real adversity.

2. Communication Is Paramount

Communication was, and always is, an absolutely essential component in all interactions – engaging, polite, constructive, inclusive of all parties, and at all times. In our own unit, this approach overcame many significant challenges including fear, panic, anxiety, and unwillingness to work, which were so prevalent at the outset. A daily full-staff interaction was initiated with all the role players involved in the functioning of the unit, where everyone had a voice. A similar session was undertaken at night so that night staff would not be excluded. This interaction initiative was enormously time consuming but so worthwhile and beneficial. Any issues were openly addressed with respect, tolerance, and resolution, which allowed for informed and decisive decisions to be made that were then easily implemented. Staff felt backed and appreciated. The initiative also allowed for ongoing encouragement and support. It ultimately led to fabulous teamwork and spirit, and allowed for duties to be performed with passion and purpose in an effulgent and excellent fashion. We even had members volunteering for extra work, which would have been unheard of at the outset. The impact of this approach spilled over to other disciplines and working partners with resultant cohesive, collective, and collaborative interactions and efforts. A similar approach with family engagement was embarked upon from the very first patient, and a cellular phone was obtained for video calls where feasible with families and patients.

3. Staff Protection Is Vital

Although there were advocated guidelines regarding personal protective equipment (PPE), it was felt that these were not optimal for front-line workers. Several staff members became infected, some with serious illness, early on in the pandemic. Staff protection was deemed to be of utmost importance and a non-negotiable issue. Consequently, we initiated our own in-house PPE training and extended the PPE requirements to what was perceived to be most desirous and adequate rather than those recommended by local guidelines. The training was incessant, and staff soon became extremely confident. Following this initiative, there were virtually no new staff infections, and many other parties started attending our educational training sessions and adopted our policy. The initiative also allowed us to reinforce exemplary infection prevention and control (IPC) measures. In addition to the physical protection of staff and safety elements, their psychological well-being and support elements were deemed essential from the outset and were further reinforced and enhanced by the daily communication sessions.

4. Challenges Also Present Opportunity – Expanding Existing Services and Facilities

The expansion of existing facilities was advocated early on and felt to be preferable to creating new independent temporary facilities, which would potentially be dismantled at the end of the pandemic. Engagement with relevant social responsibility partners was initiated and resulted in effectively substantial expansion of our ICU facility within weeks, which will remain post the COVID-19 pandemic. This initiative has probably advanced care in this domain by at least 10 to 20 years, and many thousands of patients are likely to benefit from this action for years to come. Countless lives have already been saved as a consequence of the expansion initiative. Similar projects were advocated and facilitated elsewhere in the country based on our model and initiative. A nursing upskilling program was also initiated and embarked upon to address nursing requirements. This program was a massive success, and we have retained these valuable members as part of our enthusiastic team.

5. Simplicity and Adherence to Basic Principles Is Key

Doing the simple things well is something that I have promulgated for some time as it usually results in favourable outcomes, and the general approach was no different with COVID-19. The importance of good clinical acumen was once again shown to be extremely useful – something that requires renewed emphasis. Being poor does not mean poor care, and sound practice with excellent quality care is both feasible and possible. We should and do continue to strive for excellence even in the face of adversity. It was soon realized that care should not be compromised to "do more with less" as this practice ran the risk of doing "less for more." Principled clinical direction is required and should be maintained, even under exceedingly difficult circumstances, to ensure that patient care is never compromised.

6. Flexibility Is Essential

There was upfront recognition of the need to be flexible as we went along. Flexibility involved following trends; engaging continuously with various authorities, valued colleagues, friends, and groups; insightful and objective introspection; and adapting management accordingly. Many patients benefited from this approach.

7. Privilege to Be in the Profession Is Emphasized

COVID-19 emphasized once again what a privilege it is to be in this profession – and continues to do so, as does all our other non-COVID-19 work.

8. Relevance of Critical Care/Intensive Care Is Highlighted

This pandemic has highlighted the relevance, importance, and need for critical care/intensive care services and staff, an often-neglected issue. No hospital can truly function fittingly without adequate critical care services and staff. So many benefited from just a few who gave so much. Kudos to a great team. Acknowledgement is bestowed upon all the champions out there, and we remember and salute all those fearless colleagues who paid the ultimate price in their endeavours to help those in need.

9. It Is Critical to Care

We should never forget the spirit of "ubuntu," a wonderful South African and African philosophy – always be compassionate and humane to patients, staff, and families.

10. Making a Difference Is Possible

It is possible to make a difference even in the face of adversity. During the pandemic, we suffered a major fire in the hospital requiring evacuation of all patients and staff. On our return some months later, we were beset by a flood. None of these elements or any other, however, will ever extinguish our burning passion for this magnificent profession or drown our enthusiasm and desire to assist the patients we are so privileged to treat and cherish!

17 Vaccinating Remote Indigenous Communities

Homer Tien, MD, MSc, FRCSC
President and CEO of ORNGE; Chair of Ontario's COVID-19 Vaccine Distribution Task Force

Submitted 19 July 2022

Part 1. Operation Remote Immunity

Operation Remote Immunity (ORI) was Ontario Canada's initiative to vaccinate thirty-one remote First Nations communities and the municipality of Moosonee against COVID-19. ORI officially started on 20 December 2020. But in my mind, it unofficially started on 3 December. I received a call that day from an unknown person from the government of Ontario. I almost didn't answer it, thinking it was Service Ontario chasing me down for unpaid parking tickets. When I finally picked up, Minister of Health Christine Elliott was on the other end. She introduced herself and asked if I would consider being a member of the about-to-be-announced Ministers' COVID-19 Vaccine Distribution Task Force. Of course, I agreed. COVID had been raging for the past 9 months. In Ontario alone, there had been about 125,000 total confirmed cases and just over 3700 deaths. We were all scared: scared for our own lives as health care workers and scared for our families – particularly for our elderly parents and grandparents. The long-hoped-for vaccines against COVID were about to be approved by Health Canada and represented the light at the end of a very long and dark tunnel. Apart from wiping down groceries and sleeping in the basement after clinical shifts at the hospital, I wanted to help protect my family and my community in some meaningful way.

A little voice in my head urged caution, however. Why me for the Vaccine Task Force? I'm a trauma surgeon at Sunnybrook Health Sciences Centre. I have no special expertise in public health or knowledge concerning COVID or vaccinations. I previously had served in the Regular Forces of the Canadian Armed Forces and had deployed many times to Afghanistan and the former Yugoslavia. But I was no expert in logistics; I was only a combat surgeon. The most likely reason for my appointment was that I was also chief executive officer (CEO) of ORNGE, Ontario's air ambulance and critical care transport provider, and that ORNGE was going to be tapped to play a role in the COVID-19 vaccination program. As part of our normal work, we were already moving critically ill and injured patients from remote First Nations communities to regional health care facilities in Ontario, including those with COVID. We were also now working with the Ministry of Health to transport COVID testing samples from northern to southern laboratories to reduce turnaround times for test results.

Vaccinating Ontario's remote Indigenous communities was going to be challenging. There are dozens of these small communities, accessible only by aircraft, in Northern Ontario. The distances between these communities are immense. ORNGE's major airbase in Northwest Ontario is in Thunder Bay. The northernmost community in Northwest Ontario is Fort Severn, located on the shores of Hudson Bay about 750 kilometres* away from Thunder Bay. The westernmost Indigenous community in Northern Ontario is Poplar Hill, and it's about 950 kilometres† from the easternmost community, Moose Cree First Nation on Moose Factory Island. Given the immense distances, the lifelines of these communities are their airports, many of which have only gravel runways with no de-icing facilities and are supported with only regional weather reporting. A severe winter weather storm can sometimes stop flights for 24 hours into and out of these communities. In addition, the nursing stations that provide health care to the communities are frequently understaffed and would not be able to manage the COVID-19 vaccination program while meeting the daily care needs of their community members. Most importantly, there was a real sense of urgency to vaccinate these communities. They had been locked down since the beginning of the pandemic because there was a fear that the virus would decimate the communities if it ever got into them. Houses were crowded, and there were no isolation facilities in the communities. Infection control would be near impossible.

The other major challenge was going to be vaccine hesitancy. Different Indigenous leaders were already warning me that there was likely

---

* 466 miles.
† 590 miles.

to be immense distrust of any government-sponsored vaccination program, stemming from a long legacy of systemic racism, colonialism, oppression, and broken promises. Why would any Indigenous person trust a system that allowed and propagated the residential school system that has caused so much intergenerational trauma? Between 1883 and 1996, up to 150,000 children were forcibly separated from their families and sent to these schools with the aim to "kill the Indian in the child" and assimilate them into Canadian culture.[1] This same system then allowed medical experimentation on Indigenous children at these residential schools. Malnourished Indigenous children were denied adequate nutrition to study the benefit of vitamin supplementation versus other forms of nutritional supplementation. Informed consent was never obtained. Even as children died, the experiments continued.[2] Indigenous leaders told me that this distrust had resulted in an influenza vaccination rate of about 8 per cent, and they were desperate to see higher COVID vaccination rates to protect their communities from the pandemic.

Although I had not received any confirmation of my role in the immunization program for these remote communities, in my mind, my appointment to the COVID-19 Task Force served as a "Warning Order" to get ready for this mission. The Pfizer vaccine required storage and transport at $-70°C$.[‡] ORNGE had no such storage facilities at our bases and no such transport containers for our aircraft. I immediately asked our procurement team at ORNGE to start looking for these as I imagined that they would be in short supply. Everyone in the world would be looking for them. In addition, ORNGE only has eight fixed-wing aircraft, all of which are the Pilatus PC-12, a single-engine turboprop air ambulance. These aircraft were already overtasked; they were used 24/7 for air ambulance work and performed about 3300 air ambulance missions in 2020, averaging about 1700 kilometres[§] per mission. We needed to secure other aircraft for the vaccination program. I asked my aviation group to start contacting commercial air carriers around the province and the Ministry of Northern Development, Mines, Natural Resources and Forestry (MNRF) to check for the availability of aircraft.

Former chief of defence staff General Rick Hillier was announced as the chair of Ontario's COVID-19 Vaccination Distribution Task Force on 23 November 2020. The Task Force was convened on 4 December under

---

‡ $-94°F$.
§ 1056 miles.

his leadership and had been meeting bi-weekly since its inception. At the 20 December meeting, General Hillier announced that a decision had been made: I would be in charge of Operation Remote Immunity. He announced this decision in classic military style: "Homer, you're in charge, and you're going to be the one throat we choke if this doesn't go well." That night, I didn't sleep well. I could feel General Hillier's hands around my throat, and I felt like I had swallowed a lead ball that was now sitting in my stomach. Although "failure is not an option" is a much-used line, failure was truly an option for this mission. Bad weather, human health resource challenges, and vaccine hesitancy could all result in a low vaccination uptake. Future surges of COVID infections that would decimate these communities would be the overt consequence of my incompetence and failure.

The next day, I stopped feeling sorry for myself and got to work. One of the first steps of the military planning process is to assemble the leadership team. Two separate teams would be required: one would be my headquarters staff, which would be involved in all aspects of operational planning. The second team would be the Tactical Operations Centre, which would be responsible for overseeing day-to-day operations. These teams would all come from ORNGE. Another important early step in the military planning process is to understand the restraints and constraints that we would be operating under. Indigenous leadership and autonomy were critical, so ORNGE was co-leading Operation Remote Immunity with Nishnawbe Aski Nation (NAN), the political organization representing all of the remote Indigenous communities that would be part of ORI. NAN had already contacted me to discuss a set of guiding principles for ORI:

1. Community resources are constrained. ORI should not impose further stress on resources.
2. ORI teams should be dually vaccinated, and all efforts should be made to ensure that the teams do not bring COVID-19 into the communities.
3. Teams needed to be competent in their areas of service.
4. NAN, tribal councils, and community leaders need to be involved in the decision-making process for the plans and need to approve the plans.
5. Community members who help organize and run clinics need to be compensated.
6. ORI teams should be culturally competent and sensitive to community nuances.
7. Translation must be provided.

8 Home immunization services need to be provided.
9 Supplies should be left in the community in case hesitant people reconsider.
10 Non-Indigenous members of the community should also be eligible for vaccination.

All of the guiding principles were reasonable and practical, but some were challenging to implement. For example, a very small amount of vaccine was just starting to arrive in Ontario. How were we going to ensure that all ORI team members were doubly vaccinated when we didn't even know who would be on the teams? Indigenous leadership and autonomy were the overarching principles, however, so I started to think of the guiding principles as having the force of "orders" instead of "nice to follow but optional." With that in mind, developing a "concept of ops" became easier.

Our first step was to determine with NAN and the communities how much time we had to complete the vaccination program. The communities along the James Bay coast are often evacuated in early April because of spring flooding. So the vaccination program needed to be complete by then; otherwise, extra logistical challenges would be imposed in trying to vaccinate communities evacuated to different cities across Ontario. With that in mind, we developed a quick timeline for our operation. Because it was already 20 December, because the vaccine had not yet arrived in Ontario, and because all of our vaccination teams needed to be doubly vaccinated, I tentatively picked 1 February 2021 as the start date of the mission and 15 April as the end date for completion of second doses in all communities. From this timeline, I then worked with my team to develop our concept of operations based on the guiding principles set out by NAN:

1 **ORI should not impose further stress on community resources.** From a planning point of view, this guideline meant that teams would fly in to vaccinate and fly out the same day. They would not stay in the community.
2 **ORI teams would be dually vaccinated and ... would not bring COVID-19 into the communities.** There were very few dually vaccinated people in Ontario at the beginning of ORI, which meant that ORNGE front-line staff had to be prioritized to be vaccinated starting right after Christmas 2020. Even with that, our tight timeline for completing the mission meant that our teams would need external, vaccinated health care workers. So we started to recruit physicians and surgeons from hospitals and medical schools because front-line

ICU, Emergency Department (ED), and operating room (OR) health care workers were being prioritized for vaccination. And they volunteered, even though many were working extra hours in the face of the onslaught of COVID-19+ patients at their own institutions. We recruited from Queen's, NOSM, and the University of Toronto. Because we were still short for our first rotation, which started on 1 February, I did a separate emergency recruitment drive from my friends and colleagues in the Department of Surgery at the University of Toronto.

We also obtained some rapid tests. All team members were required to have a negative antigen test and screen negative for symptoms prior to boarding our aircraft to vaccinate in the communities. The communities had protected themselves by locking their communities down at the beginning of the pandemic. The last thing we wanted was for our vaccination teams to bring COVID into their communities.

3 **Teams need to be competent in their areas of service.** We were very sensitive to guard against the idea of sending unsupervised trainees to "practise" in these communities. Medical students and residents were only allowed to participate if they were going as part of a team from their medical school with proper supervision from clinical faculty at that school. We also briefed the community if trainees were part of the team. Communities could opt out from having trainees vaccinate in their communities, but most allowed them in because they saw it as a wonderful opportunity to foster interest in Indigenous health among future physicians, surgeons, and other health care workers.

4 **NAN, tribal councils, and community leaders need to be involved in the decision-making process for the plans and need to approve the plans.** NAN and ORNGE set up an ambitious schedule of meeting with the leadership of every community (n = 32) prior to the start of the mission. We wanted the opportunity to understand their situation and their needs, and an opportunity to address any vaccine hesitancy they may be feeling. We met with NAN leadership and NAN chiefs on a weekly basis. We also set up a schedule for the tactical operations leaders and our operational planning team to fly into each community to meet with local leaders to plan each clinic at the local level.

5 **Community members who participate in organizing and running the clinics need to be compensated.** This concept was such a simple and important sign of respect for the community members. External vaccination teams would not be able to pick appropriate

locations for the vaccination clinics, set up the appropriate stations and waiting areas, roster people to come for their shots, and set up ground transport for the teams. Only community members could do these tasks, which represented a significant amount of full-time work for them. Vaccination team members were being paid to participate in the program. Why should we treat community members any differently? We started working right away with the First Nations and Inuit Health Branch (FNIHB) of the federal government and Indigenous Affairs Ontario to establish a budget for funding the community coordinators and team members for each community.

6 & 7 **ORI teams should be culturally competent and sensitive to community nuances. Translation must be provided.** All team members were required to take the San'yas Indigenous Cultural Safety Training Program prior to participating on the mission. Many of the surgeons from the University of Toronto who participated were so impressed with this training package that they asked for this training to be a part of faculty training. The university's Chair in General Surgery established a Chair's Challenge for her faculty to complete this training. We also had all of the consent and information forms translated into Cree, Oji-Cree, and Ojibway. Translation actually proved to be very challenging as it was difficult to find an approved translator familiar with all three dialects who could verify the accuracy of the translations.

8 **Home immunization services need to be provided.** This requirement was a community-focused guiding principle that protected the most vulnerable. To operationalize it, we requested the participation of the Canadian Rangers, which are a subcomponent of the Canadian Armed Forces Reserve, made up of Inuit, First Nations, Metis, and other Canadians. The Indigenous members of the Rangers are mostly recruited from the communities that they serve. The Rangers would be able to provide transportation and act as guides for many of the home visits and also help the vaccination program in community in many other ways. Some communities chose not to activate the Rangers within their communities and activated other resources.

9 & 10 **Supplies should be left in the community, and non-Indigenous members of the community should also be eligible for vaccination.** Vaccine supply was very limited at the beginning of ORI. Ensuring that there was sufficient vaccine for non-Indigenous members of the community was initially a challenge, but as vaccine started to arrive in Canada in larger quantities and more regularly, these requirements became a non-issue.

The plan was developed with NAN's guiding principles as the key requirements for the plan. Six teams were organized. Each team consisted of a team lead and second-in-command who were ORNGE paramedics. They were in charge of teams of external health care workers and administration staff recruited from diverse agencies including Queen's University, NOSM, University of Toronto, Northern EMS organizations, Georgian College, the Canadian Red Cross, Calian, and FNIHB. Forward operating bases were organized in Thunder Bay, Timmins, and Sioux Lookout. Teams were prepositioned at these locations. The normal deployment cycle included travel days to and from the forward operating bases, confirmatory training, and COVID testing at the bases. Teams had 5 days to vaccinate each community, and each day was a 12-hour day, including flights in and out of the community. The ORNGE headquarters staff and tactical operations staff organized everything seamlessly.

We had a soft launch of ORI in mid-January to the James Bay coast and Sioux Lookout because the Weeneebayko Area Health Authority (WAHA) and the Meno Ya Win Health Centre already had health care workers in the communities ready to vaccinate. The official launch of ORI was on 1 February 2021. I was extremely nervous that first week. However, as our vaccination numbers started coming in and as community leaders began tweeting the happy stories of their communities coming together with our vaccination teams to promote vaccination and to achieve high vaccination rates, I knew that ORI was going to be successful.

Respecting Indigenous leadership and autonomy was the reason why ORI was successful. By ensuring that NAN guiding principles had the force of "orders" and not "optional guidance," we ensured that the voices of the community leaders were the ones that were heard and that mattered. The plan reflected the wisdom of the Indigenous leaders and community, and their special knowledge of the situation in their community.

Part 2. Chairing the Provincial COVID-19 Vaccine Distribution Task Force

By early March 2021, my stress level surrounding ORI had diminished. Although there were still many things that could cause day-to-day operations to unravel, each successful mission added to the experience and confidence of the ORI team. I started to look forward to the end of ORI in mid-April and the resumption of a more normal schedule. Since December 2020, the ORI team had been working non-stop, 7 days a week and for 12 to 14 hours per day. During ORI, I would often only see my children when they came down to my basement office to bring me coffee or meals.

On 15 March 2021, however, two news items caught my eye. One was that both the Ontario COVID-19 Science Advisory Table and the Ontario Hospital Association declared that Ontario had entered a third wave of COVID-19. The other was that General Hillier decided not to extend his appointment as chair of Ontario's Vaccine Distribution Task Force past 31 March 2021. Both these announcements would significantly impact my ability to return to a more normal schedule over the next 6 months.

Wave 3 was marked by a surge in cases, hospitalizations, and ICU admissions in the Greater Toronto Area (GTA), particularly in Peel, Toronto, and parts of York. To deal with this influx of ICU patients to the GTA, Ontario Health established an information management system (IMS) table with ORNGE and CritiCall Ontario to coordinate the rapid movement of ICU patients from crowded hospitals to hospitals with ICU capacity. According to the CBC, this IMS table coordinated the movement of 1133 critical care patients to create ICU capacity in the GTA during the month of April 2021. At ORNGE, we created a surge response team to staff our critical care land ambulances to manage this increase in patient transport volumes. In addition, we had to increase the capacity of our dispatch centre to manage the increased call volumes.

At about this same time, I was first asked if I was interested in becoming the chair of the Vaccine Task Force. My initial instinct was to decline. ORI was daunting, but leading it was a colonel's job (which is what I was in the military) – a field officer responsible to a general (Hillier), who was responsible for developing a tactical plan and whose unit was directly responsible for conducting the operation. Leading the Vaccine Task Force would be a different beast altogether; it was a senior general's job – someone who developed strategy for thirty-four different public health units, each commanded by a chief medical officer of health, and who had to answer to ministers and the premier. Hence, General Hillier was the first chair; who was I to take over from him?

In the end, I agreed. Ontario was now fully in the midst of the third wave, and the Vaccine Task Force could not be left rudderless. Fortunately, the government, the Task Force, the Clinical Advisory Table, and Ontario's Public Service had done phenomenal work in setting the stage for a successful phase 2 of the vaccination rollout. One key achievement was the development of the vaccination prioritization matrix that guided phase 1. This matrix prioritized high-risk populations for the COVID vaccine during the period of constrained vaccine supply.

Phase 1 high-risk populations included adults aged 80 and older, health care workers, seniors living in congregate settings, and Indigenous adults. The implementation of this prioritization matrix protected the most vulnerable seniors and saved the lives of thousands of seniors in subsequent COVID waves. Another key achievement was the build-up of vaccination capacity. Public health units had established numerous hospital-based and community-based mass vaccinations clinics and were just awaiting sufficient vaccine supply to ramp up vaccinations. As well, the framework was established for enlisting extra pharmacies as another major channel for vaccinations.

I officially took over on 1 April 2021 as chair of the Vaccine Task Force. One of the first things I did was to call Dr. Peter Jüni and Dr. Adalsteinn Brown, respectively the scientific director and the co-chair of Ontario's COVID-19 Science Advisory Table, to ask for their advice. As of February, the Science Table had already unveiled modelling data indicating that Ontario was headed into a third wave, spurred on by the Delta variant, and that ICU admissions were projected to increase dramatically. As the new chair, I wanted their opinion as to what the appropriate vaccination strategy would be for Ontario as we headed into Wave 3. Their advice was encapsulated in a simple analogy: "dump the water wherever the fire is." In the case of Ontario, we should preferentially supply vaccines to the public health units with the highest incidence of COVID. This advice became our hotspot strategy. These hotspots tended to be in lower income, racialized communities. In many jurisdictions in the United States, the highest vaccine supplies and administration rates were being observed in high-income areas with the lowest incidence of COVID. The Vaccine Task Force members, government, and public service officials all quickly agreed to implement our strategy. Our plan was to reverse this trend and measure our performance against this action. Over the next few months, vaccine was prioritized to the communities with the highest incidence of COVID. In addition, we established our own provincial COVID vaccination teams – including the GO-VAXX buses – allowing us to establish pop-up vaccination clinics in community centres, places of worship, and high-risk work settings in the COVID hotspots. With this strategy, and by working with each of the local public health units, we were able to increase the vaccination rates in the hotspots beyond that observed in higher income/lower incidence neighbourhoods.

Since April 2021, I have continued for months as chair of the Vaccine Task Force, and with its dissolution, I have continued to stay on to provide operational advice about the vaccination program. Even so, April 2021 will always be special to me. My first month as chair of Ontario's

Vaccine Task Force was marked with extreme stress and worry. Wave 3 was at its height; ICUs were filling up. Patients needed to be transported quickly to create ICU capacity in crowded hospitals in Peel, Toronto, and York. Vaccines were seen as the only way out of Wave 3, and I was a brand new chair. In the end, we reached our vaccination target of administering first doses to at least 40 per cent of Ontario's adults by the end of April 2021; in fact, we hit this target 1 week early. Our hotspot strategy was working; vaccine was being preferentially administered to lower income, racialized communities with the highest risk of infection, and the incidence of cases was already starting to dip in early May 2021. What I will always remember is how government, public service, public health officials, and other health care workers rallied and were completely focused on vaccinating as many fellow Ontarians as possible. And as with ORI, I felt that each day of high vaccination rates and lower case counts in the days and months after 30 April 2021 was contributing to a feeling of confidence and competency among vaccine team members. As each new wave or new challenge emerged, I was very proud to hear vaccine team members say, "We've got this."

REFERENCES

1. The past is not the past for Canada's Indigenous peoples. *Lancet*. 2021;357 (10293):2439. https://doi.org/10.1016/S0140-6736(21)01432-X. Medline: 34175069.
2. MacDonald NE, Stanwick R, Lynk A. Canada's shameful history of nutrition research on residential school children: the need for strong medical ethics in Aboriginal health research. *Paediatr Child Health*. 2014;19(2):64. https://doi.org/10.1093/pch/19.2.64. Medline: 24596474.

PART FOUR

Stories from Forgotten Places

The media accounts of the pandemic that circulated within the Western Hemisphere focused either on the North American or European urban experience. When they expanded beyond these confines, they tended to focus on areas of cataclysm: new deadly variants ripping through South Africa, the emergence of deadly mould co-infections in India, strict lockdowns in China, and so on. But the pandemic was, by definition, a global event, and while we are unable to provide accounts from every corner that was touched by this catastrophe, in section "Stories from Forgotten Places," we have assembled accounts from locales that received relatively scant media attention. "COVID-19 Pandemic and the Fate of Indonesian Children" describes the effect of the virus on children globally and particularly on those living in one of the most populous yet ignored countries on earth, Indonesia. Similarly, "Caring for Paediatric Patients with COVID-19 During the Pandemic in Peru: Experiences from 2020 and 2021" tells of the challenges of caring for children, far too many of them orphaned, in Peru, another low-income country with a struggling health care system. "From the Four Directions: Healing on Navajoland" provides a unique viewpoint on the American pandemic experience – the account of a Diné (Navajo) physician first witnessing the devastation wreaked by the virus on the Navajo Nation and later witnessing the recovery of the nation based upon faith, family, and tradition.

18 COVID-19 Pandemic and the Fate of Indonesian Children

Kurniawan Taufiq Kadafi, MD
Faculty of Medicine, Universitas Brawijaya, Dr Saiful Anwar General Hospital, Malang, Indonesia

Ririe Fachrina Malisie, MD, PhD
Faculty of Medicine, Universitas Sumatera Utara, Adam Malik General Hospital, Medan, Indonesia

Submitted 7 December 2022

This chapter will describe the problems of the COVID-19 pandemic in Indonesian children during the first 2 years of the pandemic, the challenges we faced, and how we overcame them.

Since the emergence of a new infection outbreak was first announced at the end of December 2019, and the World Health Organization declared it a pandemic on 11 March 2020, it has spread to 210 countries. It is now 2022, and the COVID-19 pandemic has not shown any signs of ending. As of 20 May 2022, there have been 3,917,531 confirmed cases of COVID-19 in the world, including 270,720 deaths and 1,344,120 recovered cases. In Indonesia in May 2020, there were 2,302,691 active cases; most (98 per cent) were mild cases, while the remaining 2 per cent were severe cases. Children have not escaped the pandemic's impact. Cases in children predominantly (50–80 per cent) resulted from contact with the child's infected family members. Around 2 per cent of children infected with COVID-19 were asymptomatic, while the majority of infected children (91–100 per cent) presented with fever. Deaths in children have not yet occurred. However, it is feared that children are a group vulnerable to severe infections. Previous international outbreaks of MERS-CoV (Middle East respiratory syndrome coronavirus), which is also known to cause lung infections, typically resulted in asymptomatic infections in children (32 per cent) or relatively mild symptoms, yet it can cause severe illness with a mortality rate that has reached 6 per cent.

In the case of COVID-19, children have a low rate of infection. In addition, clinical symptoms in children are also often mild to moderate, and children rarely experience severe clinical symptoms. A study by Jacqueline S.M. Ong and colleagues,[1] who obtained data in China, reported that cases of COVID-19 in patients under the age of 19 only reached 2 per cent of confirmed cases, while in Italy, confirmed COVID-19 cases in children reached just 1.2 per cent. In Korea, however, the number of confirmed COVID-19 cases in children under the age of 19 was 4.8 per cent. Cases of children with COVID-19 were recorded at 12.3 per cent of a cohort of 1391 paediatric patients screened at Wuhan Children's Hospital in China in early 2020. A clinical and epidemiological study of thirty-six children with COVID-19 conducted by Haiyan Qiu and colleagues[2] in Zhejiang, China, found that 89 per cent of the children had been infected by close contact with family members; however, 47 per cent of these children had mild clinical symptoms, while 53 per cent had moderate clinical symptoms. No children in the study experienced severe or even critical clinical conditions. The most common symptoms experienced by children infected with COVID-19 were fever and dry cough; other symptoms, which rarely occur in children, were runny nose, swallowing pain, tightness, vomiting, or diarrhoea.

Researchers have advanced theories to explain why a child's clinical symptoms are milder compared to clinical symptoms in adults. The role of the angiotensin-converting enzyme (ACE-2) may provide one explanation.[3-5] ACE-2 acts as a receptor for the COVID-19 virus to enter into cells, causing infection. ACE-2 receptors basically have a protective function in several organs, including the lungs, kidneys, heart, gastrointestinal tract, and blood vessels. If the COVID-19 virus binds to the ACE-2 receptor, there will be impaired function in many organs, including the lungs, kidneys, gastrointestinal tract (the patient then experiences symptoms of diarrhoea, nausea, and vomiting), and the blood vessels. The number and expression of ACE-2 receptors increase in adults and in people with diabetes, as an example, worsening their illness. In children, the expression or number of ACE-2 receptors is still relatively small compared to adults, which makes it hard for the virus to attach optimally to children's cells and could explain why children have milder symptoms than adults. However, another theory is that children's ACE-2 receptors are less sensitive to binding COVID-19, so the children experience a protective effect. In addition, it is hypothesized that children also gain protection from often experiencing other viral infections, stimulating more antibody production and an ability to fight off serious COVID-19 infection. However, although children's clinical symptoms are usually milder than those of adults, children are also carriers of the virus, which can be transmitted to adults.

What has happened so far in Indonesia? At the beginning of the pandemic, no official data existed, which made it difficult for clinicians to create standard guidelines for diagnosing COVID-19. Around the world, transmission from children to nearby adults can and has caused fatal illness in adults, especially in those with comorbidities such as diabetes. Therefore, if a child is confirmed positive for COVID-19, close contacts must be traced and their infection status determined – whether they also have COVID-19 or not. Vice versa, if a family member is suspected of or confirmed to have COVID-19, the child must be monitored and, if necessary, a doctor consulted about the child's status, especially since children with COVID-19 are sometimes asymptomatic or have mild-to-moderate symptoms. This common, practical approach has caused significant challenges in Indonesia where diagnosing and monitoring the spread of COVID-19 has been difficult.

At the beginning of the pandemic, Indonesia was very unprepared to face this emergency situation. One problem was the limited availability of personal protective equipment (PPE). Many doctors and paramedics were forced to use modified raincoats to protect themselves when treating COVID-19 patients. COVID-19 spreads quite fast and can cause death, which resulted in a heavy psychological impact for doctors and paramedics who used raincoats as PPE, a solution very far from what is considered standard PPE everywhere across the globe. Although there were no reports of infection spread due to this practice at that time, the use of raincoats as PPE was still nerve-wracking for those on the front lines. This situation occurred in the first months of the COVID-19 pandemic. Later, the government worked to provide PPE, and finally the limits on PPE availability were overcome.

In Indonesia, another problem in handling COVID-19 in children was the difficulty at the beginning of the pandemic of establishing a COVID-19 diagnosis. Unlike in adults, the results of laboratory examinations in children with confirmed COVID-19 do not provide a distinctive picture. In a study sample of 1099 adult patients with confirmed COVID-19 from thirty-one provinces in China,[6] the haematological (laboratory blood cell) examination results showed that 82.1 per cent of patients had lymphopenia (decreased number of a subcategory of white blood cells); 36.2 per cent of patients had thrombocytopenia (low platelets, which are cells that help blood to clot); and 33.7 per cent of patients had leukopenia (overall low white blood cell numbers). By contrast, the results of laboratory examinations in children with confirmed

COVID-19 showed that 16.6 per cent had leukopenia, while lymphopenia only occurred in 12.9 per cent of patients and thrombocytopenia in 3.2 per cent of patients. Some medical centres diagnosed patients with COVID-19 using a scoring system. The scoring system contains clinical findings, haematology (laboratory blood cell) results, and radiological (X-ray and/or CT scan) results. This system is difficult to apply to paediatric patients because most of them have mild symptoms and may even be asymptomatic, and the results of haematological (blood cell) examinations are not specific. Therefore, screening paediatric patients is more difficult than screening adult patients. In paediatric patients, contact history tracing must also be carried out as it will help to establish COVID-19 infection. The lack of specific diagnostic tools such as rapid response tests or RT-PCR (reverse transcriptase-polymerase chain reaction) tests at the beginning of the pandemic was an additional challenge. Even when tests were available to establish diagnosis in paediatric patients, the turnaround time in Indonesia was long, taking up to 1 week, which required doctors to be very careful when diagnosing COVID-19 in children. As a result, many children who were suspected of COVID-19 remained in isolation rooms for a long time.

As a result of these challenges, family members of paediatric patients with COVID-19 often experienced high levels of anxiety. In fact, a COVID-19 diagnosis often could not be confirmed in some children who were being treated and experienced worsening illness, even though some of these patients eventually died. Sadly, sometimes the PCR results for these patients were only available a few days after they died, which caused many social problems. Many families of patients became angry because the wait time for the diagnosis results was too long. They worried that, if their children were not actually infected with COVID-19, they would be exposed to COVID-19 due to these delays and the limited availability of testing. This fear often led to anger and could trigger violence against the health officer, which was very concerning. Families of patients expressed their dissatisfaction with the hospital services as verbal anger towards doctors and paramedics, even to the point that some health care workers were subject to physical violence. This problem was slowly solved by procuring tools and inspection kits that were easy to obtain. At this point in the pandemic, children suspected of having COVID-19 had to go to a laboratory, health clinic, or hospital to obtain a COVID-19 PCR test. As of the last few months, the diagnosis of COVID-19 can now be determined in less than 24 hours.

In Indonesia, another problem during the pandemic concerning children was their immunization status. The pandemic has led to various policies to minimize large crowds of people with the aim of preventing COVID-19 transmission. These measures will certainly affect children's health services, especially immunization. The programs of integrated health centres (IHCs) in villages have been temporarily suspended in order to prevent the transmission of COVID-19 from person to person. One of the programs at the IHCs is the immunization of children. Consequently, the delay in these programs will cause the child's immunization status to be compromised. The low coverage of routine immunization in 2019, because immunization programs only reached 60–70 per cent of children, will continue to decline if the pandemic does not end soon. However, routine immunizations for children must still be completed. At the beginning of the pandemic, the Indonesian Pediatric Association recommended that immunization during the pandemic be prioritized for children aged 0–18 months. It is feared that, if immunization is not carried out, new problems will arise during the pandemic or after the emergence of a pandemic in the form of outbreaks of other infectious diseases, such as diphtheria and pertussis, due to low immunization coverage. This risk will certainly be a new problem for the government, as well as for the Indonesian people. Several strategies were carried out at the beginning of the pandemic to keep immunization programs running, including arranging an immunization schedule with appointments to minimize children's contact with other patients and setting up separate immunization sites and places for treatment in facilities that provide immunization, such as private doctor practices, hospitals, or health centres. If circumstances permit, the plan is to immediately immunize those who have had their implementation schedule delayed. In the sixth month of the COVID-19 pandemic, the Indonesian government is working to reactivate immunization services. Some of the strategies that have been implemented are drive-through immunization sites and mobile immunization services. As a result of these measures, immunization coverage began to increase. Hopefully, the pandemic will end soon for us and the future of our children.

After 2 years of the COVID-19 pandemic, predictions made at its beginning have really happened. Cases of clinically severe pertussis are now being reported, some even requiring treatment in paediatric intensive care units (PICUs); cases of severe diphtheria with complications of respiratory failure are also being seen. These outbreaks of infectious disease have encouraged the government and the Indonesian Pediatric Association to intensify immunization programs that had declined at the beginning of the COVID-19 pandemic.

COVID-19 vaccination is also an issue. At the beginning of the pandemic, many people doubted the value of the vaccination and even refused to be vaccinated. Various efforts have been made by the government to increase the COVID-19 vaccination coverage, one of which is to impose conditions that vaccination is required for people entering public service centres, such as transportation hubs and shopping centres. Awareness of the COVID-19 vaccination among people in Indonesia has increased significantly after so many people died from the Delta variant of COVID-19. After that, the government could more easily vaccinate the Indonesian people, including children.

Another problem that occurred at the beginning of the pandemic was that not all hospitals and doctors were ready and willing to treat COVID-19. This hesitancy caused a rise in the number of patients with COVID-19 in certain hospitals. Although there is an increase in cases of the Delta variant of COVID-19, many patients are not handled optimally due to lack of oxygen and have to remain in the emergency room or even in the ambulance because hospitals and hospital wards refuse to admit them. Many patients are lining up due to limited treatment rooms, and a lot of patients end up dying because they could not get the maximum treatment. This situation is very concerning. Efforts to sort patients in many hospitals have been carried out using a triage system. But because so many patients come to hospitals in critical condition, almost all hospitals have difficulty accommodating patients. Paediatric patients receive separate treatment priorities. However, in some hospitals, intensive care for children and adults is combined. Consequently, with the increase in the number of Delta variant cases, some paediatric patients have had difficulty accessing treatment rooms. The government is working hard to solve this problem by creating special emergency hospitals for COVID-19 patients. This step is proving quite successful in reducing the accumulation of patients in other hospitals. The Indonesian government is trying its best to overcome this issue, and slowly the problems are being resolved.

REFERENCES

1. Ong JSM, Tosoni A, Kim Y, et al. Coronavirus disease 2019 in critically ill children: a narrative review of the literature. *Pediatr Crit Care Med.* 2020;21(7):662–6. https://doi.org//10.1097/PCC.0000000000002376. PMID: 32265372.
2. Qiu H, Wu J, Hong L, et al. Clinical and epidemiological features of 36 children with coronavirus disease 2019 (COVID-19) in Zhejiang, China: an observational cohort study. *Lancet Infect Dis.* 2020;20(6):689–96. https://doi.org/10.1016/s1473-3099(20)30198-5. PMID: 32220650.

3. Dioguardi M, Cazzolla AP, Arena C, et al. Innate immunity in children and the role of ACE2 expression in SARS-CoV-2 infection. *Pediatr Rep*. 2021;13(3):363–82. https://doi.org/10.3390/pediatric13030045. PMID: 34287338.
4. Patel AB, Verma A. Nasal ACE2 levels and COVID-19 in children. *JAMA*. 2020;323(23):2386–7. https://doi.org/10.1001/jama.2020.8946. PMID: 32432681.
5. Schurink B, Roos E, Vos W, et al. AE2 protein expression during childhood, adolescence, and early adulthood. *Pediatr Dev Pathol*. 2022;25(4):404–8. https://doi.org/10.1177/10935266221075312. PMID: 3220822.
6. Guan W-J, Ni Z-Y, Hu Y, et al. Clinical characteristics of coronavirus disease 2019 in China. *NEJM*. 2020;382(18):1708–20. https://doi.org/10.1056/NEJMoa2002032. PMID: 32109013.

19 Caring for Paediatric Patients with COVID-19 During the Pandemic in Peru: Experiences from 2020 and 2021

Jesús Domínguez-Rojas, MD
Department of Critical Care, Instituto Nacional de Salud del Niño (National Institute of Children's Health), Lima, Peru

Alvaro Coronado-Muñoz, MD
Department of Pediatrics, Division of Critical Care, Montefiore Medical Center, Albert Einstein College of Medicine, New York

Submitted 6 June 2022

We are both paediatric intensivists. Even though we lived the pandemic in different countries, we have shared clinical and research experiences that started at that time. We present how we saw and lived the COVID-19 pandemic in Peru, with a particular focus on paediatric patients.

Peru was one of the first countries to implement a full lockdown, starting on 25 March 2020. Despite efforts to contain COVID-19, Peru was one of the countries in the world with a very high number of cases per capita and a high mortality rate, especially during the first year. Our country has a public health system that constantly operates at its limit. During the winter, it is not unusual for emergency rooms to be overwhelmed, with patients waiting in the hallways, and to get a general ward bed or, even worse, a critical care bed can take days or weeks. Paediatric care in public hospitals varies seasonally. The number of beds and critical care units for paediatrics is far smaller than for adult services. In order to understand our public health system, it is important to know that one-third of the population in Peru lives in the capital city, Lima, and most of the hospitals, approximately 60 per cent, are in Lima. Health services outside the capital city, and more specifically access to higher levels of care, are scarce.

One of the first measures the government of Peru took to create more beds for adults was to open paediatric units to adult patients. However, over time, we noticed an increase in the number of paediatric patients with COVID-19. Initially, most COVID-19 cases could be managed in the outpatient setting or in the emergency rooms, but care providers always feared that we would end up with positive cases in the paediatric wards. As expected, we saw a sharp increase in COVID-19 patients requiring admission to regular hospital floors. We did not have any specific isolation system for these patients; in many hospitals, they had to share rooms with other patients. We needed to screen all the positive contacts in the inpatient setting, and some kids developed nosocomial (hospital acquired) COVID-19 infections. Our next fear was that we did not have critical care units specifically for paediatric patients with COVID-19. The design of the critical care units in different hospitals did not allow for isolation, so we needed to think about adopting the same scheme that the government had taken for adult patients: create specific COVID-19 units. A "COVID-19 hospital" was created that included a paediatric emergency room, general floor, and critical care unit. As expected, over time, the number of patients in this hospital surpassed its capacity, forcing the rest of the hospitals to create designated COVID-19 areas. Patients with chronic diseases who were not managed within the primary care system were the worst affected by the collapse of the paediatric health system. Most primary care systems closed, leaving children only the option of seeking help in the paediatric emergency rooms, where they were exposed to COVID-19. Consequently, numerous paediatric patients with comorbidities and increased risk factors became critically ill with COVID-19, increasing the length of occupancy of critical care beds as well as our mortality rate.

As mentioned before, the general feeling during the first few months was fear – a generalized fear of the unknown and fear that we health care providers would get sick ourselves. The lack of personal protective equipment (PPE) transformed that fear into panic and anxiety. PPE was our only tool that could make us feel reassured when we were taking care of COVID-19 patients. However, as with many other resources and similar to many countries, we didn't have enough PPE, and many health care providers stopped taking care of these patients. The reality in Peru concerning the lack of supplies created a generalized panic in the hospitals and the society. The country was running out of oxygen supplies. We did not have an oxygen generator in every hospital – generators needed to be distributed by a private company, which did not have enough supply for the demand. The system was in shock, and the country was hypoxemic! As described by various studies and reports, the mortality rate in Peru during the months of oxygen deficit was the highest we saw. Oxygen needed to be prioritized for critical care units, depriving even emergency rooms or floors. Family members of patients with chronic conditions or oxygen requirements at home had to stand for hours and days in long lines at oxygen plants to have their tanks filled. The price of oxygen and oxygen concentrators skyrocketed. The situation started slowly and reverted when donations and international help funded small oxygen plants in various important hospitals. Our units throughout the country had a limited number of ventilators and medical supplies for critical care patients. We had to limit therapies such as renal replacement therapies (dialysis) or surgeries. Furthermore, we have a limited number of paediatric intensivists in the country. We needed to get help from hospitalists or general pediatricians and train them in basic critical care medicine, such as ventilator management, so they would be able to help in emergency rooms and critical care units. We built a hierarchical model of medical care led by the intensivists. We were receiving referrals from different hospitals around the country, and many of them did not have a pediatrician on staff. We did not have a telemedicine system. We sometimes used videocall, but communication was difficult due to the volume of patients. Most of the time, patients were transported by ground since finding air transport support was difficult. Due to the large volume of adult patients who needed to be transported, the paediatric cases had less chance of being transported to Lima. Additionally, some transport from remote areas could take up to 2 days. These referrals were often delayed due to lack of personnel, the transport personnels' fear of not being able to return to their place of origin, and the lack of oxygen or transport equipment such as a mechanical ventilator. Some patients were manually ventilated by a physician or nurse during the transport. In most places, children were being managed by adult intensivists or providers, and we needed to redirect them on how to treat paediatric patients, how to stabilize the children and transport them to us. Medical care for children is different from that for adults. Paediatric lungs are still developing and changing in their functioning and anatomy during the first years of life. Therapies are calculated on the basis of weight, and not using appropriate dosing can result in more complications than benefit.

In the paediatric COVID-19 critical care unit, every time we had a patient with cardiac arrest and the "Code Blue" alarm was activated, we all had to take care of that patient, even though we were afraid of not being protected enough and not being able to reach the patient soon enough. What decisions should we make in that moment? We were afraid of being infected ourselves and of making medical decisions that would increase that risk, such as disconnecting the patient from the mechanical ventilator. Those fears made us feel restrained in our practice. Looking back, the lack of knowledge about the virus, including the outcomes and therapies, may have led to mistakes. It was extremely difficult to make decisions for children in critical care. When to intubate? Should we intubate? If we do it soon, are we improving or worsening the outcome? We were literally praying when caring for these patients – struggling with the combination of making the "right" decision and not getting infected at the same time. We already knew how many health care providers, nurses, and doctors were dying in our country and that our mortality rate was one of the highest in South America.

One of the most difficult issues to deal with during this time was control of close contacts. The government designated public areas to isolate adults, children, and whole families in these quarantine areas. As adult cases worsened more frequently and with higher severity than children's cases, those families needed to be separated. We could not cheer or console the children while wearing all our protective equipment, which was particularly hard for younger preschool-age children. It was very difficult to distract them, and we did not have enough support to play with them or take them out of bed. We knew they were separated from their families. We also had to keep ourselves isolated from the families of our patients. We only communicated with them once a day by phone call, and it was very difficult to call so often to deliver bad news. One glimmer of hope was to discover over time that the outcomes in paediatric patients were not as grim as with adult patients. Every child saved gave us hope and moments of happiness. However, from the paediatric perspective, we also saw a heartbreaking reality: many of the paediatric patients hospitalized with COVID-19 who were separated from their families never got to see their parents again. According to some journalistic reports[1] based on the Peruvian Department of Health, up to 98,000 children lost both parents during the pandemic. It was particularly hard for us in critical care to see children, who had spent weeks on mechanical ventilation and who had finally made a full recovery, discover that their parents had died.

Accepting and processing death is difficult at any age. For children and teenagers, to lose their parents is particularly hard; it causes a shift in their life that will be extremely difficult to overcome. Many of them did not understand what had happened. They were not only losing someone they loved; they were also losing their safety, their life structure, and their guide in emotional, psychological, and economic aspects of their life. The likelihood of continuing their education and having psychological and emotional support is very low in a society like ours. The mark that the pandemic will leave on this generation will be seen throughout the coming years. We don't have a real measurement of the stress disorders generated from being hospitalized for so long, surviving the disease, and finding themselves alone in this world. The lack of socialization during their developing years will probably have an immeasurable impact. Certainly, we had to learn not only how to manage this disease in all its forms but also how to cope with the emotions stemming from fearing death, fighting death without resources, and saving many of our patients. Currently, the government, with the help of different international groups, has created support groups and programs for children who have lost their parents, which will provide psychological and financial support. However, the outreach of these programs is still limited considering the large number of children and families affected by these heartbreaking outcomes. Different programs have also been created to support health care providers who dealt with patients and families going through these difficult times.

One positive aspect of these past 2 years is the support and collaboration we have been able to develop with colleagues working in different parts of the globe. Medical news travelled very fast. The entire medical community was facing the unknown, and many therapies became experimental. The only way to help each other was to share cases, experiences, fears, and treatment plans. Initially, when cases in Peru began to have bad outcomes, we saw the opportunity of sharing those experiences by publishing these cases and other research studies regarding our experience. We need now to look to the future and discover how to continue contributing to science and be prepared to face any future complex medical situation like the one we have lived through since 2020. Paediatric research groups and paediatric advocacy groups are being created to find solutions and to understand the consequences of the times we have lived through. Continuing to share these experiences can help create awareness of the medical needs resulting from these pandemics in children from our country and different places around the world. Many of our colleagues in different countries have faced the realities we share. We hope we will continue to improve the lives of children, of COVID-19 survivors, and help develop awareness about the efforts it will take to keep improving their lives in the coming years.

REFERENCE

1. Hurel L. In Peru, more than 98,000 children have been orphaned due to the pandemic. *France 24*. 8 January 2022. Accessed 30 May 2022. https://www.france24.com/es/am%C3%A9rica-latina/20220108-peru-huerfanos-pandemia-ayudas-sociales

20 From the Four Directions: Healing on Navajoland

Melissa Begay, MD
Assistant Professor, Division of Pulmonary, Critical Care and Sleep Medicine, University of New Mexico School of Medicine

Submitted 16 September 2022

On a midday spring afternoon in the high desert of New Mexico, the local tribal radio station discusses the daily toll of coronavirus cases in the cities of Los Angeles and New York. These cities appear eons away from the radio station based in Window Rock, Arizona. The radio announcer tries their best to translate how the virus is airborne and causes an acute respiratory syndrome, but the Navajo (Diné) language for words like "spike proteins" and "illness" seems woefully inadequate. The announcer states that the virus is "invisible" and people should "cover their mouths," and also discourages people "not to curse at the virus" because it is a "living thing." The Diné perspective on balance or *hozho* and reverence for all living things extends even to the coronavirus.

Perhaps it is because Diné is a naturally picturesque language rooted in balance and multitudes of time, distinguishing objects based on living or not-living forms, that makes it incredibly challenging to convey what was occurring: pandemic, emergency, disease, and death. I recall that afternoon distinctly and am reminded of my own community perched atop the North Rim of Canyon de Chelly, a National Historic Park and cultural stronghold of the Navajo. The epic tall rock spire named Spider Rock is often the centre focus on postcards to Instagram reels, capturing the pink glow of the evening desert light against magnificent canyon walls. Canyon de Chelly is the cultural home of many Navajo deities, and its many rugged slots and caves hid the Navajo people during the US Army Inquisition in 1864. US military General Christopher "Kit" Carson was tasked to capture and enslave the Navajo and proceeded to march them hundreds of miles on The Long Walk (known as *Hweeldi*) to Fort Sumner, New Mexico. From 1864 to 1868, the Diné lived in internment camps until their release in 1868, when the Treaty of Bosque Redondo between the United States and Navajo tribal leaders permitted them to return to their homelands, called *Dinétah*. The *Dinétah* landscape appears desolate and vast – 27,000 square miles* centred on the Four Corners region of the American Southwest, roughly the size of the state of West Virginia. *Hogans* and trailers form an extensive network of rural neighbourhoods connected by dirt and gravel roads. Would the low population density of seven people per square mile† shield most from the virus? If the history of infectious diseases such as smallpox and influenza among Indigenous people since New World contact were to be referenced, there was indeed much to fear. The Navajo Nation is recognized as one of the largest federally recognized tribes, and on 20 May 2020, the Navajo Nation was the US epicentre of the pandemic with a higher per capita rate of COVID-19 infection than any US state. The etiology for this rate is not one dimensional, as there is not a single explanation for how it occurred. Rather, it is the consequence of a long history of socio-economic marginalization, chronic immunosuppressive disease, health inequities, and extreme poverty. All of these factors played pivotal roles in the pandemic experience of the Navajo people and Indigenous peoples worldwide in the global outbreak.

Native Americans, often referred to as American Indian/Alaska Native (AI/AN) or the Indigenous People of the Americas, were disproportionately affected by the COVID-19 pandemic. According to recent US Centers for Disease Control and Prevention (CDC) data, AI/ANs were 2.8 times more likely to be hospitalized with and 2.1 times more likely to die from COVID-19. Throughout the 574 federally recognized tribes and 100 state recognized tribes in the United States, Native communities faced enormous barriers and relied on key organizations and stakeholders to mitigate COVID-19. At the forefront was the Indian Health Service (IHS) as well as tribal councils/governments, urban tribal health centers, university hospitals, and local non-profit organizations who collectively used their resources to enact prevention and treatment protocols, disseminate information and essential supplies, and assist in the vaccine campaigns. Many organizations were faced with overcoming the historical mistrust of health care systems, unresolved trauma inherited though centuries of genocide, and the interplay

---

* 69,930 square kilometres.
† per 2.6 square kilometres.

of extreme poverty and persistent health inequities. The heavy burden of uplifting communities through a pandemic that affected many tribal members and instilled fear, anxiety, and often post-traumatic stress disorder (PTSD) and physical trauma only compounded the urgency and challenged often poorly funded social services.

High rates of chronic medical disease created a nidus for increased COVID-19 infection and hospitalizations across many tribal communities. The average life expectancy of an AI/AN is currently one of the shortest in the United States at 67.1 years, having fallen roughly 6.5 *years* during the pandemic. High rates of comorbid diseases that increased the risk of being hospitalized with COVID-19 are widespread: for example, Native American adults are more than twice as likely as white adults to be diagnosed with diabetes, and as of 2018, 48.1 per cent of Native American adults had a body mass index (BMI) of 30 or greater. Further, one in four Native American adults live in extreme poverty in the United States. Yet, per capita expenditure for IHS health care is $2834 compared to $9404 for Veterans and $12,744 for Medicare. There are extreme physician shortages, with a 25 per cent provider vacancy across the national IHS system and a high rate of physician turnover (an average stay of less than 3 years). Inadequate access to social services, underdeveloped health care infrastructure, and lack of tribal government funding to prepare adequately for and during the pandemic presented a time capsule of injustices that have persisted for centuries.

On the Navajo Nation, the conditions of living without basic human necessities such as water, electricity, or proper plumbing have persisted for decades. Recent data show that 30 per cent of tribal members do not have access to water, electricity, or plumbing, and 85 per cent of members do not have access to natural gas. The lack of a telephone and "street address" creates a disproportionate reduction in access to emergency services, effective monitoring, and early warning systems. Over half of the 110 Navajo communities lack access to broadband. Over 1.2 million people on tribal lands lack basic mobile LTE. Poor access to the internet limited families' access to both remote learning and remote working opportunities, and was also a barrier to receiving timely and accurate information on COVID-19 prevention strategies.

Although this lack of access to modern necessities continues regardless of living during the pandemic or not, Navajo people are industrious and creative in ensuring a continued livelihood since, for many, going without water and electricity is just a part of living on the reservation. A visit to a typical rural Navajo home in the winter reveals people stocking up on firewood and preparing food security and conservation water management for both humans and livestock. As a child, I recall hauling water to my grandparents' home and using a homemade water filtration system my Grandmother made out of a Bluebird Flour sack to filter the debris out of water before it was siphoned into drinking tanks. It's not until you learn to live without the essential services we often take for granted that you realize the depth of the issue and how events like the pandemic direct a large magnifying glass on these inequities.

While the traditional lifestyle on the reservation is a source of resiliency, it also increased the threat of spreading the virus. Many Navajo households are multigenerational and consist of many families living together. Taking care of elders, revered as the language and culture knowledge keepers, is a duty many adults value. Children under the age of 18 are four times more likely to live with a grandparent. There is only one nursing home on the reservation and a lack of professional caregivers. Similar to concerns of multigenerational homes during the 2014 Ebola outbreak in West Africa, these close living conditions not only increased the incidence of outbreaks in large family clusters but also presented difficulties with self-isolation and quarantine. It wasn't unusual during the pandemic to learn that many tribal members were in quarantine in the old *hogans* often used for traditional ceremonies or even living inside vehicles. Further, many Indigenous people hold large gatherings to celebrate life events and to honour key milestones and seasonal activities such as coming of age ceremonies, personal prayers and ceremonies, and harvest gatherings. These large events posed a threat for outbreaks in families and communities, and eventually were prohibited during the pandemic under public health orders, along with establishing curfews and closing tribal borders.

With the odds of a good outcome increasingly stacked against many tribal communities, what can we learn from these experiences, and how can we identify the most salient factors to improve the likelihood of surviving the COVID-19 pandemic? From my perspective as a physician and a Navajo tribal member, there were three key factors in strengthening the fabric of survival in both individual families and communities. First, looking inward into the strengths of the Navajo culture, spirituality, and history provided a much-needed protective role in displaying hope and tenacity of spirit. There was an immense return to, and education on, traditional food ways and systems such as traditional gardening and the growing of heirloom varieties of traditional foods. Further, many traditional medicine people were actively cultivating herbs and providing education on how to care for oneself through the pandemic with mental fitness and immune-boosting medicines and compounds. Access to these traditional practitioners in the community through the pandemic gave many the connection to a health care system they trusted and sought guidance from. Elders and cultural teachers provided a reminder of Navajo history through oral storytelling of the Navajo Creation Story and of humans and animals journeying though the Four Worlds to this modern world, the Glittering World, and of the Twin Warriors slaying monsters to protect the Navajo people in arduous times. The passing on and providing messages, especially to Navajo youth, of the historical knowledge of their ancestors surviving genocide, historical trauma, cultural assimilation, and The Long Walk were important reminders in navigating the loneliness and anxiety of the pandemic – all resulting in a sense of empowerment and heightened resilience. Second, the roles many Native American and Navajo physicians took on the front lines and as advocates for their patients ensured health competence through a cultural lens was incorporated into all emergency preparedness programs, pandemic surveillance, and vaccine strategies. Although Native American physicians comprise less than 1 per cent of all physicians in the United States, their key leadership roles in IHS hospitals, urban tribal health centers, and national organizations like the Association of American Indian Physicians were essential in establishing culturally aware prevention and management strategies. Lastly, an overall utilitarian approach and sense of beneficence to fellow tribal community members in safeguarding elders and children were pivotal in mitigating the pandemic's toll in tribal communities. The sense of urgency and the knowledge of how previous infectious diseases such as smallpox, tuberculosis, and influenza decimated entire tribes were instrumental in embracing social distancing protocols and obtaining the vaccine, and the Navaho achieved a vaccine acceptance rate that has surpassed any other ethnic group in the United States. It is worthy to note that the vaccine strategy was heralded by many stakeholders alongside the IHS including grassroots communities and organizations like the Diné Medicineman Hatalthi Association, which endorsed the vaccine as a safe and appropriate "medicine" (since the vaccine was often described as a part of water), an essential tool for fighting COVID-19.

It's a cool fall morning in September 2022, and the local radio announcers are set up against the 3.5-mile-long‡ line of hundreds of

---

‡ 5.6-kilometre-long.

parade goers at the 74th Annual Navajo Nation Fair in Window Rock, Arizona. Just a year ago, the tribal capital was in lockdown, and curfews were in place. Vehicles were lined up for food delivery and essential supplies. The crowds of people are the same, but the season of change is in tow. The theme for this year's celebration is "Honouring Our Front-line Workers," and many parade floats have painted pictures of first responders and health care workers wearing masks and smiling. The crisp air carries the scent of coffee and breakfast burritos filled with spam, green chile, and potatoes. The sounds of children laughing and people on horses and four wheelers echo off the sandstone cliffs. There is much anticipation after a 2-year hiatus. The local tribal radio announcers are enjoying the sights and discuss the daily schedule of events. They don't talk about the daily toll of COVID-19 anymore but instead remind people to wear their masks, be kind to one another, and enjoy themselves. As we gather and greet each other, many for the first time in years, I am reminded of the devastation and all that has transpired, the lives won and lives lost to COVID-19, and it feels a bit surreal. As of this week, Navajo Nation *Dikos Ntsaaígíí* Situation Report #874 reports 73,365 confirmed COVID-19 cases and 1896 total confirmed deaths. The daily case rate thankfully continues to trend down.

I sense in myself cautious optimism. Yet I continue to have many questions looming in my mind. What does the future hold? How can we prepare for the next pandemic? How can we strengthen ourselves as a community and tribal nation? What is our global Indigenous responsibility in this outbreak? The answers aren't quite as clear as the blue desert sky I'm sitting under, but there are data and clear waypoints to peruse. The lessons learned point to an overwhelming responsibility as an individual and community, an urgent sense to prepare, to build key infrastructure, to utilize existing resources, and to move forward intently and with a renewed sense of spirit and purpose: to use traditional knowledge passed on from our ancestors since time immemorial and to gather our global and local community, exchange ideas, and learn to integrate intercultural practices to create tools and develop policies that strengthen the health and socio-economic status of Indigenous people worldwide.

We can and must prepare for the future generations to come.

PART FIVE

Learning Under Fire

The pandemic disrupted every aspect of health care, but few areas experienced disruption as significantly as health care education and training. At the start of the pandemic, medical students were prohibited from even entering hospitals, and physicians-in-training were removed from their established training rotations in order to care for the deluge of COVID-19 patients. This section, "Learning Under Fire," describes some of the experiences of becoming a physician under these unprecedented conditions. "Waiting in the Wings: A Medical Trainee's Pandemic Experience" shares the story of a medical student exiled from her training facility, experiencing what should be the core of her medical education "remotely." "Becoming a Psychiatrist During a Pandemic" recounts the difficulties training in a specialty that is fundamentally based upon human contact when human contact was prohibited or, at best, extremely limited. "PANDEMIC RITES: Rites of Passage as an International ICU Fellow and the Journey Back Home" tells of the particular challenge of being caught between two worlds and medical systems at a time when neither was functioning anywhere near its best and shows the struggle to find a place within systems in chaos. "Resident Training in COVID-19 Times" attempts to explain from an administrative viewpoint the difficulties in reworking training schema during the pandemic years to provide adequate instruction while balancing safety concerns, physical limitations, and unsettled medical training facilities.

21 Waiting in the Wings: A Medical Trainee's Pandemic Experience

Gabrielle Karlovich, MD
General Psychiatry Resident, Temple University, Philadelphia

Submitted 18 June 2022

After receiving my acceptance to medical school, I distinctly remember the wisdom a professor offered me: "Nothing can prepare you for this, Gabrielle, so don't even try."

I was one member of medicine's vast Type-A club. So, contrary to his advice, I was up for any challenge and attempted to get ahead of the curb, regardless. I scrolled through online forums, reviewed college coursework in anticipatory studying, peppered current and past trainees with questions, but to no avail. He was right. Nothing can prepare *anyone* for "the next four years," even when they do not encompass a global pandemic. They are brutal and exhausting but also transformative and inspiring. Looking back, I realize students are moulded month by month into better, more self-aware thinkers and healers, and no one leaves the same as they entered. Like many trainees, I dabbled in "the real world" after my undergraduate education, but my heart was irrevocably set on this lofty goal of becoming the first physician in my family. As I walked across the dimly lit stage and ceremoniously donned my white coat for the first time, I felt in my bones that I would heal with my words and my hands – and I would do good in this world.

The reality of our first year was not rosy, even as it began with the status quo. I was taken aback by the rapid-fire pace of our course load, which my family affectionately deemed drinking from the firehose. The entirety of my Ivy League education, a hundred science credits, was neatly summarized in our first few weeks. And on top of the mountains of book learning – biochemistry, immunology, microbiology, genetics – we were constantly "doing." We interviewed standardized patients in mock encounters with actors feigning rage, grief, or anxiety to test our bedside manners. We practised skills in simulation labs, keen-eyed physicians sliding our stethoscopes *just so,* so we could hear an aortic regurgitation murmur for the first time. We were absorbing information around the clock, and it was not unusual for me to stay in the library cubicles well into the night, running to the subway station to make it home over the river in the nick of time. The facts we learned in the morning would come alive in the afternoon to keep us completely engaged with the material. Yet, in the same way that I was struck by the deluge of medical school – unready and unprepared – the world was struck by the COVID-19 pandemic.

The first time I heard of coronavirus outside of one measly lecture slide in our infectious disease unit was a *New York Times* podcast in January. I was interested in global health, having worked in Cambodia prior to medical school, so I brought up the topic in one of our small learning groups the next day. Unsurprisingly, it elicited minimal commentary then; we predicted COVID would run its course like Ebola or Zika: completely devastating but confined geographically.

As the weeks rolled on, this notion was tested. We began receiving updates from our medical school dean, ensuring us that our institution would be following state and local guidelines and keeping us apprised of the situation in the meantime. The administration's demeanor was calm and reassuring, so we resumed life, calm and reassured; there was certainly enough to keep us occupied. However, my girlfriend who lives in Europe hurriedly called me one afternoon with a completely different tone. I could tell she was panicking.

"Go wherever you can," she insisted. "Get as many masks as possible for yourself and lots of bleach. The masks – they're called N95s."

I knew what an N95 was because in medical school we are all fitted with protective equipment in case we ever work with a patient positive for tuberculosis, on air droplet precautions. I had never actually worn one in a clinical setting.

I assumed she was being a typical Greek hypochondriac until venturing out to seven different pharmacies and convenience stores throughout Philadelphia. I remember looking dumbfoundedly at the shiny white aisles. Even before general knowledge of COVID in the United States had reached the masses, all had been quietly, surreptitiously emptied of their supplies.

We had one final exam before spring break, ironically, on infectious diseases. Over one hundred students crowded into the school auditorium with our laptops, like we had every other month before. Our class president demanded we take a collective selfie because we were unsure when we would be back. In the photo, there is a sea of faces, all grinning. We guessed it might be a couple more weeks at most before "normalcy" resumed: a small, very welcome extension of spring break. Many were looking forward to having a little more time with loved ones, me included.

The next series of events occurred in such a brief span of time I did not have the wherewithal to process much in the moment. I flew to Greece to see my girlfriend on a Friday night. I was planning on staying in her apartment for the week. We received word on Sunday that the country would be shutting down its air service: no flights in and no flights out. On Monday, the school announced it would be starting virtual lectures, with no expected date to resume in-person learning.

I was stuck in a foreign country, watching my own crumble from afar.

Having witnessed the devastation occurring in Italy, Greece took extremely proactive measures. Its population was dually vulnerable: largely elderly and without appropriate infrastructure on the islands to care for an influx of intensive care unit (ICU) patients, not to mention teetering on the brink of financial ruin after declaring bankruptcy in 2011. There were 89 confirmed cases on 13 March 2020 with 0 deaths, but the government's reaction was swift. All non-essential movement was restricted. There were seven reasons one was permitted to leave their home, and we needed identification and signed attestation for the purpose of such travel. Many people did not leave their homes for any reason at all, petrified of the consequences. For the first two weeks of my stay, I was like a deer in headlights. I did not go outside, but my girlfriend had to for work, and she was met with over five checkpoints to get downtown on the days that she ventured out.

In the meantime, the apartment complex smelled putrid. Pets relieved themselves on balconies, so stale urine hung in the air, while the café society crowd that typically reserved cigarettes for social scenarios began adapting the practice as a sole hobby. It was physically and mentally stifling. When I finally had gone stir crazy on day 14, I volunteered to take the dog down to the yard. There were dewdrops frozen on the grass that parted under my sneakers. I walked to the edge of the property, behind a white fence, and peered around the street. Police vehicles roamed by every few minutes, and aside from the sound of their cars idling, it was so quiet. In these early days, existence was like sleepwalking through life.

After the week-long break ended, our virtual classes began. Due to the time difference, my 8 a.m. class now occurred at 3 p.m. Greek time. I recall sipping bialetti coffee after coffee that morning, impatiently waiting in the Webex session to see my friends' faces flicker onto the screen – to not feel as alone. For a while, we all just sat in our designated learning spaces, breathing. I don't remember who broke the ice, but suddenly we were talking, and we did not stop for the designated 2 hours.

Now, in these sessions, we largely ignored the learning objectives we were supposed to meet for our units on haematology, oncology, rheumatology, and the musculoskeletal system. We checked in with one another. We swapped theories on what was going to happen next. We devoured crumbs of news from our professors who worked in the hospital. And in the last 15 minutes, we begrudgingly finished some work. I dreaded each sign off, as the rest of the day I was glued to the couch, expected to sift through the same amount of school work with none of the support. My girlfriend's dog, who was then still a puppy, took up residence on my lap.

The COVID situation in the United States began to drastically diverge from that in Greece. While Greece's hospital numbers stayed primarily below 3000, the United States was riding its first wave. Three thousand, five thousand, seven thousand, ten thousand, *thirty thousand.*

I watched my professors – many who had been on the front lines of the HIV epidemic – grow weary. The bags under their eyes and stilted expressions were still discernible in low-resolution webcams. There was a quiet knowing among us that, after each sign off, many returned to COVID units: hallways of beeping machinery, ventilators, and motionless bodies. In the mornings, they taught us, and come midday, they were on the front lines. Paediatricians and family medicine doctors were also thrown into the deep end to help manage the load of ICU patients – performing tasks and thinking in ways they had not done since they were in medical school. Everyone was on edge.

In Greece, it was a dystopian existence, but it was safe. The lockdown lasted for 42 days. Eventually, the civilian restrictions relaxed, and I was able to go for runs in the mountains each day. My sneakers slammed against ochre rocks, and I stared down at fields of olive trees and the glistening sea. In my newfound freedom, I felt guilty, and I grew frustrated. I had been accepted into medical school at the worst time: too young with too little experience to be of any use in the hospital setting. All I could do was watch and wait.

Everyone always wonders what they would do in a time of crisis – what kind of person they would be. We are taught by the media that there are only two camps: the moral, brave souls who acted and the cowardly who did not. We think of the radicals immortalized by history: though their names are not well known by many, the friends and employees who helped Anne Frank, her family, and the Van Pels family hide from the Nazi regime as red flags waved in the Netherlands;

Frederick Douglass who escaped slavery and proceeded to go back and fight for abolition; Malala Yousafzai, barely a teenager, who faced down an entire regime for a chance to get an education… But what if the crisis of our lifetime was occurring right in front of us and we were in the wrong place at the wrong time? Even if my education were timelier, how could I possibly augment the response to the tragedy occurring 5000 miles* away? This situation made me realize that so many of us are simply helpless to affect change, no matter how deeply we are impacted by it.

My inability to contribute also drove my resentment to fester. I grew angry at the complacency from politicians and civilians: the United States largely accepting its catastrophic failure, its preventable loss of lives. I raged when health systems did not offer hazard pay and provided personal protection equipment (PPE) to their administrators over their residents. I seethed when cities threw parades for health care heroes but refused to do the one thing we asked: mandate masking. I boiled when they attacked the front line for being complicit in genocide: alleging that this pandemic was all just a set-up to kill off the elderly. I grieved when an idol of mine in holistic reproductive health care succumbed to conspiracy and became a mouthpiece for the anti-vaccination movement.

Come second year, I alternated between the United States and Greece: two apartments, two very different realities. Either way, I engaged in my education through a screen. The second year of medical school is notoriously the most intellectually challenging: the material shifts to organ systems' anatomy, physiology, and pathology as we simultaneously prepare year-round to take the first of a series of 8-hour national exams. My lectures were mostly old recordings from the year prior, and my anatomy cadaver lab was replaced by a virtual 3D program that crashed every 10 minutes. I found it difficult to care.

My dissatisfaction was temporarily swayed by encouragement from professors. I buckled down and got to work. How could I not when they were living the horrors day in and day out? One professor raised the idea that we may still be fighting the pandemic when my class would become interns in 3 years; he was only slightly joking. I yo-yoed between adrenaline-fuelled study sessions to hopelessness and paralysing anxiety.

It also took a personal toll. My aunt passed away after 11 days in a COVID ward in October 2021. Up until that point, it was the deadliest day of the pandemic. Three days prior, her nurse held up an iPad

---

* 8046.7 kilometres.

to facilitate our FaceTime conversation. Even though my aunt was convinced I was in my final year of law school, she was *finally* somewhat lucid. I had hope that she might bounce back, but everything crumpled after that conversation. Organ systems shut down one after the other like dominoes. I got The Call while hovering over the tomato section at Trader Joe's, debating whether the extra $2 for Camparis was worth it. It hit like a gut punch over and over and over again. My second year of medical school was stained with grief.

There were other blows. We did not do enough to protect those who wanted to protect us. As provider suicides slowly ticked upwards, I was grimly reminded of the wars in Afghanistan and Iraq. We cheered for these kids, told them they were patriots, shipped them off to witness horrors most people could not imagine, and then tossed them aside when they returned to us damaged. I thought of my friends fresh out of nursing school or the ones starting their internship years. They were not prepared for the endless trauma, and they suffered for it, mostly alone. Wasn't this the same thing? I began to see cracks in our system I hadn't paid much attention to in the past. I became fixated on new, important issues surrounding mental health, and my priorities shifted.

The pandemic fundamentally shaped me and the kind of medicine I want to practise. Prior to medical school, I had worked in Cambodia and, throughout, had partaken in paediatric sepsis research. I was convinced that I would graduate, finish residency, and pursue a career in the international arena: establishing sustainable public health care initiatives abroad for the most vulnerable populations with the least amount of political power. Yet my idealism about doctors' roles in society and my faith in achieving good health policy was irrevocably shattered in the wake of COVID. We refused to do the bare minimum to promote the health of us all. We did not listen to scientists. We did not distribute vaccines justly. I was disenchanted with our systems' limitations and recognized a career in policy would only frustrate me. I wasn't cut out for it – not in this cultural climate.

My wavering certainty about my career path came at a time with my newfound love of psychiatry. During the pandemic, I continued leading a virtual tutoring initiative for at-risk youth in our city, and I watched as these children fudged smiles, withered, and became apathetic. We physically drove to do check-ins on a 9-year-old boy whose parents were both suffering from long COVID; for 3 weeks, he was entirely on his own. We delivered snacks, and sat 10 feet[†] apart, him on his

---

† 3 metres.

porch, us on scattered lawn chairs. Between my interactions with these kids and our emergency rooms' statistics exploding with increased paediatric suicide attempts, I saw the United States's burgeoning need for mental health providers. I thrived, healing by forging connections with others, and realized there were elements that we *could* control in our patients' lives. I felt like I had some power back. I finally felt of use.

What did that professor tell me all those years ago? Nothing can prepare you for the next 4 years? While I am writing this chapter, I am finishing up my third year, and I do not know how my time in medical school will end. We have continued to see waves of cases and are in the middle of another "level red." The United States just surpassed one million COVID deaths last week.

As I reflected upon my experience, which was largely atypical, I wanted to consult my peers. I asked them: describe our pandemic world as medical students in a few words. Here were their responses:

Isolating.
Nerve-wracking.
Eye-opening.
Emphasis on frustrating.
Being in the medical field now means you could die doing your job. And that's accepted.
Paranoia.
Racial reckoning.
Crisis after crisis.
We deserve better.
Alone.
Netflix and survive.
Relentless.
Still no universal health care?
Overwhelmed.
What mental health?
Such a disappointment.
Enlightening… good and bad ways.
Motivating?
Would anything change if it happened again?
I wish I knew less about my patients' beliefs.
Roller-coaster.
BURNOUT.
Missing milestones.
How do we "just move on"?
Privileged but still mad.

Empty void.
Guilty – I didn't do enough.
We never learn from our past.
I know myself now.
I want to care but I can't anymore.
Rage.
Blind leading the blind.
Marathon after marathon.
Where are the adults?
Trying.
Surviving.
Eternity.
We'll never be the same.

22 Becoming a Psychiatrist During a Pandemic

Houman Rashidian, MD, FRCPC
Psychiatrist, Trillium Health Partners, Mississauga, Ontario

Sabrina Agnihotri, MD
PGY5 Resident, Department of Psychiatry, University of Toronto

Submitted 18 October 2022

The COVID-19 pandemic dramatically altered the landscape of medical education, and it is not yet clear what the ramifications of these changes will be. Residency represents a unique time in our professional development, perhaps akin to late adolescence. We are joyously on the verge of independent practice but still require experience, mentorship, and demonstration of critical knowledge before breaking out on our own. As residents training within a subspeciality program, these transitional checkpoints are achieved through direct clinical encounters and observation that were significantly reduced during the pandemic due to necessary infection control practices.

Beyond these clinical aspects, residency also represents a time for exploration of future career goals. As such, given that we were both passionate about leadership skill development, it seemed like an exciting challenge to pursue the role of co-chief residents in psychiatry at the University Health Network (UHN) during a global pandemic. Our journey started in July 2021. We were well into the second wave

---

At the time of writing this chapter, Dr. Rashidian was a Postgraduate Year Five (PGY5) Resident, Department of Psychiatry, University of Toronto, but is now Psychiatrist, Trillium Health Partners, Mississauga, Ontario. Dr. Agnihotri was a PGY4 Resident at the time of writing, but is now a PGY5 Resident in the Department of Psychiatry, University of Toronto. Dr. Rashidian and Dr. Agnihotri were Co-Chief Residents in Psychiatry, University Health Network, Toronto, at the time of writing.

of the pandemic, and the excitement of virtual learning and Zoom socials had worn away to make room for severe peer isolation. We were ready for the challenge of finding ways to engage our fellow residents and to strengthen a sense of community again. Although this optimism was challenged throughout our tenure, the resilience of our resident body, coupled with strong site director leadership, allowed us to navigate through the COVID storm. More than 2 years now into our COVID-laden training, we reflect back on the collective experiences shared by our peers in training, as well as on the leadership challenges and opportunities we encountered as co-chief residents.

Maintaining Emotional Boundaries

Compounded with our personal pandemic experiences, we also, as resident psychiatrists, felt the devastating impact the pandemic had on our patients. Job loss, relocation, isolation, and death became common stressors, leading even those with the strongest support systems to reel in mental and physical anguish. We remember the story of a young boy who presented to Toronto's Hospital for Sick Children (SickKids) seeking psychiatric support, having last seen his father alive as he was leaving to get a COVID polymerase chain reaction (PCR) test. How could we provide comfort and perspective in such situations where shock and uncertainty were overpowering us as well? The fourth wall between patient and physician began to crumble, as the world was truly experiencing shared trauma. Although feeling emotions with our patients can sometimes serve well as a demonstration of empathy, maintaining mental boundaries is key to retaining an objective therapeutic perspective.

Learning the Basics

Diagnosis and treatment processes also became more complex. There were questions regarding overpathologizing patient experiences. For example, whereas before a diagnosis of depression and/or anxiety would have seemed obvious, we now had to consider what normative responses one would have while adjusting to a worldwide pandemic. Behavioural treatment recommendations were obsolete during the citywide curfews and lockdowns. Group therapies that create routine and encourage individuals with depression to leave their home were cancelled. The pandemic placed enormous pressure on an already fragile mental health care system in Ontario, which trickled down to the increasing volumes we encountered on our emergency call shifts.

Fortunately, through the loosening of lockdown restrictions over time, we slowly began to witness a recalibration of coping responses as society became active once again. This resilience in our patients was inspiring to witness.

Virtual Reality

In psychiatry, the switch to virtual care represented an immense barrier to training. Without years of experience behind us, we rely on dynamic interactions between ourselves, patients, and our staff. Feedback on our interviewing skills became limited in the outpatient setting, which has largely remained virtual to this day. Teaching opportunities were reduced to virtual slides, with endless days of sitting in front of our laptops at home or having patient encounters infiltrate our own homes. The interactions and nuances in body language that were once part of our rapport-building tool set were removed. Our chief office hours and resident lunches became virtual, eliminating the community-building and informality of destressing with colleagues over a bento box. However, as the weather permitted, we organized individual outdoor socials for each year of our program to try and foster these critical connections. Especially meaningful to us was being able to witness some of our postgraduate year (PGY) 1 and PGY2 colleagues meeting each other in person for the first time at these events and supporting this blossoming peer support network.

Resident Wellness

The most drastic effect of the changes to our learning environment as residents was that of burnout, and this issue became much of the focus during our chief residency term. One of our most important and time-consuming tasks was to develop the daily call schedule for the psychiatric emergency department. At UHN, we create this schedule for 1 year. Each night there is one resident on call overnight, in addition to one on back-up in the event that the primary resident cannot attend due to an emergency. As wave after wave of COVID struck our residents, back-up resident activation became the norm, and the demands placed on our peers often significantly outweighed their capacity. Some individuals even left the call pool indefinitely due to wellness-related accommodations.

This situation often left us scrambling to find coverage for shifts even on the same day. We took turns making the dreaded "you are being activated" phone call. Call coverage was the most challenging aspect of being a chief resident, as we were constantly balancing individual versus collective wellness. However, the collegiality of our colleagues shone through as many residents stepped up time and time again to cover each other. Our postgraduate leadership also took notice and organized increased financial compensation for call coverage. UHN staff on call often covered back-up shifts as well. These changes ensured that our call pool was available to help patients while allowing residents to obtain the rest and time they required to take care of themselves.

Through the desire to support our peers and maintain an image of resilience, we did not fully appreciate the stress we ourselves would experience and our own need for support. Fortunately, as co-chiefs, we had one another to rely on. We would call each other during stressful times and help each other vent and work through various logistical, administrative, or communicative problems. We also had a strong protective force in our site directors, who were always there to guide us through various problems but also to provide positive reinforcement and emotional support. Furthermore, we had a monthly meeting with the psychiatry program director as well as the associate program director, who provided us with key mentorship and insight regarding their own techniques for protecting personal wellness in leadership roles. Ultimately, it took a collaborative team effort to survive and thrive throughout the year.

What started off as a year fraught with isolation and loneliness ended with a sense of renewed faith that we are truly all in this together. We look back with a mixture of grief for lost opportunities but also with gratitude for being able to support our patients and front-line efforts, pride for pushing ourselves in ways we never imagined, and hope that these unique training challenges will only make us stronger, more empathic physicians.

23 PANDEMIC RITES: Rites of Passage as an International ICU Fellow and the Journey Back Home

Onion Gerald Vergara Ubaldo, MD, MBA, FRCP, FPSCCM
Emergency Medicine, Critical Care Physician, Philippines

Submitted 26 June 2022

EPISODE 1: The Beginning

It was mid-February when I first heard the news of COVID-19 entering the Philippines. I was finishing my second year of an adult critical care fellowship in the Philippines and had my future planned out. I had already been accepted into the University Health Network (UHN) adult critical care fellowship training in Toronto, which was slated to start in July. Even though the world was already feeling the COVID wrath, the Philippines luckily remained rather secluded from it. I can still remember that day when we had our first confirmed COVID case. I was in a different hospital doing my cardiothoracic surgery elective when my department head sent me a text message saying that we had a confirmed COVID case admitted to the intensive care unit (ICU) of my home hospital. Slowly, the number of cases began creeping up, and most of my colleagues were quarantined, either because of exposure or actual clinical illness. My elective was cut short. I was pulled out and reassigned to man the ICU due to personnel shortages. It felt as if I were going into battle blindfolded. I guess most of the world felt this way since COVID is a novel virus associated with a novel disease. I went in the ICU intending to use what I had learned from my almost 2 years of ICU training.

I have always believed that the intensivist program is one to marvel at. It gives clinicians the opportunity to take a holistic perspective into patient management. That was something I always admired about intensivists and probably the reason why I got into the field in the first place. I always dreamed of being a complete physician – a multi-organ doctor and not a single-organ doctor, which most Filipinos have been accustomed to. The ICU, for me, was more than just a bed space where "closer monitoring" can be done. I think the ICU is a living, breathing environment with its own atmosphere geared towards holistic care from head to toe, avoiding the fragmentation of care brought about by having numerous single-organ doctors for one patient. I say this because it may be the reality for some well-off first-world countries but not, unfortunately, for the Philippines. For me to take up intensivist-level training post–internal medicine residency was surely a big risk as a career path because the culture and the environment in the Philippines was, and still is, a single-organ physician–dominated arena where the ICU, sadly, is still seen as a bed space rather than what I hoped it to be. But one thing was certain: the COVID pandemic exposed the necessity for intensivists in the Philippines.

As I stepped back inside the walls of my home hospital's ICU, I was greeted by smiles, albeit underneath their masks. My colleagues surely welcomed additional warm bodies to help them take care of the sick patients currently residing in the ICU. At first, the workload was manageable, with one or two patients being admitted in a day. However, as the days went by, we saw the first surge of COVID patients coming into our unit. My home hospital was one of the well-off and technologically advanced centres in the country. However, COVID really strained the health care that we, as an institution, could deliver. I could see in the eyes of my colleagues the fatigue from handling too many patients at a single time: nurses who had 1:2 to 1:3 nurse-patient ratios and residents, who had never seen the ICU, having to learn skills as fast as they could – ventilator management, sedation, hemodynamics, fluid responsiveness, heart-lung interaction – most of which was well beyond their actual knowledge expectation. The Emergency Department became an extension of the ICU. Patients were lining up outside of the hospital waiting to be seen. People were dying left and right.

As a graduating fellow in the critical care program, I was expected to be able to handle multiple sick patients, having to insert multiple central lines, prone and paralyse patients in a night. Because of staffing issues, we were asked to go on consecutive night calls for ten nights at a time to preserve our other colleagues from exposure. On top of these demands, the Philippines, being a third-world country, eventually lacked enough personal protective equipment (PPE) to be able to supply our health care team. We resorted to recycling our N95 masks and buying respirators out of our own money to lessen the burden on the hospital providing for us. But I guess one of the most, if not the most, terrible things that happened was our isolation from loved ones. Being a critical care fellow on call during the first wave of the pandemic, where most of us were still blind about how to manage sick COVID patients, I had to live within the hospital, away from my loved ones, for our tour of calls. Instead of being able to focus on my health and those of my loved ones, I was asked to look after other people's loved ones. To say that it was a scary time was an understatement. After the call shifts, it was mandatory to self-isolate, which meant less time to spend with family even after work was done. To put it into perspective, the usual call shift for an internal medicine resident and a critical care fellow spanned from 24 to 48 hours in the hospital. During normal times, such a stretch of call was not allowed due to the extreme risk of fatigue and the potential for error events. However, in our setting, there was no choice.

To be honest, when I set out to become an intensivist, I really did not expect a pandemic to happen. But perhaps being an intensivist-in-training and eventually an intensivist in the Philippines during the first wave of the pandemic did teach me a lot. Not only did I gain the pathophysiological knowledge of different disease entities that ranged from COVID to the comorbidities that patients had, but I also developed the attitude necessary for an intensive care specialist to be able to provide the best health care possible given the resources available at that time. Often, as most of us know, it is as simple as holding the patient's hand when they need someone the most. If there is one thing I learned from being an intensivist in the Philippines during the pandemic, it is that patients and their relatives often needed my intensivist heart more than they needed my intensivist mind.

EPISODE 2: The Flight

As I graduated from my program in Manila (having been immersed in COVID responsibilities during the last few months), I began to think about my next steps. On the one hand, there was this great opportunity for me to train in Toronto under the #2 ranked critical care program in the world. On the other hand, there was this call to stay in the Philippines and try to help as much as I could since the country's health care delivery system was being ravaged by COVID. Although sometimes it is hard to admit, the Philippines, despite being laden with government corruption, will always be my home, and often my nationalistic self will control my decisions. With that being the case, I sought out job opportunities, however small, in order to be able to try and ease the burden on my intensivist colleagues. I sent out applications and went to tele-interviews, but unfortunately it seemed that no one was willing to hire me. Was it because of a lack of funds or some other political scheme? I would never know. I was ready to give up my dream of training abroad to be able to help with the COVID fight in my country. But, as fate would decide, the latter was not the option given to me. I then prepared to leave the country and go to Toronto.

My family is a very tightly knit one. We are a family of four – my parents, my sister named Ginger (hence my name), and me. Growing up, I was taught to put family and religion first above anything else. It was no surprise to me that my leaving them was one of the hardest things I had to do, especially during the time when they needed me the most. I seriously considered not flying out to Toronto anymore to receive additional top-notch training. I talked with my family about it, and if they were being honest, they would have preferred me to stay in the Philippines where I could keep an eye on them and they could keep an eye on me. I had no relatives and no friends in Toronto. If I decided to go away for one whole year, it would be just me. But again, no one was willing to offer me work at home, and I could not help if the Philippines would not let me. I shifted my focus and decided that I would be able to help more once I had acquired the skills and know-how that no one in the Philippines could teach me – I could only acquire those things in Toronto. My family, especially my sister, were very supportive of this decision. They told me that it was a great opportunity for me, something that might not come by again, and that I had to grab hold of it while it was presenting itself. So, I flew away.

The car ride to the airport was a heartbreaking one. It was the first time in my life that I would be away from family this long. I remember holding back my tears while I was saying my goodbyes in our living room. As I got inside the car (I was alone when I went to the airport because of COVID restrictions), I felt the tears gushing down my cheeks. It marked the start of 365-plus days during which I was without family in a country I have never been to with people I did not know. Was I scared? Of course. I was scared that I might get sick while I was away, and I would have no one to take care of me. I was scared that my parents and my sister would get sick, and I would not be there for them. I was scared to underperform in the critical care program that I had applied to. I was scared that I would not measure up to the first-world standards, me being from a third-world country. These were the thoughts in my head.

I arrived in Toronto at night. The fifth day of August marked my first of 14 days of quarantine. Upon landing, I already felt the loneliness of being without family. I settled down in my rented apartment about a quarter past midnight. I can still remember, as if it were just yesterday, the exact same feeling I felt a year ago – a mixture of excitement, fear, anxiety, and loneliness. But, as it turns out, that day was day 1 of a life-changing journey for me as a "padawan" of the intensive care order.

EPISODE 3: The Work

My year of rotation started at the Toronto General Hospital. I remember stepping into the ICU and feeling in awe of how massive the place was. It dwarfed any ICU we had back in the Philippines. I ran down the list of patients with their diagnoses; I have never worked in such a high acuity setting in my life. The General was known to be the ECMO (extracorporeal membrane oxygenation) and transplant centre. That being the case, I was really excited to learn from the people who ran the unit.

The first few days and weeks were rough. I was still trying to get a feel for the place and trying to catch up with how things were done in Canada. The health care system was very different, and the "way of doing things" was definitely very different than how things worked in the Philippines. Back home, most of the health care was paid for out of pocket, meaning that the patient pays for most of their expenses. I have never worked in a setting where the government, via taxes, pays for most of the health care. Another thing that brought a pleasant surprise for me was the intensivist-led design of the ICU. This practice was the ideal set-up for an ICU, something that is really lacking in the Philippine setting. I was also surprised that most of the COVID patients admitted into the unit had been there for a long time. Back in the Philippines, our patients could not afford to stay that long in the ICU on organ support. Most of them would expire because interventions are limited due to lack of funds. That was a sad reality I experienced back home but not in Canada. I consider Canadians very lucky to have such a robust health care system geared to take care of them whenever they need it. Such is not the case in the Philippines. To put it bluntly, if you do not have money in the Philippines saved and allotted for health care, you will die, because you won't be able to afford the life-saving interventions. It was such a breath of fresh air to be able to work in a clinical setting where I rarely had think about the costs – the use of gloves, the recycled masks and gowns, the subpar interventions that we ended up doing because we must consider the finances of our patients in the Philippines. We ended up having to prematurely discontinue most of our life-saving interventions because of the financial aspect of health care – our patients could not afford them.

My experience as an intensivist working and training in Toronto was very different from my experiences in the Philippines. As I wiggled my way through the daily routine of ICU work in Toronto, I sometimes caught myself asking, "When do we stop? When is it enough?" This question came up because I had never experienced so many interventions for one single COVID patient in an ICU setting. They ranged from ECMO, to transplant intensive care, to advanced mechanical ventilator interventions, to renal replacement therapy, to inhaled nitric oxide for one single patient. In the Philippines, that would never happen, but in Toronto, often it was the norm. Back home, we worry about many things: Where do we admit the next COVID patient? Where do we get our PPE? How many times do we have to recycle our masks? Do we really need to intubate the patient since we do not have any ventilators left? But I found myself wondering, What life would they have after going through all of this? These are questions I never had to ask as I trained in Toronto.

My training was a joyful experience yet a painful one. The former because training and working was easier. It gave me the liberty to focus on learning and helping our patients get better. The latter because it made me realize how the Philippines was lagging far behind in terms of optimal health care delivery, and that was the sad reality waiting for me.

As the days went by, I felt that I was slowly getting my rhythm. I felt more comfortable doing the rounds, leading the team as we went through the problem lists, the issues, and formulating the plan for our beloved patients in the ICU. The "Canadian way" of doing things was slowly being inculcated in me. I learned to appreciate how brilliant my ICU attending physicians were. They were rockstars in their own respect, and if I wanted to be a good contributor in the unit, I had to follow suit. Because I never had to worry about the financial aspects of the patients and there were no resource limitations, unlike ICUs in the Philippines, I was able to focus on learning – not only from a medical and pathophysiological perspective but also from a professional aspect. During COVID, I felt that the ICU team was a well-oiled machine. We all knew where our roles started and ended. We all were aware of how the person next to us was feeling. Constant communication with everyone in the unit was paramount – between nurses, physicians, students, and allied health care workers. This aspect of work I loved very much. We all knew that we were tired and fatigued from taking care of our COVID patients and from the strain the pandemic brought to us (endless lockdowns, not being able to enjoy our social life as much as we had before), but we never let these difficulties get to us, and we treated each other with respect. Ultimately, we loved each other, which made life as an intensive care specialist working and training in Toronto such an amazing and life-changing experience for someone who came from a third-world country.

Being an international critical care fellow, I had the pleasure to work with other physicians from different parts of Canada and the world. Apart from sharing all our ICU experiences, we also bonded and shared parts of our own culture with one another. Often it was through food and cooking. I still remember that, as we went home from a call shift, we would individually cook one of our local dishes and bring it in the morning to share with the others. This practice made me realize how much a hub for international culture and cuisine Toronto really is, and it made working and living in Toronto alone for a year more exciting.

It is true that I failed to experience Toronto as advertised because of the restrictions mandated by the pandemic. But my life as an intensivist-in-training in the ICUs around Toronto will always be one of the highlights of my career. Not only was it fulfilling from a knowledge standpoint, but it made me a better person, a better doctor, and overall, a better human being. It also made me realize how un-ideal the Philippine health care setting was and how far behind we were in terms of optimal health care delivery, especially when strained as it is during the pandemic.

EPISODE 4: The Return

I landed back home on 11 September 2021. Because the Philippines was still in lockdown, I was greeted by unknown faces rather than the faces of my family. I got inside a van and made my way to a hotel quarantine facility. A week went by, and then I was able to meet with my family. Lots of kisses and lots of hugs were given. After more than a year of being away, of mostly having breakfast, lunch, and dinner alone, no feeling even comes close to the happiness of being able to share a meal with your loved ones.

To be honest, not much had changed with the Philippine situation when I went back home and did the rounds looking for work: COVID cases were still up and down; ICUs were still somewhat full. But I found that Filipinos were sick and tired already. Our response to the pandemic was suboptimal, probably because of the lack of funds. We could not implement serial lockdowns because the Filipino people needed to go to work to be able to provide for their family – they would not be able to do so if the government were to put work on hold again. It was reported that fewer deaths were happening in the hospitals, but that was only half true. Because Filipinos did not have money anymore, they did not have the spending power to be able to pay for their health care needs; hence, they deferred going to the hospital, even if they needed to be admitted. Most of them, especially the financially challenged, would just end up in the emergency rooms or, worse, outside the hospitals, and they would die there – never seeing the inside of a proper hospital room or an ICU bed.

My nationalistic self went into overdrive as I went out, resume in hand, and applied for work as an intensive care specialist to the different hospitals in my area. Armed with the knowledge I had gained from training with some of the best and remarkable people in the field of intensive care medicine, I thought most of the hospitals would welcome me with open arms. I wanted to help in the hospitals and bring "the Canadian way" of doing things into the realm of Philippine intensive care medicine. I thought it would be a no-brainer – hiring a well-trained young buck coming back home to help where help is needed the most. But I was wrong.

I underestimated the politics and the inherent Filipino culture. I felt that most of them saw me as a threat rather than an asset to be had. Months passed by, and I was rotting at home. "We do not have a need for an intensive care specialist" or "There is no gap in our service delivery" or "We already have a cardiologist and a respirologist" were some of the top replies I got when I went out looking for my place in the Philippine health care setting. The fragmentation of health care is a pandemic in the Philippines. If a patient has a cough, they would automatically see a respirologist. If they have chest pain, an automatic referral to a cardiologist will happen. Abdominal pain? A gastroenterologist would be called in. It is not unusual to have twelve doctors handling a single ICU patient, all because of this fragmentation of care, which is the standard of care in the ICU setting. To say that I miss the intensivist-led design in Canada is a huge understatement.

The experience of applying for work back home broke my heart. I really wanted to help and to elevate the Philippine intensive care scene. However, the circumstances I went home to were still the same as when I left. I remember, as I was about to make my way back home, receiving a lot of messages urging me to come home, telling me that the knowledge I had now acquired and the experience I had garnered would be a welcomed addition. But that was not the reality I saw when I tried to reincorporate myself again into the mix. It was and still is such a sad experience for me. It truly was heartbreaking. Whatever love I had for my country sadly went away.

I tried to make my way back to Canada where I felt I would be more appreciated. However, certain circumstances hindered me from doing so – my family's health (as most of them acquired COVID for a brief period), my personal health, and responsibilities that I now carry. Going back to Toronto is easier said than done. I really do hope things change, but this experience showed me that my country, the Philippines, prioritizes certain things more than the important ones, which is probably the reason we are at a standstill instead of moving forward, or worse, we are moving backwards. It is probably why we are still a third-world country, and why, if a next pandemic happens, we will probably respond in the same way – unequal allocation of resources, poor governance, recycling of PPE and masks, and having people die without seeing the inside of a hospital.

The Philippine health care setting is something that should not be regarded as ideal. Being able to experience working and training in Canada showed me that. The Philippines is not yet ready for the ideal setting. Will it ever be? For my children and the children of my children, I hope so. As for me, I will continue trying to work using the standards instilled in me from working in Canada. The "Canadian way" of doing things has now become my norm. Hopefully, by being able to work in the ICUs in the Philippines, I will be able to show the Filipino people the standard of care for ICUs. Hopefully, one day, it will become the Filipino standard of care as well.

24 Resident Training in COVID-19 Times

Pamela H. Orr, MD, MSc, FRCPC
Professor, Internal Medicine (Infectious Diseases), Medical Microbiology, and Community Health Sciences, University of Manitoba, Winnipeg

Submitted 17 May 2022

In one way or another, the COVID-19 epidemic overwhelmed all of us who work in health care in Canada. When I say "overwhelmed," what I mean is the visceral experience of the gap between the needs of individuals, families, and communities for care and our ability to provide care. The cries for help came from those with COVID-related illness and those with other health needs that were not met due to COVID demands. Many cries for help were silent, silenced, ignored, dismissed – the suffering of those who no longer received preventive care, timely care, cancer screening, social support, surgery, in-person care, diagnostic or therapeutic touch, or attention. But we heard them.

I served as the head of education in the Department of Internal Medicine at the University of Manitoba from 2017 to 2021. I took the job because I could see the growing fault lines in our health care and education systems. Some of these tensions were old, dating from well before my residency training in the 1980s, and some were new. Internal medicine residents are physicians who have graduated from medical school and are now in training to become specialists in the various disciplines that comprise internal medicine. I wanted to protect, support, and promote our residents as learners and as practising physicians. Ultimately, it is in order to provide the best care for those we are called upon to serve.

In Winnipeg hospitals during the peaks of the pandemic waves, COVID patients were admitted to specialty service units such as obstetrics, surgery, or intensive care, but the majority of hospitalized patients were looked after on designated isolation internal medicine wards. Care was provided primarily by internal medicine attending physicians, not "core" (the first 3 years of postgraduate training) residents. That was unusual, as normally core internal medicine residents work alongside attending physicians in a form of "apprenticeship." Several residents volunteered to work more directly with COVID patients, and at one point when staff physicians were overwhelmed, several subspecialty residents (in their fourth or fifth years) were redeployed to work on the COVID wards.

This policy was instituted by the dean of our medical school at the University of Manitoba. In other Canadian training programs, internal medicine residents were integrated into the care teams on COVID wards. Opinion varies as to whether the decision here was the right one. Some residents and staff thought that all physicians, including those in training, are called upon in times of crisis to look after those in need, despite personal risk. Is that not part of what it means to be a physician, part of the covenant with the people we serve? Others thought that we should protect and shield residents from a little understood illness associated with considerable mortality and, at the time, for which there were no preventive or therapeutic interventions. At the beginning of the pandemic, this approach may have been influenced by the ethical concept of "fair innings," which promotes the idea of giving advantages to those who have not had an equal opportunity to live and thrive.

No matter which approach was chosen, or the underlying philosophy, the pandemic has certainly impacted the quality of resident education. The dual role of residents, as both learners (students) and employees providing service, is a source of tension that has always existed in medical training but which has been exacerbated by the pandemic. Residents are licensed to practise medicine as learners, working within accredited training programs. In the role as health care workers looking after patients, they are employees of health authorities (in most cases), which are arms of provincial governments. Their salaries therefore derive from taxpayers. Alternatively, in their role as learners they are fee-paying students registered in university postgraduate medical training programs. Learning takes place while looking after patients at the bedside, in the emergency room, walking in hallways, talking to families. It is an immersive process with supervising and mentoring physicians and other health care workers who have a responsibility to teach, correct, and model professional behaviour, roles, and responsibilities. Additional learning throughout training is also carried out in classrooms, small group seminars, conferences, rounds, alone or in groups at night and on weekends. These dual roles reflect an old and honoured tradition of apprenticeship, of learning and developing skill through working alongside members of the profession, receiving feedback and evaluations, being challenged with increasing responsibility and expectations.

Tension has always existed between the voracious demands for service (looking after patients) and the need for time to study and learn. The latter does not just refer to time spent sequestered during the day in a real or virtual seminar room. It also means time spent with supervising physicians and other health workers wherever we see patients. However, academic supervising physicians are also obligated by their university contracts to meet scholarly requirements of their own in terms of research, administration, and other professional activities, all the while maintaining overarching responsibility for patient care and teaching.

In Manitoba teaching hospitals during the peaks of the pandemic, staff physicians significantly increased their workload to care for patients on COVID isolation wards, while internal medicine residents continued to work primarily with non-COVID patients on regular wards in order to keep care for these patients as functional as possible. Previously structured teaching sessions, many of them online, continued as much as possible. However, while the residents' hours of work were limited by their contracts, the workload of ward physicians in sections like general internal medicine was not limited or controlled. Most of our staff physicians are independent contractors, not employees. Nevertheless, appointments and privileges depend on meeting patient needs for care and academic performance.

My observation is that the massive number and complexity of patients needing care during the COVID pandemic has adversely affected the amount and quality of resident teaching, knowledge, and skills. Supervising physicians are exhausted. Residents are exhausted. Time for, and focus on, teaching is drained by the incessant demand for the care of very ill people. Online teaching is not conducive to engagement of teacher and learner, and is an inadequate medium for learning clinical judgment or technical and crisis management skills.

The Royal College of Physicians and Surgeons of Canada (RCPSC) requirements for residency training programs, developed pre-pandemic, have continued through the pandemic with little to no respite. These include the need for programs to move to a new method of evaluating residents, called "Competency by Design," and the accreditation processes that programs must meet. The pressure on residents and staff has been enormous. In many cases, the ability to meet the RCPSC requirements lies not with the teaching staff and academic departments but rather in health systems and those who lead those systems: the hospitals and clinics and health authorities that are responsible for the conditions in which we all work.

I have felt a kind of wonder that is hard to describe to be living through such a great crisis. I believe that this feeling of wonder is shared by many physicians, whether in training or post-training. It is one thing to know that the world is subject to recurring pandemics, but it is another thing to live through one.

In conditions of conflict, epidemics, and disasters, health care workers, in training or post-training, have always been called upon to serve those in need. I recall the time I spent teaching in Laos. Physicians there told me about their experience as medical trainees sent to the border between Laos and Cambodia. They were taught to perform field amputations for mutilated refugees fleeing from Pol Pot's regime. That is what is meant by performing the extraordinary in an ordinary way and the ordinary in an extraordinary way. That is what we have been asked to do during the pandemic.

Appropriate pride, confidence, the well-being that comes from working together for a higher purpose, the building of strength though the exercise of physical and moral courage: these are the experiences that residents and staff have communicated to me. However, I also hear of and see exhaustion, distress, disappointment, burnout, depression, anxiety. The distress covers a spectrum: moral, emotional, psychological, physical, spiritual. Many older physicians recall their own training as being much more onerous in terms of workload, hours, and responsibility compared to the workload of residents now. This argument is not a good one when we consider the need to support and promote the well-being and health of those who care for others. The changes in working conditions and employment contracts that have come about in recent years through advocacy and resident union negotiations have appropriately tried to place limits on workload, to provide healthy environments, and to protect and promote group and individual learning.

During the pandemic, additional mental health resources have been made available through health care and professional organizations. However, both residents and staff are often reluctant to access such resources due to worry about stigma and what it will mean in terms of their ability to practise medicine. Many do not find them helpful, particularly if they are generic in nature and don't speak to actual experience. The increasing focus on physician (resident and staff) well-being began pre-pandemic but is now a matter of even greater urgency. The fear, anxiety, and anger provoked by the pandemic has led to aggression turned inward (self-harm) and outward (lateral and vertical aggression against others) among health care workers. Training programs need to do more in terms of creating environments free from harassment and abuse of residents by teachers. However, it is a two-way street. A growing body of literature and experience demonstrates that faculties also need to do more to protect teachers and supervisors from abuse by learners.

The RCPSC accreditation teams put a great deal of emphasis on resident well-being. This emphasis is appropriate. All programs want their residents, and staff, to be well physically, emotionally, and psychologically. The well-being of residents is tied to the well-being of their teachers. They are bound to each other, and their mutual health is a necessary but not sufficient requirement for successful educational programs. However, neither can be well in the broken health system that we have now in the third year of this pandemic.

Whether the current balance in terms of workload and education, work as education, is correct is widely debated. There are those who believe that every interaction in the care of patients is a learning experience. Others define certain types of work that are imbedded in clinical practice, for example, completion of forms and discharge summaries, as devoid of learning. If a resident has looked after a certain number of patients with problem "X," should they be exempt from seeing or looking after any further such cases? If certain days or parts of days are set aside for study, what is the effect on the continuity of care for the patients whom they are following when they leave the ward or clinic? Isn't continuity of care an essential skill and practice? If an increasing proportion of resident time is set aside for sequestered study, will training programs need to be lengthened in order for residents to gain sufficient clinical experience and skills to qualify as competent medical practitioners? Furthermore, has the epidemic curtailed the exposure of some residents from the necessary diversity of clinical exposures to such an extent that their training must be prolonged?

I have posed a lot of questions here but answered few, if any. At least in my centre, one thing that is clear to me is that we have to stop thinking of residents as an unlimited resource to look after however many patients requiring care day and night. We must define the most appropriate patients for residents to care for and have a workforce of attending physicians, house officers, nurse practitioners, and physician assistants to look after all the other patients. In this way, the workload will be better distributed for teachers as well as learners. There must be call schedules and responsibilities and payment methods that will ensure that all patients are well cared for (in all the dimensions of what makes care "good") and that there is not the kind of "patient creep" that I experienced during my residency – the call in the middle of the night instructing me to do work outside my remit, that is, to do someone else's work for them.

My thoughts here are rooted in my own experiences and observations. I was a medical student at the University of Toronto in the 1970s. Our class was huge, and the experience was alienating until I became a clinical clerk and rotating intern at St. Michael's Hospital. Dr. Peter Kopplin mentored us, by which I mean that he cared for us, respected us, taught us, showed us what it was to be a wise and caring physician. He was a bright light in a widespread "shame and blame" culture of medical training. I left as soon as possible, meaning after internship, to work for a year as an emergency room doctor in a community hospital, where I learned that I actually had skills and knowledge. I met another visionary mentor, Dr. Jack Hildes, who sent me to the Arctic, where I worked for several years as a general practitioner. I was embraced by the Inuit people, and my time there tested me at my very limits as a physician and a person. Returning in the mid-1980s to residency training in internal medicine at the University of Manitoba was a very positive experience. The work was hard but not nearly as hard as being the only physician in a remote region larger than the size of Germany, with few resources other than a microscope and an X-ray machine very capably operated by the nursing station janitor.

I experienced great solidarity among the residents in my program. We cared for each other. The chief residents were highly respected leaders, not only knowledgeable but wise and devoted to their patients and to us. They were our models, and we wanted to measure up. I could not believe my luck in having other staff physicians and teachers around me or, at the end of a phone at 3 o'clock in the morning, to give me advice when I was on call. What was not to like about residency? Well, there were elements of misogyny, racism, sexual harassment, antisemitism, homophobia, bullying, and abuse in greater or lesser degree, reflecting their presence in society as a whole at the time.

The thread that runs through my own experience of medical training and has guided me since has been the search for mentors, models, and like-minded physicians with whom I could form a "clan," bound together with respect and caring, curiosity and learning, skill and wisdom.

I think one of the most important things we have learned, relearned, in the pandemic is the moral imperative of advocacy. It is surely one of the physician roles that has been most needed during this pandemic. Although we are taught that advocacy for patients and communities is part of our role as physicians, the "hidden curriculum" of health systems often teaches us that silence, compliance, and rule following is expected. Nevertheless, we have seen notable examples of advocates among teachers and residents during this pandemic. They have held us together, motivated us, inspired us. They have taught us to speak up for those without a voice, to be wholly present for those in need, to question and seek answers, to be physically and morally courageous. We must advocate for each other, both staff and trainees, support each other, create better and more sustained mentoring while holding each other to account. We have known this for a long time, but COVID has made the need for systemic change more urgent and evident.

PART SIX

Systems on the Verge of Collapse

"Systems on the Verge of Collapse" provides several insiders' view of the health care system during various phases of the pandemic – flaws, failures, and all. "Anticipation, Dread, and Worry: Preparing for the Arrival of Sick Patients" tells of the anxious days waiting for the arrival of the virus – preparing for the unpreparable. "'The War on COVID-19': Reflections from the ICU Front Line" describes the siege mentality of the COVID-19 front lines with its tumult of emotions – camaraderie, fear, uncertainty, anger, determination. "Seven Days in the ICU" recalls the day-by-day activities of a physician in the ICU at the height of the pandemic, the horrors seen, emotional rollercoaster ridden, and lingering effects only to be guessed at. "The Pandemic Was a Powerful Teacher: Ramping Down Services" details some of the administrative lessons learned through the pandemic of the capacity of a health care system to expand and the consequent challenges involved in returning the system back to its previous size, while leaving plans in place for future pandemics. "COVID-19 Seen from a Preventionist Physician's Point of View: Will We Be Able to Draw Lessons for the Future?" gives a unique perspective: a physician whose primary role is to prevent the spread of infection within and beyond the hospital setting addresses the shortcomings of the current health care system and speculates on whether we truly will, as we have promised repeatedly, not be as unprepared "next time." "Treating the Unvaccinated During COVID-19: Did I Sign Up for This?" wrestles with one of the major internal conflicts faced by health care workers in the later waves of the pandemic – providing high-level compassionate care to those who, due either to ignorance or hostility, refused to take appropriate preventative measures and became infected with COVID. And "Siloed Still…" bemoans the failure to adapt on a larger scale as each COVID wave hit. This chapter discusses the perpetuation of what became a new "business as usual" approach in the health care arena, where unproductive divisions and compartmentalization between the health care system and society at large remained.

25 Anticipation, Dread, and Worry: Preparing for the Arrival of Sick Patients

Matyas Hervieux, BSc (Hons), DHS, MA, MD, CCFP(EM)
Department of Emergency Medicine, University Health Network, Toronto

Submitted 18 October 2022

Preparing for the COVID-19 pandemic was demoralizing for many, if not all, front-line health care workers. Yet, for many of us who have lived through other infectious disease scenarios, we were initially optimistic that our previous experience in similar situations would provide us with the knowledge and skills to navigate this terrifying pandemic. We believed our expertise would be invaluable, given that, unlike governmental leadership that frequently changes, we offered lived experience that would be crucial to managing the impact of this pandemic.

In hindsight, our response to previous threats such as severe acute respiratory syndrome (SARS) was relatively remarkable. While it was a much smaller event, we rapidly and successfully limited exposure to SARS and analysed our response both in real time and after the outbreak, learning from, and responding to, our mistakes while creating clear isolation policies and enacting strict public health measures designed to protect our population and our workers in anticipation of future events. We also knew from our experience with SARS the consequences of a poor response, lack of preparedness, and inappropriate access to personal protective equipment (PPE). We had learned that the consequences could be dire and that the lives of citizens and health care workers would be lost if these issues were not taken seriously.

Indeed, with SARS we had gained confidence in our ability to rally quickly to such an "all-ready-out-of-the-gate" scenario. For these reasons, when the COVID pandemic arose, it was initially reassuring as Canadian front-line workers to be working within a socialized, public health–oriented health care system that had experience with dealing with a viral outbreak. Given the universality and prioritization of our health care system for the fundamental values of health and well-being in Canada, we also believed that, despite the looming pandemic, our approach would be to adhere to the general principles of public health while smoothly implementing our previous lived experience.

Initially on the front lines, there seemed to be only one appropriate response: all our preparation should be directed at identifying and containing this virus before it spread throughout our population, knowing that any delay in such a response would have disastrous outcomes. These thoughts made an extremely stressful situation somehow more palatable.

Unfortunately, we were wrong due to several limitations beyond the reach of front-line workers. The initial response to this looming pandemic brought to the forefront the disheartening reality that we had inadequate governmental and public health leadership that failed to implement the lessons we had previously learned from dealing with SARS. The failure to swiftly commit to these strategies meant that appropriate public health protocols and institutional protocols designed at containing COVID were never implemented. As a result, our health care system remained relatively unprepared to deal with a global pandemic, and we, as front-line health care workers, would assume much of the negative consequences of a disorganized system in which we have little voice or control.

The most telltale sign of the systemic disorganization found throughout our intersectoral health care partnerships was demonstrated by the fact that we began to prepare for this pandemic so late in the game. Indeed, there was never a unified intersectoral action plan to address our anticipated first steps of early identification and prevention of spread. Rather, at times, it seemed that various intersectoral agencies were at cross-purposes. For example, it was disheartening that mandatory testing, isolation, and travel bans were not implemented quickly for travellers arriving from abroad. Equally disheartening was the lack of a system-wide attempt to recruit and train intersectoral partners on containment. Right from the start, the reactive, rather than proactive, manner in which pandemic preparations were made, across seemingly all intersectoral agencies, meant that any opportunities to control speed and spread, and to strategize appropriately, were lost.

That is not to say that significant efforts were not made to establish communication and a cohesive approach among intersectoral stakeholders. Federal, provincial, and municipal governments, public health, and stakeholder organizations including health care unions, front-line workers, hospitals, care homes, and so on were all called upon to contribute to our pandemic response. But these efforts at collaboration were mostly uncoordinated, reactionary, and failed to acknowledge or implement the lessons learned from front-line workers during SARS and our exposure to other pandemic/infectious disease–related events.

Instead, there seemed to be a prioritization of governmental and institutional issues – partisanship, budgetary constraints, cross-border relations, and the like – rather than population health, public health, and front-line worker safety. When effective communication was possible, there were simply too many players, too many political egos, and too much political posturing to broker any response that forefronted public health, population health, and front-line safety.

Similarly, even when public health initiatives were implemented, these efforts were either poorly implemented, dismissed, or misinformed. Evidence-based approaches seemed to be sidelined and treated as merely one "perspective" on how to prepare for COVID. As such, decision-makers disregarded many public health warnings and recommendations during the preparatory stage and throughout the pandemic. For emergency department front-line health care workers, it was shocking to see the manner in which our provincial premiers dismissed public health recommendations and how our federal government failed to enact appropriate public health policies to ensure Canadians were protected. Many of us watched in horror and disbelief as our federal and provincial governments lost precious time squabbling with each other and public health officials about what policies or procedures to implement that would best protect our population. Lives were lost as a result. Yet, regions like the Northwest Territories and other countries (notably New Zealand) took the opportunity seriously to limit entry of COVID at their borders and fared much better.

The deprioritization of public health initiatives in Canada was all the more frustrating given that the media was bombarding us with international images of hospitals and cities overwhelmed by COVID patients. The lack of preparedness in other nations to COVID made our lack of preparedness even more frightening, especially given the alarming number of deaths experienced by other nations. To many front-line workers it felt like our Canadian leaders and many other leaders around the world, likewise, did not seem to grasp the significance or the extent of what was coming.

In time, it became painfully obvious to us that there would never be more aggressive attempts at containment. Hopes of containment were, perhaps, never realistically achievable given our governmental, corporate, and public desire for ongoing global interconnectedness coupled with the virulence of this new virus. As a result, it became increasingly clear that we had to prepare ourselves for the inevitable reality that COVID would spread throughout our communities, our hospitals, our nursing homes, and our public institutions, and we were forced to accept the eventuality that COVID would cross our front line and that many of us would fall ill and – in view of what we were seeing in the media and what we were coming to know through health care grapevines – possibly die. It was also clear that this eventuality would mean that many of us would also infect our loved ones who could also die. Worse yet was our understanding that the fallout of this ineffective response would have disproportionately disastrous consequences for our most vulnerable populations.

Impact on Emergency Departments: Variability, Vulnerability, and Animosity

This poor global and Canadian pre-pandemic planning created some unique challenges for emergency physicians as we were often put in impossible situations. Emergency rooms across our country were very often the first point of contact with people sickened by COVID. My colleagues in all sites had similar experiences. We were frequently being approached by nursing and other allied health staff with questions regarding COVID: How transmissible is it? Is it aerosolized? What is appropriate PPE? Will it affect my pregnancy? What risks would there be to their immunocompromised children/family members if they contracted COVID? How will it interact with my specific comorbidities? How should we protect ourselves during procedures? Will our hospital and public health policies be ineffective? What about the mismatch between our hospital policies, public health policies, and the available research? Emergency physicians were bombarded by myriad questions that we not only did not have the answers to but that were also equally applicable to our own lives, our families, and our friends, which heightened our own sense of personal vulnerability.

There was also an expectation placed on front-line emergency physicians that we were somehow to be leaders during this process, when in reality, we were for the most part voiceless at the tables that had the most impact on directing the health care system response throughout this process. We had no voice or control about how to prepare or respond to the anticipated masses of the population who were likely to become acutely, and severely, ill. Instead, we, like all front-line workers, were navigating our way through the dark: trying to find Town Hall meetings for updates and searching for daily or even hourly updates on how to safely perform our jobs based on news from colleagues around the world, how to best treat the COVID-positive patients who would present in respiratory distress, and how to protect patients in our institutions without COVID so that they were not exposed during their stay in hospital. This last challenge was especially difficult, given that our emergency departments have been universally designed to have wide-open spaces separated by cloth curtains, which are clearly ineffective in isolating patients from each other.

In sum, these were all impossible scenarios presented to front-line workers and, perhaps especially, to hospital-based physicians because we simply did not have any real power to be heard in a significant way and had little to no influence on decision-making in our institutions at the community level, provincially, or nationally. It became readily apparent that, despite our expertise, we were not "stakeholders" with a clear, unified voice. Instead, each hospital, each institution, and each level of government seemed to take their own unpredictable and solipsistic approach to COVID preparedness and responsiveness.

As the COVID pandemic began to unfold, emergency departments across the world witnessed inter-agency differences in COVID preparedness. This variability in practices and protection from site to site became apparent early on because many front-line workers are employed at multiple sites. Those who worked in urban areas found that the academic hospitals they worked at were eager and willing to develop and implement changes to flow and the physical workspace early on. Some of these institutions seemed keen to develop contingency planning and to devise a stepwise approach to implementing successive phases of institutional change to adapt to the ever-increasing needs of the pandemic. Front-line workers in these types of centres felt better protected and respected by this proactive approach: many front-line workers were consulted to help design and redesign throughput, which helped to lessen fears of the looming onslaught of patients.

For those of us who also worked in rural hospitals, the inconsistency of the rural approach was all the more apparent: pandemic planning seemed to be more like the wild west, where experienced front-line workers were shamed and silenced when suggestions for improvement were made to non-academic leaders and clinicians. Similarly, suggestions and/or the provision of information we shared from our experiences working at other sites, which we hoped would help with local planning, were perceived as criticisms. This divide between academic larger hospitals and rural centres further contributed to the sense of helplessness of front-line workers, perhaps especially those working in rural hospitals where, despite fewer resources, institutional attitudes prevented us from adapting approaches to fit local needs and improve safety for patients and staff.

This lack of autonomy and sense of vulnerability was heightened by cross-agency discrepancies. For example, paramedics in our area were not given N95s early on. Moreover, when vaccinations became available, our paramedics were put at the end of the queue behind other front-line workers. Insultingly, paramedics who were denied access to vaccinations were asked to wait outside psychiatric and prison facilities while vaccination clinics were proceeding inside for residents and administrators on the off chance that someone receiving a vaccination may have a serious reaction! This disregard further demoralized all front-line emergency workers, whether we worked in or out of the hospital, because differences in approach across agencies ultimately demonstrated that different front-line workers – all of whom played an essential role in our pandemic response – were being valued differently. These inconsistencies in practices and recommendations gave rise to further uncertainties and animosity.

The Issues of Resources and Supply Chains: Patient and Front-Line Staff Safety

Pandemic preparation also made us increasingly aware of the lack of resources, in Canada and around the world, that we would have to fight the pandemic. We were constantly being informed that we would likely face PPE shortages because we rely heavily on oversees suppliers, such as China, to provide us with PPE. We watched in horror as colleagues in the United States were forced to recycle their PPE or use bandanas as PPE (many of whom fell sick or died) and as competition between countries to secure supplies drove hoarding and increased costs. Our hospitals were constantly locking down PPE, and workers themselves felt the need to hoard and "steal" PPE in order to ensure their own protection.

Other resource limitations also became apparent. Canada's supply of ventilators and ICU beds per capita is staggeringly low compared to that of other developed nations. A competition for ventilators also arose with similar consequences to those seen with shortages of PPE. The promise of vaccine development and availability likewise raised questions as to whether Canada would be able to produce its own vaccine when the time came or whether we would rely on foreign supply chains and their prioritization of Canada over other populations. These concerns were even more significant for those living in low-resource settings.

In addition, pre-COVID we were already experiencing human-resource shortages including nurses, registered practical nurses, physicians, and personal support workers. Realizations such as these made it clear to all front-line workers that the lack of resources we were experiencing before the pandemic would make the course of the pandemic all the more stressful and unbearable.

In the face of so much uncertainty and lack of necessary resources, it is not surprising that the majority of front-line workers felt it was safest to err on the side of caution, to be over-diligent rather than under-diligent with our attempts at containment, self-protection, and the protection of our patients. Yet, despite our own beliefs in proactive policy and procedure, as front-line workers we were subjected to "policing" of our practices by clinical and non-clinical managers.

Our safety became a negotiated issue, where the need to take a very cautious approach to protect workers was in tension with official policies that prioritized resource allocation and budgetary considerations and therefore tended to be subjective, arbitrary, and non-evidence-based. Adoption of policies to effectively protect front-line workers and patients from COVID was also being influenced by the optics of these approaches: administration seemed more concerned over what messaging adopting overly cautious approaches might send to colleagues, officials, patients, and families.

The most demoralizing part of this decision-making, for most of us, was that the decision-making was being performed by non-clinical policymakers who, for the most part, had never been and never would be on the front line. Even prior to COVID, it was clear that these policymakers did not understand the intricacies of front-line work, such as workflow and risk management. This procedural ignorance meant that advocating for more cautious policies and procedures, both within or external to our workplaces, was for the most part ineffective, as a top-down approach to policymaking limited negotiation and our input, especially in the preparatory phase.

But it was not simply that our inclinations and desired level of protection were incongruent with emerging governmental, public health, and hospital policies. In many ways, it felt like front-line workers were being managed with an intentionally heavy-handed and authoritarian approach by our policymakers. Our voices were being systematically ignored; it seemed that we were not supposed to speak at all. For example, it became scientifically apparent early on that COVID was aerosolized, that the droplet precautions recommended at that time were not sufficient, and that PPE against aerosolized virus was necessary. When concerns like these were brought forward, our policymakers decided to risk our health and safety. They relied on unclear evidence and decided that we did not need protection against aerosolized particles: we were not allowed to have N95 masks (let alone N99s!) and other appropriate PPE unless a patient was coughing and sneezing in our vicinity or we were engaged in aerosol-generating procedures. Of course, it is unpredictable when a patient will cough or sneeze next to you! As a result, our workplaces denied us access to PPE such as N95 masks, for example, either by locking them up or rationing their use, and implemented inferior-level masking policies that would inevitability lead to exposures and infections for staff and outbreaks among patients.

The result was that many of us felt very vulnerable, scared, and scrutinized: scrutiny directed at us not for lack of a willingness to engage in safe practice but because we questioned the logic of not being allowed to wear appropriate PPE or to engage in practices that made us feel safe, including making our own assessment of what level of mask to wear, when we would choose to engage in aerosolized protection, and so on. During one of our first outbreaks among staff and patients, it was hard to not feel abandoned and angry: we had asked for safer policies and procedures but were being falsely reassured that ineffective policies were safe.

Worse yet, we were kept in the dark about our own exposures: we were not informed if we had worked with a provider who became ill, and, therefore, we were not able to make any independent assessments about our own exposure risks. Learning days later that you had been exposed to COVID in a lunchroom or workstation further undermined our sense of security and made many realize our health and safety were simply not a priority.

Emergency Department Designs: Issues of Workplace Safety

A similarly heavy-handed approach was evident when front-line workers started to advocate for safer workplaces. Indeed, in many sites the physical construction and the throughput of our workplaces put patients and staff at risk. When concerns were raised at many sites, there was reluctance or outright refusal by our employers to limit exposure by attempting to physically modify these workspaces or by redirecting flow through them. For example, many of us worked in facilities with no negative pressure rooms, a single negative pressure room, or a negative pressure room that was inappropriately situated in our workspace (the only way to access a negative pressure room would be to transport infectious COVID patients through other clinical areas, waiting rooms, and other public places).

A logical approach during the preparatory stage would have been to redesign our workspaces to create isolation and negative pressure rooms close to points of entry and to reimagine the flow of our departments to limit exposure to other areas and to protect workers and patients from COVID-positive patients. Yet, for many of us, these types of initiatives were inconsistently implemented within or across institutions, or our suggestions were ignored. Many centres took a "wait and see" approach with unspecified determinants for when flow or structural changes should be implemented. Some workplaces even shamed workers for raising concerns about throughput and lack of preparedness. These reactive-type institutions left their front-line workers feeling disrespected, disillusioned, and vulnerable. Animosity directed towards administration and clinical decision-makers unnecessarily intensified, morale plummeted, and many staff members began to look for other employment or chose to work at the better of their two worksites.

Even in academic centres that seemed onboard with redesigning throughput, front-line workers' safety was neglected in other ways. While some sites did conduct air quality and air filtration studies, and emphasized the need for social distancing and reduced occupancy, it was demoralizing to visit many other sites and witness the conditions in which workers were forced to eat, take breaks, and change. None of these rooms had negative pressure units, and the most effective air filtering rooms were reserved for those struggling with highly contagious airborne illnesses. None of these rooms were adequately cleaned. Instead, workers' spaces were overcrowded, and there were no sinks available in lunchrooms, break rooms, or change rooms to ensure appropriate donning and doffing of one's PPE. In other sites, where occupancy was considered, the consequences were a lack of available space to take a break, eat, and grab a few moments of precious respite. I personally witnessed workers changing in a toilet area in the middle of a busy Emergency Department! If nothing else, the pandemic has made it salient that hospital design must consider and prioritize worker safety with respect to having safe places to eat, change, work, and take a break during infectious disease outbreaks.

Even before the first patient walked through the door, the treatment health care providers received in this preparatory phase set the stage for significant, and severe, institutional (sanctuary) trauma (trauma that results from institutional acts of omission or commission that can worsen the effect of a traumatic experience or cause trauma as a result of violating the dignity or safety of a worker). Indeed, the notion that the institutions we had devoted our lives to could act in such a cavalier manner with our health and well-being was distressing. It is hard to put into words the sense of despair, betrayal, and helplessness many front-line workers felt as we were not heard and were confronted with the seeming reality that our health and safety were simply not valued by our policymakers. As it became increasingly apparent to front-line workers that the lessons we had learned from SARS were not being respected or implemented, this sense of disillusionment deepened.

Most of us to some degree felt betrayed by our governmental decision-makers and also betrayed by the institutions that we worked for – hospitals, nursing homes, paramedic services, fire departments, police services, ambulatory care centres, and other similar institutions. The maltreatment we received from community-based special interest groups intensified these betrayals. Many of us looked for ways out. Many of us have abandoned or are abandoning our callings because of this betrayal. This phenomenon is not only seen in nursing staff or in hospitals as reported extensively in the Canadian media. Indeed, across the board we witnessed an early exodus in nurses, registered practical nurses, personal support workers, and nurse practitioners. Physicians started reducing their hours or leaving their positions in ambulatory care centres, nursing homes, and home care.

The sense of being devalued, vulnerable, and not respected in our workplaces, I believe, is one of the most significant reasons for current burnout rates among health care workers. The betrayal health care workers felt as our employers left us vulnerable to COVID, and possible morbidity or death, inflicted severe institutional trauma. It is this type of mistreatment that prompted so many of us to leave emergency medicine, precipitating our ongoing crisis of increasing staffing shortages, long wait times, longer admissions to the Emergency Department itself, and poorer quality of care. We need to find ways to hold those accountable who inflicted this kind of trauma on health care workers and fix this abusive system. Creating a responsive and respectful work environment is the only hope we have of encouraging health care workers to return to the front line and stay there.

26 "The War on COVID-19": Reflections from the ICU Front Line

Peter G. Brindley, MD, FRCPC, FRCP
Professor of Critical Care Medicine, Adjunct Professor of Anesthesiology, Adjunct Professor, John Dossetor Health Ethics Centre, University of Alberta, Edmonton

Submitted 5 July 2022

It's important for me to stress that, regardless of my COVID-19 experience, my life is ludicrously fortunate and blessed. Accordingly, I am merely writing this chapter as an effort to explain what it felt like being an intensive care unit (ICU) doctor during the pandemic. It is categorically not my intention to complain, whinge, or claim special importance. After all, for the last two decades it has been a thrill to work as an intensive care doctor and a delight to pontificate my way around the world as a professor of critical care medicine. Nonetheless, COVID was hard, darn hard, but not just because of long hours with little time off. In fact, the hard work was a doddle compared to the existential angst.

What was far tougher and somewhat unexpected for health care workers – perhaps you can relate – was how it was profoundly draining to experience so much preventable death, to receive the accusations of anti-vaxxers, and to endure bureaucratic crackdown. It was also – as strange as this word may seem in the setting of a pandemic – profoundly tedious because things dragged on and on, and because the

---

This chapter is adapted from a 31 March 2020 newspaper article by Peter G. Brindley in Canada's *National Post* entitled "'Life in the Trenches': An Edmonton ICU Doctor Describes the War against COVID-19" (used with permission); and from "Health Care Workers Are Scared but, in Some Ways, Also Lucky" by Peter G. Brindley, published in the *BMJ Opinion* on 31 March 2020 © 2020 BMJ Publishing Group Ltd. All rights reserved.

lack of beds and the isolation requirements made everything harder and slower. This job is challenging during the best of times, and that's why most of us like it. The difference is that 2 years of COVID felt like 5 years of regular work. It also felt like the first time we went to war as a profession. Let me try to explain without causing too many eyes to roll as I describe "medicine's war on COVID."

Health care workers – including this author – have been guilty of throwing out gratuitous military metaphors when describing our work. For example, we talked about being "on the front lines" despite, previously at least, minimal risk of personal danger. We argued with our funders about equipping us for the "war on disease," while realizing we were probably laying it on a bit thick. But in 2020 – *a year that shall live in infamy* – when it came to combating the COVID pandemic, the analogy of "total war" finally seemed fit-for-task. Moreover, politicians used the same language, and for the best part of 2 years, just like in war time, activities were cancelled unless vital to the "war effort." Finally, everyone knew why my "industry," namely, intensive care medicine, mattered. Heck, even my opinion was sought after, and for a brief period I was invited onto TV and radio in order to share what it was like to be enrolled "in the unit."

As numbers increased, like you, we health care workers were scared. After all, we were preparing to "go over the top." Like many elderly people, we health care workers presumed that we were considered expendable. We suspected – and were often right – that our needs would be given little more than lip service from administrators, who remained far from the "action." Similarly, the relationship with administrators and politicians felt like "command and control" rather than engagement and empowerment. Heck, it felt like a full-time job just keeping up with all of those two-page emails, ever-changing protocols, and seemingly contradictory edicts.

Meanwhile, at the bedside, at least we had each other's backs. I mean this statement both literally and figuratively, given the need to "buddy-check" gowns and protective equipment. Hyperbole aside, I was never prouder of our staff and prouder to do this job. Moaning was replaced, at least temporarily, with meaning, and many of us were surprisingly happy not being "resigned to barracks." We discovered a lot about our comrades, and we were reassured that most ran in and few ran away. We had a renewed sense of purpose and saw each other's strengths. This unity was in contrast to more placid circumstances, when for reasons that now seem inexplicable, we constantly found ways to find fault or take umbrage. It was strangely liberating to focus on the bedside job and nothing else. Fake bravado notwithstanding, we were up for this challenge.

Humour and common sense returned to institutions that were previously – in my opinion at least – held back by excessive political correctness and bureaucracy. Regardless, my heroes were not doctors or nurses or administrators but rather those in the "logistics corps." I am talking about those who swept floors, made sandwiches, served coffee, directed pages, and brought in supplies. After all, we health care workers were the regular troops who had signed up willingly for this "fight" years ago. These other members of the battle group might have been less eager conscripts, but there is no doubt that they were (and always will be) vital to morale. We worked hard to give these colleagues a smile and to regularly ask them (albeit from a distance of 2 metres*) how they were faring. Many of these everyday heroes looked scared, so we tried harder to make them feel visible. I rapidly learned names and looked forward to offering grateful hugs the second this "battle" was over.

If years of reading military history taught me anything, it is that battle plans rarely survive contact with the enemy and that combat travels with denial and propaganda. We spent an inordinate amount of time dealing with virus deniers (the so-called COV-IDiots) who believed this fight was a phoney war and that the vaccines (when they arrived truly in the nick of time) were the problem, not the solution. I was (and remain) a huge vaccine proponent, but I always struggled with the lockdown. However, it is worth remembering that the predictions were that COVID could kill 2 per cent of all those it infects and that it was expected (in the pre-vaccine days) to infect at least 50 per cent of the population. In other words, we can look back with the retrospecto-scope, but there was every likelihood that it would be horrible: mathematically, economically, socially, and medically. I would use the term "unprecedented," but that word became so hackneyed during the pandemic.

The "bulldog spirit" of health care workers, and in fact all workers, was massively challenged by the expectation of ventilating hundreds, of staff falling ill and dying, and because of the constant fear of taking this infection home to loved ones. Just like any war, this one would ultimately be won or lost on the home front, so it was important to engage the public. We were already low on blood, so we pleaded for donations; and food shelves were at risk of emptying, so we begged the public not to hoard. We asked people to be patient with the blood banks when

---

* 6.6 feet.

depositing and with the food banks when withdrawing. We all needed to find a way to pull together, even while being physically ordered apart. This battle was also social media's first war. We needed to learn when to tune in because we craved information and connection but to power down before we all lost our minds to information overload.

Those who have seen actual military service were quick to remind us not to panic, to slow down, and to prepare for a long campaign. Similarly, we needed to unleash the incredible creativity and tenacity that exists throughout society and to explain that these characteristics were definitely not the sole preserve of doctors and nurses. Engineers and truckers and bus drivers played a huge part. It was important to me that society did not divide into health care workers and others. Instead, the better distinction was between those who found a way to help and those who found a way to complain or obstruct. We all had a part to play. In this regard, it was comparatively easy being a doctor: I just kept doing what we were trained to do.

Emotions spread like viruses, so we asked the public to keep a check on theirs. On a more personal level, sometimes I succeeded, and sometimes I failed. For example, I was livid the day I discovered that hand sanitizer had been ripped off the hospital walls and masks had been stolen by the public. In keeping with the war theme, a colleague of mine suggested it was like guns being taken away from soldiers by the very people expecting to be defended. We pleaded with people to stop doing this STAT.

Ultimately, the COVID battle was to regain the simple pleasures of life rather than to collect medals or glory. It was and is the chance to become a better or worse version of ourselves. There were many lessons to be learned, and each of us had this time of relative shutdown to listen to greater and lesser degrees. For example, we learned that the economy matters, but it is not all that matters. We were reminded that we are all vulnerable, and none of us is truly a nihilist or an island. I am more convinced than ever that life always has something to teach, and the offer of a cup of tea is always a good idea.

We health care workers were scared, but we were also lucky. We had the chance to relearn that human contact is lovely, that caring for others matters, and that finding humour in the everyday is glorious. These things should never have been previously taken for granted, and your doctors and nurses were as guilty as anyone. Hyperbole and overstretched metaphors aside, it was a war worth fighting and one that might one day be seen as our finest hour. Like you, we didn't want this war, but we were ready, willing, and able. I look forward to one day telling my grandkids.

27 Seven Days in the ICU

Laura A. Hawryluck, MSc, MD, FRCPC
Professor, Critical Care Medicine, University of Toronto

Submitted 19 May 2022

I have fractured memories of my initial contacts with doctors as a child. I remember the waiting rooms and the toys – and Mom warning me not to touch them. I remember the defining moments of the cold of undressing, the crinkly uncomfortable paper of the examining tables. I remember the otoscope looking into my ears and sticking my tongue out solely to be forced to gag on the tongue depressor. I remember the vaccines. And I remember the fear of the needle. Yet what I also remember even more vividly is, when tearful, being handed a stethoscope, the earpieces oh-so-carefully-placed, and being told, "Shhh… listen." And hearing the sheer magic of my heart beating, of my breathing for the first time. As I was born with some orthopaedic issues, I remember having to wear leg braces that constantly needed adjusting as I grew, the mocking of other children, my absolute hatred of the special shoes I had to wear. Yet maybe it was because of this mockery that, from an early age, I refused to let any health issue define me, refused to let them limit me. I always had an overwhelming curiosity and a deep-seated need to explore the Canadian woods, the lakes, and the mountains – a *need* to see what was around the next bend in any trail. I remember how the doctors, picking up on my natural curiosity – likely, in part, due to my not-so-subtle barrage of "why?" "why?" – would go out of their way to explain, to show, to teach, a lot of their patience aimed at decreasing my fears. I remember them talking with me about not letting the comments of others ever define who I was, that I was the only one who could ever do that. I remember them telling me at each visit, "One day, *you* will *be* a Doctor." I started medical school at 18 years old.

I wanted to help people heal, and perhaps even more subconsciously, I wanted to help them be less afraid when facing any health issues.

Maybe all this is what ultimately drew me to treating life-threatening illnesses and to one of the newest and scariest fields of medicine: critical care. I finished my training to become an intensivist at 27 years old.

> In the span of 7 days I live many lives,
> As lines etched across hands join and entwine,
> With mine.
> Intimate short stories, complex chapters, though sometimes just significant verse;
> Sometimes for better,
> Too often for worse;
> As lines etched across hands join and entwine,
> With mine.
> What will fortune's teller make
> Of all the lines so gently layered in time;
> Of that ever important life line,
> Altered now and poorly defined?

The intensive care unit (ICU) is a very intimidating place – from all the machines and constant alarms, to the aggressiveness of the treatments, to the realization that sudden life-threatening illness may unexpectedly rob us of the ones we love and all that we care the most about in life. One of the most important parts of working in the ICU is understanding who we are treating, who their family is, and their inter-relationships – both to understand what matters to them, what it means for them to live, how medical science can help them, and crucially, how to help them navigate the fears of the uncertainties and unknowns. This all-important understanding is gained, as so many things are, through stories. The stories shared are often those of the moments that stand out to others, those that, in the collage of a life lived, resonate in that they, in some uniquely personal way, define who we are and what we believe in. Life-threatening illnesses have a way of quickly stripping life down to what is crucially significant for any one of us. For the ICU team, the stories shared can make us laugh, make us cry, make us understand what love and courage truly are, and can make us want to fight for justice within the health care and/or broader social systems. The range and depth of vulnerabilities exposed – the what ifs, the regrets, the fears – are rarely known by many others in any person's life, even within a family or among those who may have been friends for years. It is in the stories that the bonds between the patient, family, and ICU team are forged, wherein another less well-appreciated aspect of the intensity of care within the ICU is created. The stories give us the drive and strength to continue forward. The stories are never forgotten. For it is in these stories that our humanity lives within the stark, sterile, harsh physical spaces and aggressive treatments that are otherwise far from humane.

> In the span of 7 days I live many lives;
> Whether happy or sad;
> Whether with or without;
> Whether in or out of love;
> Torn asunder,
> With the flash of lightening and the roar of thunder.

Typically, in the ICU we work a week of 7 days and 7 nights. The intensity of what we live through with the people who need our help, with their families, with their stories is such that 7 days and nights are normally the most we can work in a manner that lets us be truly present in the ways needed to provide the care our patients and families deserve. In this span of time, we can live many lives indeed, as their stories become entwined with ours. Even after the week of call is over, the stories remain, sometimes to be resumed after only a short break in on-call schedules when we pick up the ICU once again. Sometimes the stories disappear into the ether, needing to be tracked down so that their end, at least that of the ICU part, is understood and either celebrated, mourned, or to be continued with the hopes of the ICU team that their future will indeed be better. Sometimes people return to see us once they are able. More often though, the most important part of the stories' endings cannot be known, and the uncertainty of whether we have been able to help or not remains forever shrouded. Still the stories are not forgotten.

> So many lines, so tangled and confused.
> Can any be rejoined – even fused?
> And if… if… repaired once again,
> What will fortune's teller now make
> Of the paths these delicately etched lines take?
> Of the strength of the mend;
> If… well… what then?
> Will the story resume?
> Or, will history subsume…

When the COVID-19 pandemic really hit the ICU, there were so many people sick, so many who couldn't breathe – people who came with massive heart attacks, massive strokes. The ICU teams were overwhelmed by the sheer number, yes, but more by the sheer magnitude of suffering, the sheer severity and spectrum of its destruction. The horrors of seeing people not being able to breathe unless deeply sedated, pharmacologically paralysed, and proned are impossible to un-see. And even then, still the desperate fight for every breath to be able to get enough oxygen in for them to stand a chance to survive. The worldwide medication shortages to take away the struggle to breathe followed, as did shortages of those needed for us to assume control of their breathing with our machines. The shortages extended even to a lack of oxygen, the most fundamental treatment in all of medicine in some settings. The need to expand the ICU team's abilities to care resulted in fewer staff for more patients, resulted in newly redeployed physician and nursing staff joining the ICU team – all with varying strengths and skills. Yet still the need seemed never ending. ICUs surged into spaces we were never designed to be in, posing their own set of challenges as spaces were transformed to meet our most essential needs. Equipment needs soared, and machines were redeployed from wherever they could be grabbed. Day became indistinguishable from day, night from night, week from week. The ICU teams would move from one person to another to tend to their needs, to deal with their crisis, to try to stop them crashing through all the efforts being made to keep them alive. Life too often reduced to a minute-by-minute struggle, while the ICU team held its own breath to see if what was being tried would finally work… just a little… please… just a little. Something, anything in the right direction, the thinnest threads of progress brought hope, and hope mattered so much to all of us. Yet the uncertainties of what survival would look like remained. The certainty that life would be altered, sometimes forever, was often far too clear. Yet there was not enough time to do more than try to keep people alive. The hours were long, very long. The efforts were sustained, without any periods of slowing of activities during which ICU teams usually recharged. It was exhausting. And still the losses were heartbreakingly high.

For the first time ever, no visitors were allowed in the ICU – this measure because of infection control policies to reduce the risk of spread and because many of the patients' family members were themselves sick with COVID, some also in hospital or even in the ICU. The memories of those video calls, the words "I love you," the last ones before someone was intubated, their knowledge that it may be the last time ever to speak, will haunt us all for the rest of our lives. Words heard so many times as the whole ICU and anesthesia teams prepped the medications needed to sedate and intubate, discussed the plans to get life support started, and then waited, spectators to most intimate words said and moments lived, all the while hawkishly watching oxygen saturation levels, all the while being briefed on problems with others in need, before swooping in and around to seize as much control as possible of the brain, heart, lungs, and body. A short phone call to the family would follow to say it went "well." Video calls would be set up by the nurses for families to speak to their heavily sedated loved one – often to the back of their head as they lay proned, the ventilator, infusion pumps, and beeping monitors more visible than the person they love. These calls were monitored so that, at their end, the equipment could be cleaned and moved to the next patient. Brief status updates were given by overstretched bedside nurses, working long overtime hours, caring for multiple *sick* patients. Doctors would only have time to reach out during usual hours with bad news or when gut-wrenching, tough decisions needed to be made. Otherwise, short calls would be made in the evening, answered by families, voices caught in their throats in fear over what the updates may hold, what the doctor would say, and what was left unsaid. Fear was always thick in the air and could not be alleviated, no matter the message. The cycle repeated. And for the first time, the stories stopped.

> If there are no more stories here,
> Not even those over which to weep,
> There are no more secrets to keep.
> If life is reduced to tasks,
> It is such a simple ask;
> If... well... no longer a doctor, simply a shell,
> Who can hear her own echoing death knell;
> With each and every wave,
> Less and less chance of her being saved.

During the worst of the "waves," the care in the ICU became robotic and task-oriented in an increasingly noisy, sterile environment inhabited by high efficiency particulate air (HEPA) filters and strangers difficult to identify, never mind hear, under layers of personal protective equipment (PPE), and with even more alarms going off than usual. We experienced so many deaths in such a short period of time. We had no specific treatments to turn anyone around. We had no real chance at all to get to know the people we were trying to help. Nor could we get to know and help support their families; we could often do nothing to allay their fears. Over and over, we could only clutch the phone while they cried. We were offered psychological support, wellness programs. We were offered help communicating and connecting with families, creating even more distance between the who and the what/how of treatments. These attempts to help us fundamentally failed because they did nothing to address the sense of profound loss of who we were, a sense that necessity and exhaustion had robbed us of our abilities to provide the depth of care we so valued. At its worst, COVID robbed us of knowing the stories, even if painful, even if cut close to the bone, even if haunting, that teach us about what it *is* to *live* and that therefore sustain us. For so many of us, it was ultimately not the exhaustion nor the long hours that vanquished our ability to go on, that resulted in our own struggles for resilience; it was the descent into the robotic, the perception – real or not – of the loss of our own humanity.

The ICU is a field of intensity in so many ways, in treatments, in its search to push the boundaries of medical science, and in its quest to understand who we are treating and how we can help. The intensity is always focused outward to those who need us. Inadvertently, what the COVID pandemic has brought to the ICU is an appreciation of who we really are, what matters to us, and an understanding of the humanity that we seek to give to our brutally austere spaces and equipment. It has taught us to *know* the value of the stories. For a field that is feared by those both within and outside of health care, that has seen itself publicly attacked for a perceived desire to "play God," for being impersonal and uncaring, a field that is deemed too powerful and often too expensive, this self-understanding and new-found clarity is a very unexpected and remarkable gift. It allows us to truly understand the need and develop the means to keep the stories alive, to stay connected to the most important aspect of who we are as professionals and, even more fundamentally, as people. Within the stories in which we live, even the ones that break our hearts, we can and will find the paths to heal ourselves, to train our future teams, and finally, we will find the ways in which to retain them so that we can all continue to still *be* right here for this ongoing pandemic and for any future crisis.

> Will the doctor in me prevail?
> Or will there be only echoes in an empty shell…
> As it shatters,
> And razor-sharp pieces scatter;
> As lines etched across hands join and entwine,
> With mine.
> What stories will be there then to tell…
> With every wave,
> Within the doctor is there a person left to save?

As I write this chapter, it's the start of a new year, and the Omicron variant is raging. Its stories – for the ICU – are as yet largely unknown.

Its anticipated impact has us receiving messages from our hospitals' leadership to prepare for Armageddon. It's a time full of threat for ongoing ICU team attrition and burnout, and yet it's also an opportunity for us to learn from our very recent past. Let us hope we can hear and heed what our own history has to teach us; let us hope we have reached a point of truly understanding who *we* are – for if not now, when?

> In the span of 7 days I live many lives,
> As lines etched across hands join and entwine,
> With mine.
> Intimate short stories, complex chapters, though sometimes just significant verse;
> Sometimes for better,
> Too often for worse;
> As lines etched across hands join and entwine,
> With mine.
> What will fortune's teller make
> Of all the lines so gently layered in time;
> Of that ever important life line,
> Altered now and poorly defined?
>
> In the span of 7 days I live many lives;
> Whether happy or sad;
> Whether with or without;
> Whether in or out of love;
> Torn asunder,
> With the flash of lightening and the roar of thunder.
>
> So many lines, so tangled and confused.
> Can any be rejoined – even fused?
> And if… if… repaired once again,
> What will fortune's teller now make
> Of the paths these delicately etched lines take?
> Of the strength of the mend;
> If…. well… what then?
> Will the story resume?
> Or will history subsume…
>
> If there are no more stories here,
> Not even those over which to weep,
> There are no more secrets to keep.
> If life is reduced to tasks,
> It is such a simple ask;

If... well... no longer a doctor, simply a shell,
Who can hear her own echoing death knell;
With each and every wave,
Less and less chance of her being saved.

Will the doctor in me prevail?
Or will there be only echoes in an empty shell...
As it shatters,
And razor-sharp pieces scatter;
As lines etched across hands join and entwine,
With mine.
What stories will be there then to tell...
With every wave,
Within the doctor is there a person left to save?

28 The Pandemic Was a Powerful Teacher: Ramping Down Services

Fayez Quereshy, MD, MBA, FRCSC, FACS
Vice-President Clinical, Surgical Oncologist, and Minimally Invasive Surgeon, University Health Network, Toronto; Associate Professor, Department of Surgery, University of Toronto

Submitted 24 November 2022

It is too soon to know exactly how the pandemic has changed us. The truth is, we are still *in it*, and we may be for *quite some time*. Throughout the pandemic, the science of this deadly virus has revealed itself in small increments. In the beginning, we had challenges that were previously unencountered. Like many places around the world, the threat of limited hospital capacity and care providers, insufficient personal protective equipment (PPE), and constrained critical care resources were very real. With those factors weighing on us, coupled with the speed of the spreading contagion, the University Health Network (UHN), a quaternary care teaching hospital in Toronto, Canada, began planning to take dramatic measures to respond (*and brace ourselves*) for the unknown. The pandemic challenged us on several levels, with a burgeoning threat to the health system as well as to the personal safety of providers and their family members. Admittedly, what was most ominous is that *all of us* were vulnerable.

Perhaps even the most experienced leaders might have been stunned at the sheer pace of this global event and the complexity of the decisions we were being faced with. At the time, I was only a few months into the role of clinical vice-president when the World Health Organization declared COVID-19 a global pandemic. The learning curve was dramatic as I unlocked parts of the organization while still evolving in my own leadership style and understanding of health care management.

As a surgeon, I find joy in unravelling complex problems and working with teams to come up with creative solutions. The more challenging the scenario, the more it fuels my drive to find an answer. But I have to confess, the early days of Wave 1, where uncertainty was rampant and the fear of the unknown unprecedented, were a serious test of my inherent optimism.

We had to balance risks and benefits, stewardship of all our resources, efficiency and equity, all while keeping the well-being of patients at the heart of everything we do.

As we pivoted from "regular business" into full planning mode, while balancing the impact to patients awaiting intervention with those urgently and emergently seeking care, we also had to contend with the fear and anxiety of our health care teams and providers. People were scared for themselves and their families. Naturally, there were many impassioned conversations, as all of us wanted to ensure we did everything we could to protect our teams and our patients.

Maybe it's the surgeon in me, as I have been trained to focus on the immediate, to manage any range of consequences, including resuscitating the patient in front of me. My surgical training prepared me for managing uncertain moments and doing whatever is needed, even with limited information. In a strange way, I was as ready for this challenge as I could be, from a clinician and leadership point of view.

Ultimately, I wasn't scared to make imperfect decisions, knowing we might be wrong sometimes. The personal fear that was a constant companion was based in the worry for my wife's safety, working in the intensive care unit (ICU) as an anesthesiologist, and great concern for my father, who had significant health concerns that could have worsened at any time.

At the start, what we knew about the virus was changing almost daily – in fact, what we knew was eclipsed by what we were learning. And in the space between those two realities, fear grew. Every patient coming to UHN was treated as if they were a potential positive case, and risk assessment became extremely important. We very quickly mobilized and established a Personal Protective Equipment Committee, knowing that, regardless of how many positive patients appeared on our doorstep, we had a duty to protect our teams and our patients. The committee was instrumental in creating policies, processes, and education that were pivotal to ensuring the safety of UHN staff and patients throughout the pandemic; now, 2 years later, this team has set the course for new and innovative ways to manage PPE supplies and use at UHN and across the province.

We very quickly took a leadership position beyond our network. We felt confident we could, and should, support the broader definition of the public health benefit. I was rooted in the moral compass of doing the best for all our patients, inside UHN and outside. We are so used to thinking of the patient immediately in our orbit, but we now needed to look past our hospitals. This outreach was a new challenge for every single one of us, and it was OK to be vulnerable and say, "I don't know the answers; I don't know what's next."

One thing I believe we did effectively was to ensure a diversity of voices were heard around the leadership tables. We listened to a range of questions from all different parts of the network, elicited great feedback, and employed important learnings that everyone could benefit from. I believe we gave confidence to our teams that they weren't alone and that we would see this difficult time through together. I was a new leader, but I didn't look at any of my colleagues any differently than ever before. Leadership is not vertical for me; input from colleagues was critical, and we are lucky at UHN to have so many wise leaders with deep experience managing complex challenges.

We then very quickly started discussions about how we would augment our physical capacity, manage our human resources, and critically, how we would keep everyone safe. I was tasked with leading UHN's clinical ramp-down strategy in response to a provincial mandate "pausing scheduled care." In March 2020, I sat in a room with some of the most capable leaders in the organization, and we created a plan that would reduce our surgical and procedural services and outpatient clinical by 75 per cent overnight. There were three reasons why we needed to ramp down at that point: to make space for potential patients coming in, to decrease foot traffic in order to reduce possible exposure, and to safeguard our supply of PPE.

The weight of the conversation and the decisions was palpable to everyone in the room. We had a responsibility to ensure we kept our patients and staff safe. We also recognized our role of being strong public health partners with neighbouring institutions and the need to create capacity for the expected tide of patients who were not yet in the system. Ironically, when many decisions were first made, the case counts were less than 100 in Ontario, a number to be eclipsed in weeks and months to come. While we were initially faced with small volumes, we were epidemiologically bracing for something much greater. It was a painful paradox for everyone involved – creating capacity for *"what may come"* while pausing on care *"for those already waiting."*

Naively, when this pandemic started and we made the decision to draw down our services, I thought we were talking a month, maybe the summer at the latest. We truly thought the pandemic would be short lived and contained, and many of us were working with assumptions based on our experience with severe acute respiratory syndrome (SARS). We did not imagine it could go on this long.

Even as I sit here now, just past our third-year anniversary, we still haven't fully quantified the magnitude of the impact on population health, people who have deferred regular check-ups, people with disease who lost mobility, suffered decreased quality of life, and disease progression. It'll take up to a decade to realize what has happened. Three years later and it's kind of scary; what the pandemic has revealed is a deficiency in health human resources, physical capacity, and the use of leveraging technology.

In the summer, we then optimistically began increasing our services with the expectation that adherence to public health measures would shield us from the "worst case scenario" modelled by national and provincial experts. In an environment with limited resources, in the absence of provincial direction, how would UHN prioritize who needs urgent care and who can delay their procedures or use different kinds of treatments? And how do you do it in a compassionate and equitable way? With the input of an interdisciplinary team, UHN's ramp-down plan morphed into UHN's clinical activity calibration road map that allowed us to enable a safe, ethical, measured approach to increasing and decreasing scheduled surgical, procedural, and outpatient activity throughout the pandemic.

We took a system-wide lens and asked ourselves, "Where does UHN fit as we make these decisions?" If we were the exclusive provider of some kind of treatment or if the illness severity compromised life and limb, then that, of course, took priority. We were very good at life-saving procedures. However, for those with functional disability, their quality of life was necessarily deferred. It is not lost on me that these people greatly suffered, and continue to do so, as our backlog is still sitting at 3000. Living in a country like Canada, with publicly funded health care, we shouldn't have to have cancer in order to receive treatment.

This plan was used as an organization-wide guide for balancing available space and resources to enable UHN to provide routine care, provide care to patients in the backlog, protect regional and priority programs, and respond to the pandemic.

Every time we had to make the decision to decrease scheduled care, it was distressing to all of us, and especially to my fellow clinicians who had patients that could be negatively impacted by our decisions for the presumed "greater good." There is no doubt there were some people who became sicker because of the need to delay or defer their care. I remember waking up on more than one night fearful for the impact of our decisions – for my patients and those of my colleagues.

Ultimately, it was a fine balance of providing care for an individual patient versus being stewards of public health resources for the entire system. While we often talk about managing resources as a part of our training, known as the Royal College of Physicians and Surgeons of Canada's CanMed core competencies, never have the resource constraints been of such a magnitude that required seemingly impossible choices.

As we tell stories about the pandemic, it is important to acknowledge that everyone has grieved some kind of loss during the pandemic: a loved one, a job, a routine, human connection, life celebrations, and everything in between. However, the optimist in me, and the leader who witnessed so many extraordinary victories in the face of extreme obstacles, believes the pandemic has been a powerful teacher. We have seen how quickly we can navigate change inside our own hospitals – in many instances overnight. We have seen how breaking down historic barriers between institutions can lead to increased access to care and to innovations that ultimately result in better care for patients and improved environments for care providers.

What I often think about, and am in great awe of, is how uniformly understanding patients were – not one individual refused to accept the decision to reschedule their surgery, citing a recognition that others needed the resource. Human beings' capacity for psychological resilience and adaptability is more remarkable than we think. I personally have leaned hard on my faith to keep moving through it – faith in my family, my colleagues, and in my religion. This faith has allowed me to see many pandemic silver linings, but I know it is not the case for everyone. As we move forward, we have to acknowledge the painful sacrifices made by patients, care providers, and more broadly, the citizens of Ontario throughout the pandemic.

Anyone waiting for surgery might find it difficult to understand or accept how we balanced the resources we had to care for patients. From the outside looking in, it may seem as though we wrongly prioritized one patient group over another. I fully acknowledge that challenging decisions, with incomplete (and rapidly evolving) information, are rarely perfect. Hindsight is 20/20, but what I do know is that patients remained at the heart of every decision we made. Putting the needs of the patients first implies creating new models of care and leveraging technology to reach our patients both in person and virtually, and we did just that to provide access to care to as many patients as possible in a time of great resource constraint. We had to ask our health care providers to work in ways that were not optimal. I could not be more proud of, and inspired by, UHN team members who courageously show up every day to serve patients, families, and communities in the face of what feels like insurmountable challenges.

One very important learning shined a light on what we could do better, and that was in the area of communication. If I could do things differently, I would certainly make sure I was visiting units and seeing people more. We made the decision to discourage too much foot traffic in our buildings as a necessary precaution, but over time, it became visible how much our people needed to be seen and given the opportunity to share their experiences.

The pandemic continues to challenge us at every turn. Most of us have never had to deal with uncertainty on this scale before. Looking back on the last 2 years, we all learned a sense of permanent uncertainty, which, while challenging in the moment, brings us closer to realizing that life always entails some measure of risk. Ultimately, the next challenge is to learn to coexist with risk rather than to eliminate it.

We are by no means at the end. There will be new challenges related to the pandemic that will require ongoing collaboration and cooperation from the health system and the public. There are about a million patients awaiting surgical and procedural care in Ontario. The health care workers who have dedicated their professional lives to caring for Ontarians are burning out at a rapid pace, and the pandemic exacerbated the severe shortage of trained health care professionals and physical capacity across the province.

In the context of these complex issues that face health care leaders in the years to come, I remind myself of how well we were able to come to consensus on principles and coordinate a strategy in the face of uncertainty. What we have learned from the last 2 years might just allow us to transform a system that was in desperate need of fixing *if we all work at it together.*

I am proud to be part of the team that led this world-class hospital through a once-in-a-generation health care emergency, and I will forever be inspired by the dedication, compassion, and poise of UHN team members.

# 29 COVID-19 Seen from a Preventionist Physician's Point of View: Will We Be Able to Draw Lessons for the Future?

Jean Ralph Zahar, MD, PhD
Professor, Infection Control Unit, Microbiology Department, Assistance Publique, Hôpitaux de Paris, France

Submitted 30 June 2022

Introduction

The COVID-19 pandemic, which has already lasted 2 years with many waves and twists, has exposed us to many reflections and contradictions, both at personal and collective levels. It is obvious that a historical episode of this magnitude requires a freeze frame in order to draw conclusions that will help future generations.

Without wishing to deny or minimize the mobilization of nursing staff and all the efforts and good will that animated this period, my critical look aims at leaving a reflection for future generations. I hope that it will be useful to them in order to build and elaborate an approach that will avoid the "mistakes" or, better still, the "hesitations" that we experienced during this period.

The objective of these few lines is to evoke all the problems encountered during the pandemic as a man, a citizen, a physician (that is, as part of a body of health care workers), and a preventionist (a physician whose objective is to protect first the patients, then the health care workers, and finally, the institution). It seems important to me to describe my experience as an infectious disease prevention risk manager in a French hospital that has served one of the populations most affected by this pandemic phenomenon.

The Pandemic, a Great Period of Solidarity and Opportunity

It is important to underline that this exceptional period was the origin of an immeasurable surge of generosity – not only between different professions within the hospital structure but also between generations on the scale of entire populations and, further, on a worldwide basis. It is important to highlight the investment of companies, families, and individuals fighting against this pandemic. From a scientific point of view, the almost instantaneous exchange of information allowed not only the advancement of research but also, and above all, the improvement of daily patient care.

Never in my 30-year career have I experienced such a supportive and fascinating moment, both humanly and scientifically. While my teachers had taught me the rule of Saint Benedict, "Never go to bed without having learned something new," it had never made so much sense as it has during these 15 months and now. Scientific articles and textbooks have been scrutinized, read extensively by all members of the team with a single goal: to understand this virus – this pandemic – better and faster for the sole interest of the patient.

While this period was very rich, it was also full of contradictions, hesitations, and fears. Sometimes, it led us to make questionable decisions, both on individual and collective levels. In my opinion, it seems essential to highlight all the questions, doubts, and interrogations that a certain number of us have gone through, while keeping in mind the stakes in the profession I practise.

Nothing Before: No Problem, It Won't Happen to Us

One of the first questions this pandemic raised was our lack of preparation. Even though my generation had lived through the H1N1 flu episode, and we had previously worked at the local, regional, and national levels on various pandemic control plans, our level of unreadiness for an event of this magnitude was glaring.

It is obviously difficult to master all aspects of this pandemic. However, I was nevertheless surprised by the "cognitive bias," which consisted of denying the phenomenon as long as we were not directly concerned. Indeed, although the occurrence of an emerging disease in Asia had been acknowledged at the national and local level since mid to late December 2019, we can underline a noticeable denial of the problem, characterized by the positions taken by many decision-makers and colleagues in the media, who suggested the absence of risk in France. As expected, this stance has resulted at the local level in a lack of will to anticipate the risk. Thus, and despite numerous requests, we have not noted any willingness to provide information and training within our establishments.

But beyond the lack of preparation at the national level, I was strongly struck by the determination, sometimes fierce, of many colleagues to deny traditional knowledge concerning the modes of transmission, control, and treatment of viral infections. Colleagues rejected previous findings based on a partially true principle that SARS-CoV-2 (COVID-19) was different from all other viruses. In addition to this rejection, we believed that what our scientific predecessors had demonstrated and proposed was not applicable to the present situation. I have wondered all this time, and still do, about the sociological reasons for such an approach, which seems to start from a principle that I would summarize as follows: "Before me, there was nothing; the story begins now." How can we approach a situation such as this one without taking into account the past, even if the latter certainly could not provide all the answers?

Thus, the exclusion of past knowledge and experience, and the refusal of training and information, have led to a certain delay in the preparation of health care workers. Many of them with insufficient knowledge about infection prevention found themselves infected at the beginning of the epidemic. It took alerts not only from national surveillance structures but also from ministerial authorities for the medical and paramedical profession to accept the idea of training. Unfortunately, it was probably already too late due to the acceleration of the pandemic and the large number of patients under care, which made training more difficult and less efficient.

Reducing Risk and Accepting a Degree of Error versus "Zero" Risk

While some of us were trying to propose feasible applicable measures to control the risk of infection based on previous literature data, we have seen an overkill of prevention means motivated by fear and by ignorance of the specific consequences linked to "this" virus. I do not wish to polemicize here – nor to question the measures taken in terms of prevention or to criticize the need to put in place exceptional measures. I would like to consider the necessity for any decision-maker, especially as a scientist (I draw a distinction here from a politician), to base reflection on already known and proven scientific data. Indeed, I was hit by the initial discussions about the prevention measures to be implemented.

These initial discussions totally occulted past scientific data, whether they concerned viruses in general or the coronavirus. From these discussions, preventive measures were taken that could have exposed (in fact, did expose) patients and families to a higher risk of infection. Moreover, these preventive measures were the origin of dithering and contradictions, and especially heterogeneity of practices, and therefore created doubts as to their effectiveness among both the public and the health care system throughout the pandemic. That was the case, for example, in making recommendations for the type of mask, for the level of individual protection, and for air treatment of hospitalized patients' rooms, to name but a few points of contention.

The justified fear of the virus, its specificities, and the characteristics of our society, which refuses all uncertainties, led to the belief that there was a possibility of "zero" COVID, leading to excessive measures and misunderstandings.

Throughout the pandemic, we have experienced a contradictory debate, unfortunately often announced and relayed by the media, on the modes of transmission and the means of prevention. Fear and the lack of knowledge of historical data relating to different pandemics have accentuated a phenomenon of non-confidence among health care providers and the population. Moreover, our field recommendations based on scientific data, clinical common sense, and adapted to the specific working conditions were constantly contradicted by the recommendations of multiple learned societies (each one had issued its own recommendations) and various ministries (health, labour, and others). All these contradictions were "acclaimed" in the media with a volatility similar to the stock market during the Wall Street crash of 1930.

Communication, Social Networks, and Immediacy

As pointed out above, I was, on the one hand, pleasantly amazed by the accessibility of medical information and its immediacy but, on the other hand, unpleasantly astonished not only by the lack of control over medical information and misinformation but especially by the vehicles disseminating this information. Throughout the pandemic, the "scoop phenomenon" dominated, and a certain amount of information was first announced in the media and social networks before it was scientifically validated. I don't know how it happened in other countries, but in France we were overwhelmed by "experts."

How could I not mention the heavy influence of the media and social networks during this crisis; how could I not mention our "EGO"? It has made many of us (including me) rush to give our "expert" point of view without contradiction, to publish our small study without verification of data, leaving the field free for media and social networks to muse about and expound on both right and false interpretations. Results and comments were then disseminated through social media and taken up by health care workers (both paramedical and medical) as scientific truths, which could be used to oppose any "reasonable" proposal, without any validation by journalists and/or hosts of the various television news programs. Reflecting on this issue seems essential to me in order to make it clear that we "health care workers" are inseparable members of the society and that our words and actions, which until now have only had a local and limited impact, are being amplified by these 24/7 information channels.

The rapid display, almost instantaneous, of the results of studies (not yet published and therefore not validated by our peers) has made understanding the COVID phenomena more complex, even prolonging doubts and accentuating hesitations.

All in all, although this period was rich in publications, whatever the type of activity, it was especially striking in impeding the field of prevention from noting some disturbing elements.

The Homogeneity of Measures, the Policy of Searching and Isolating

A disturbing phenomenon probably linked to social media was the homogeneity of prevention measures throughout the world. With no intent to criticize the measures taken, I was surprised when I visited my home country (Lebanon) in the middle of the pandemic to see that, despite the economic and political crisis and financial difficulties, the governmental recommendations were strictly identical to those of high-income countries; that was also the case for many low- and middle-income countries. Not that we had to do things differently or that these populations did not deserve the equivalent of what was being done elsewhere, but I wondered about the effect of media coverage on government decisions. Indeed, did the decision-makers have the choice to consider their local problems and to adapt their policies to their specific conditions, either economic, social, or religious? Wouldn't such measures be the most effective? Wasn't there a media pressure, especially from social networks, that made some of us feel forced to do what was being done elsewhere to avoid any criticism and further judgment? How can we, in a world where information is instantly shared by all, make choices adapted to our specific situation?

Uncertainty and Fear Have at Times Led Us to Radical Measures without Any Discernment

Probably both fear and non-acceptance of uncertainty influenced Manichean decisions. I knew about fear in everyday life; it is a phenomenon that leads us to make unreasonable and sometimes unethical choices. But I could not imagine that fear would influence my professional activity and even less during a period of "war" (our president announced to the population at the beginning of the pandemic that we were at war). Indeed, thanks to my medical training (as an intensivist), I was used to overcoming fear, weighing pros and cons, and making decisions while taking the least risk for patients. This usual practice was not the case during the crisis.

I am not suggesting that decisions were made at the expense of patients, but our fear of being infected by the virus and our desire to protect ourselves sometimes led us to forget the meaning of our profession and, especially, its risks. Consequently, during the different phases of the pandemic, I asked myself the following questions:

- Were we right to isolate patients in negative pressure rooms and risk exposing them to other specific risks (such as isolation, failure to recognize they were getting sicker, failure to rescue them)?
- Were we right to protect ourselves from head to toe and risk forgetting the simple importance of hand hygiene and exposing patients to the risk of acquiring resistant bacteria and health care–associated infections?
- Were we right to interrupt visits, not accompany our dead, and even prohibit the presence of family at funerals and burials?

These topics have been on my mind throughout the pandemic because I came from the world of intensive care and had worked, throughout my initial training and my residency, to open up the intensive care wards to families. Indeed, I had started working in units limiting visits to 2 to 4 hours per day and had seen them evolve from closed services not welcoming families to totally open services, where families and sometimes friends were present, even in the most difficult moments of patient care. During the initial phase of the pandemic and up until now, we have forbidden visits, not only in the acute wards but also in the long-term care (LTC) facility and the intensive care unit (ICU). More surprisingly, a large number of us were not able to support the patients' relatives. What was "worst" for me was the refusal of some health care workers to take care of patients only because their nasopharyngeal test was positive, even when the patients were asymptomatic. This situation is still going on as I write these few lines.

At times, I did feel like a soldier going to war with the sole intention of protecting myself. I am probably exaggerating a bit, but I think it is important to highlight some facts that we will probably have to discuss again.

These Questions and Reflections Must Seek Answers

The question that has been in my mind since the end of the nth wave is to know why all these things happened. Indeed, I am among those who think that our problem was essentially sociological and that our refusal of uncertainty was one of the main elements in our decision-making. I don't know if the time for debate has come, but it seems important to me to rediscuss certain points linked to our decisions and to rethink with a clear mind our choices as a society.

In my opinion, two points in particular should be addressed:

- *The ethics of our profession and consequently our relations with the media and the importance of contradictory communication.* Indeed, I am afraid of the days that lie ahead with the prominence of "experts" who would be elected on multiple criteria but probably not based on competencies. The period we lived through was one of "experts" appointed only to tell us what we wanted to hear. Medicine is an inexact science – it makes us humble on a daily basis; it feeds on our doubts and uncertainties, and above all, on our rigour and our honesty towards our patients.
- *Training that would allow us to manage crisis situations.* In my opinion, training during "peacetime" to acquire skills that allow us to adapt to all crisis situations and to accept a possible margin of error in order to protect ourselves as best we can and not harm our patients is too often neglected.

If the points raised above seem negative, it is important to me to insist once again on how rich in learning this period was. On the human level, it was a moment of collaboration and exceptional solidarity (at least the first wave), which saw the bridging together of different scientific and health care workers from different hospitals, departments, and specialties.

But one question will persist in the upcoming months: How will we get out of this situation and move on with our lives while drawing conclusions from this event? Indeed, our policies have led the population to be tested at the slightest signs of infection, to isolate themselves and stop all activities in case of positivity, even in the absence of symptoms – all in a society that remains hyperconnected but distant and that is now exsanguinated.

Conclusion

The COVID crisis has shown the limits of the medicine we practise, but above all and especially, it has revealed a societal problem. Indeed, doubt does not seem to be tolerated by the population and even less so by the decision-makers. Many national and local recommendations have been based on the will to totally control the phenomenon (that is, to have "zero" COVID) at the expense of many other factors. The cost has been tremendous (the French government evokes the sum of 480 billion euros) without any time spent thinking of the future. The "whatever it takes" policy advocated by some people will probably have consequences in the short, medium, and long term, so the questions I am asking myself at the moment is how to get out of this situation and how to rebuild a risk management policy and a more reasonable health policy by accepting

- our limits (that is, the limits of medical science) in a world that has not and will not accept them;
- reduced means, but still maintaining quality medicine for all, which is crucial;
- a share of error to get out of a policy of "search and isolate" in order to develop a little more upstream prevention.

Could we have done things differently? If this COVID crisis allows us in the future to redefine our profession as one that avoids, or rather tries to avoid, illness and not one that cures/treats it and lengthens life, we will probably have drawn the right conclusions from an unprecedented and devastating crisis.

30 Treating the Unvaccinated During COVID-19: Did I Sign Up for This?

Peter G. Brindley, MD, FRCPC, FRCP
Professor of Critical Care Medicine, Adjunct Professor of Anesthesiology, Adjunct Professor, John Dossetor Health Ethics Centre, University of Alberta, Edmonton

Submitted 5 July 2022

People claim they want straight talk from their doctors, so here goes. The fourth – and subsequent – COVID-19 waves were largely a "pandemic of the unvaccinated" and courtesy of the unvaccinated. We finally had the vaccines, and so it didn't have to be this way. In brief, much of the 2021 COVID experience was because too many were obsessing over their rights, while they ignored their responsibilities: the other r-value, you might say. It is one thing to experience death as an intensive care unit (ICU) doctor, but it is quite another to experience so much unnecessary deaths and to be on the receiving end of so much anger.

The milk of health care kindness soured during COVID. It's because the science – and more about that abused term below – was not in doubt. The skating scores were in – no need to await the Russian judge. These vaccines were/are safe and effective, and you, the unvaccinated, were twenty times more likely to get COVID compared to the jabbed. Health care workers always cared – obviously we did – but those who did the right thing (rather than the "rights thing") did lose empathy and lost the ability to distinguish vaccine-hesitant from outright anti-vax. Loss of compassion, on both sides, was and is dangerous and may never return to baseline. Unfortunately, everyone suffers if we retreat into "us

---

This chapter is adapted from "Peter Brindley: An Open Letter to the Unvaccinated," published by the *BMJ Opinion* on 3 September 2021 © 2021 BMJ Publishing Group Ltd. All rights reserved.

and them." Many highlighted a pandemic of mental health, but I was similarly concerned about the r-value for selfishness, self-harm, and science-denial. A "don't-care strain" alongside the Delta strain.

The issue was not complicated. The goal was to get enough arms jabbed so that COVID would be more likely to downgrade from a crippling storm to a manageable swell. We would transition from pandemic to endemic, and while some would still get sick, the numbers would be fewer and the severity less. In other words, we had the power to save lives, economies, heck, even those overseas trips. That would have allowed us to more rapidly address everyone's battered sanity and the medical waitlist. Instead, it felt like some wanted to punch a hole in the life raft and have others do the bailing. If you don't care for maritime analogies, I can be blunter. Many of us underneath our personal protective equipment (PPE) just didn't get why others seemed hell-bent on giving us a belligerent middle finger and a stroppy f-you. We've performed mental gymnastics to understand where you were coming from, but we did not understand where you've ended up. Answers on a postcard, please. Alternatively, abuse us via Twitter (now X).

I've spent – maybe misspent – years bragging about where I live. I like Canadians because I am also a stubborn bugger and a big believer in liberty. In other words, I was no different from my patients in mindset, but the conclusions I reached were worlds apart. I support rights because I cherish them too. Again though, I accept that rights come with responsibilities – right? Moreover, I knew that people around here go to extraordinary lengths to help their neighbours, so this truculence made no sense. For 2 years, health care workers have not only worked our bums off but have tried to engage, persuade, plead, and, yes, even scare: because COVID was/is scary stuff. We did our compassionate best not to shame, but it didn't work.

This doctor tried not to claim any moral superiority. Eventually, we will review the ICU survival data, and I fear what we will find. COVID has been the most nihilistic ICU disease I have ever faced. Once we needed to wheel in the machines, the horses had often bolted, along with the patient's lungs. The goal is always to keep people out of the ICU because, once in, you may not come out. COVID was a stark reminder of why life support is called life support, not treatment. It maintains life but does not make you stronger. It reliably made our COVID patients weaker.

Trust me, COVID care in the ICU was not cool. It consisted of deep sedation, twiddling a few nobs, adjusting a few drugs, and managing all manner of excretions. We flipped patients on their front (aka proning) and tried plenty (likely too much) heart-lung bypass (aka ECMO).

However, we definitely did not sprinkle magic dust. Moreover, we failed to communicate that the patient's premorbid status was the more important factor in that they needed to have the "right" immune system: not too hot, not too cold. Sure, young fit people usually did better, but we could not always predict how long motors would last when pushed to the red line. We are all bookies, not prophets. Fortunately, there was always a great way to increase odds – follow science.

Too many people claimed to support science when what they were doing was scrambling for anything to support unsupportable beliefs. That was not science. I also witnessed too many reject science right up until they reached the hospital doors and then suddenly demand science STAT. After all, the same scientific method that made vaccines made the drugs and tubes and machines. I have always accepted the science of medicine (imperfect as it is) because I also accept the science of gravity (indisputable as it is). I don't pick and choose whether I believe in science based on tribal loyalty or the latest YouTube video.

Rather than put up with me spitting feathers, I'll end with the words of an ICU nurse. She said it best through tears, right as she threatened to quit: "I gave my all for 2 years ... Why didn't these people care about me or my little boy?" Sure, I'm tugging at heart strings, but that lovely boy was eleven and had significant health care issues. He couldn't get the vaccine at that time, and regardless, he might never mount a protective response. In other words, he needed the public to do him a solid and get the vaccine on his behalf. If so, then he was more likely to live, and his Mum was more likely to stay at work to help others. That and she could do what every parent must: protect their child. None of us are really heroes or villains; that language is overdone. During COVID, however, we all had an opportunity to make our corner of the world just a tad better. It still bothers me that not everybody did all they could.

31 Siloed Still ...

Laura A. Hawryluck, MSc, MD, FRCPC
Professor, Critical Care Medicine, University of Toronto

Submitted 27 September 2022

In Canada, many take pride in our health care system – the fact that it's universal, accessible to all at any time, integrated into their lives as a safety net, and "free" insomuch that our collective taxes cover its costs. Perhaps more than the system itself, it's the underpinning values that bind Canadians: protection of those made vulnerable by illness and knowing there will be health care teams who will help, people who, in their professional roles, will care for them when their personal integrity (physical or mental) is under threat, people who will simply be there in their times of need no matter who they are. Indeed, as any Canadian knows, the controversy over a public versus a public-private hybrid versus a private only model only engenders heated debate, the biggest concern being the maintenance of equity (not equality) and social justice in the provision of health care services. The Canadian health care system is not perfect; its challenges have been well described and include long waiting lists for investigations and surgeries, overcrowded emergency rooms, poor access to chronic care facilities, and so on. Yet, having travelled the world and been honoured to assist, work with, and consult on health care systems in many countries, I know that no system is perfect. All are, for the most part at least, striving to serve their people better within the means available to them. Yes, there are those who try to take advantage of current systems or propose system reforms for personal gain, be it financial or power in nature. In our world, there will seemingly always be such people. Yet there is advocacy from both within and without health care systems to try to prevent, curb, or reverse such reprehensible practices and to make health care access a foundational principle of international justice whereby everyone will know that they will/can receive timely quality health care in their times of illness and need. Such efforts continue every day to seek to improve health care systems in every country, through times of greater or lesser success. The COVID-19 pandemic has tested them all.

At the start of the pandemic, people around the world hailed health care workers as heroes and looked to their hospitals and health care systems to save them from the virus. There were clanging pots and pans, crowds clapping them in and clapping them home from work. People looked to public health professionals for guidance on how to stay safe, for how to protect those they loved. Initial recommendations included masks indoors, social distancing, and handwashing. Social distancing became physical distancing from each other, whether related or strangers. Then came washing and sterilizing of every and all deliveries. Then masks were everywhere. Then we had lockdowns and shuttering of businesses for extended periods, all in the name of "protecting" our health care systems – the health care systems that have always been meant to be at our service, not "protected" from us. For the first time, health care systems weren't "there"; they weren't in the background of our thoughts, the comforting safety net we rarely think about because the majority of us don't have to, for we rarely need such services. Now, for the first time, *everyone* was really asked directly for something – an ask *from* our health care system, a reversal of the natural order as it was. And the ask wasn't small. In return, information was confusing and sometimes contradictory without consistently clear public explanations of why it was changing, and changing rapidly. Even worse was the refusal of some to acknowledge emerging scientific knowledge and to accept that the new understanding meant changes in approaches were needed, and needed quickly. For the first time, innovative financial assistance programs were quickly assembled in Canada and other countries for those struggling to keep their businesses going, for those with reduced work hours, for those who were "temporarily" let go. Their success was variable, and many programs were heavily critiqued as insufficient and/or for lacking accountability without any grace accorded for these programs having never been required or instituted previously on such short notice and in such a widespread manner.

Hardships and financial ruin were felt by far too many people. Social inequities deepened still. Far too many had to go to work sick in order to be able to sustain their families. Far too many had to work in unsafe environments with no exploration or guidance of what would be required or any mandated requirements to make these workplaces safe, even when it became clear that the COVID-19 virus is airborne – meaning it is more infectious and can spread more widely than the initial presumption of droplet transmission. This new understanding was not acknowledged by many in public health or infection control for considerable time and is still not acknowledged by some – adding to the distrust. Far too many people were too afraid to come to the hospital to seek help, whether for COVID-19 or other illnesses. By the time they did, many went through much more than they would have if their illness had been caught earlier, and for many, it was too late.

Next came the development of vaccines, hailed as the next global saviours despite attempts to temper expectations by repeated messaging that their greatest impact was on severe illness and death (and now, recognition of a decrease in spread and protection against long COVID syndrome). Vaccines too had risks of complications. The perceived speed of their development was seen as a scientific success by some and viewed with deep suspicion and fear by others. Suspicion was compounded by medicine's past history of inflicting trauma by experimenting on marginalized peoples around the world. Strong polarization developed, and misinformation proliferated as people argued their viewpoints; a balanced perspective between the for and against vaccination groups became increasingly hard to find. Each viral surge, met with the same approach of restrictive health care measures, now worse for those who were not vaccinated, made the overall situation deteriorate even more. At times, there was simply no end in sight.

People were hailed as resilient despite research showing the significant impact of the pandemic on their mental health, feelings of isolation, loneliness, symptoms of depression, anxiety, and post-traumatic stress disorder. The concept of "resilience" became an ask through repeated lockdowns and restrictions. Resilience then became an obligation and an expectation. Who was making resilience an expectation? While resilience was a frequent request of politicians, they were making it clear that they were following advice and guidance from health care professionals. Health care systems were (still) being increasingly overwhelmed and had to be "protected." Protection now meant that access to services such as surgery needed to be triaged so as to try to save people in more urgent need, those with COVID-19 virus. People stayed away or could not get needed treatments from hospitals. They suffered more, and some died because they came in too late to be helped. Health care professionals went from heroes to being those responsible for all this suffering, to the shock of many who could not fathom why. Working in the intensive care unit (ICU), I have been constantly impressed by the resilience of people. Yet resilience is finite, and when requests for it are unreasonable, it is quickly exhausted. Then comes the backlash. This backlash was seen in countries around the world; for example, in Canada, it was seen in the so-called Freedom Movement and protests, in attacks on and refusal of public health mandates, and in social media attacks on health care professionals, even on those trying to provide balanced information. Perhaps most telling of all, it is now seen in the current celebration of the "end of the pandemic" by politicians, journalists, and the public, when the reality is that, as I write this chapter, the ravages of the pandemic are far from over.

What have all these experiences really taught us as health care professionals? What should our health care systems take away from all this polarization, the ripping apart of families, of society as we thought we knew it? The COVID-19 pandemic has revealed that health care, including public health, is far from being integrated in our society, is more siloed in ways that are important to societal health and well-being than perhaps any of us really understood.

Integrated health care systems would have acknowledged from the start that, while the goal was/remains to prevent as many people from getting sick as possible, to cure and to prevent as many deaths as possible, there were and are a lot of unknowns. What we needed and need to do will change until science can piece together the puzzle. There will be missteps needing to be corrected. Few health care professionals admitted/actually said "we don't know" to the public or to their own colleagues. Yet this response was (and, in some cases, still is) the most honest answer to many of the questions that arose. Most people can handle the fact that there are unknowns in life, especially around new emerging diseases; what they can't handle is being falsely reassured with unmerited overconfidence in the validity of such assurances. That is a lie. Lies quickly lead any rational person to distrust any current or future statements. And distrust undermines resilience.

Moreover, some challenges could have readily been predicted. These are/will be the trade-offs: challenges to global societal and individual mental health, financial losses, poverty, worsening addictions, further harms to vulnerable populations, rises in domestic and interpersonal violence, to name but a few. An integrated health care system would have understood and anticipated them. There could and should have been more planning so that these issues were better mitigated. Instead of only working internally on redeployment and wondering who could help *within*, there should have been an ask of how we could help *without*. An understanding of the anticipated trade-offs should have meant leadership from the health care system, from its hospitals in outreach – outreach to work with existing community groups tackling these challenges on a daily basis, such as long-term care facilities and children's aid societies, to promote greater safety, to develop/help man existing resources and shelters.

Integrated health care systems would have sought to use public health teams along with human factor teams to go into workplaces to provide guidance and advice suited to the particular work environment on how to keep people safe from illness. At the very least, such outreach should have been done for all workplaces considered essential during the government-imposed lockdowns. In Canada, a debate and pressure raged over the provision of paid sick leave. Yet, why do we have to accept such a low standard for a social safety net when we could have tried to form teams to really give people the best chance of not becoming ill and prevent the virus from spreading through families and societies? Surely such an approach could have been tried across industries (perhaps with greatest impact in factories/food processing industries that were hard hit) and, if successful, could have mitigated some of the mandatory shutdowns – perhaps not in the first wave but at least in subsequent ones. That public health was initially overwhelmed by efforts at contact tracing is the counter-argument. Yet, if we look at our society as a whole, we could have trained those on "temporary" employment leave to do contact tracing, thus giving them a source of income at the same time as support from other financial assistance programs.

Furthermore, people on "temporary" employment leave could have been trained to work in the hospital settings to alleviate overworked health care teams and/or to help health care teams focus on using the knowledge and skills that they had trained more extensively to acquire to help patients in need. For example, restaurants were very hard hit, and many never recovered. Many chefs and restaurants went out of their way to support health care teams by feeding them. Some were sponsored to do so, but many were not. Some health care teams came to view this kindness as an expectation, which was simply wrong. Instead, an integrated health care system could have sought to have and pay for a certain number of meals provided to patients and staff from local restaurants. Any one of us who has been in hospital would have welcomed such variety in food offerings. I am sure financial issues could have been worked out between current food services and such an alternative plan in the short term with sufficient cooperation within and between the health care system and government agencies. Personal trainers, athletic and physical therapists in gyms and clinics could have been recruited and paid to help sick patients in hospitals regain their strength, their ability to move, to walk. Such recruitment would have helped both overworked hospital-based physiotherapists and eased the burden on overworked nurses caring for so many patients yet still charged with facilitating and continuing patient physiotherapy once such plans had been developed.

Instead of triaging/shutting surgical services, alternative models of care could and arguably should have been developed. Innovations that arose from the COVID-19 pandemic included the development of mobile hospitals, some of which (for example, Fero International) permitted the provision of high-quality surgical and ICU services at lower costs than existing brick and mortar hospitals. Such models could have been used concurrently to mitigate the shutdown of surgical services and prevent the morbidity, mortality, and sheer backlog that we are currently facing in Canada and around the world. Concurrent training and recruitment of staff to work in such facilities could have occurred, since the staffing shortages now faced globally were entirely predictable. Going back to the food industry, if such facilities had been operationalized (within the public system in Canada as an example), the food industry could have been harnessed to feed both their patients and staff.

Returning to the concept of resilience and the research that showed the significant impact of the pandemic on mental health: while virtual visits with physicians and health care teams were made possible in many regions and countries (though not all) to an extent and at a speed that was previously unheard of, more open access hotlines could have been created for those who were really struggling with isolation, anxiety, and depression – those who previously had no contact with professionals for such symptoms. Telling people it's OK to reach out for help are empty statements if they can't be actioned. Furthermore, telemedicine support to geographically distant teams struggling to help communities they served could have been expanded to greater extents. And if health care systems were integrated on a more global scale, telemedicine could even have been harnessed to help overworked, overstressed, overtired teams around the world who sometimes just needed some guidance from a second set of fresher eyes.

Health care workers themselves are overworked and are now simply exhausted. Research has shown high rates of symptoms of anxiety, depression, and post-traumatic stress disorder, and most concerning, increased consumption of alcohol, sleeping aids, and suicidal ideation nearly 3 years into the pandemic. Burnout and mental health were already problematic before. Attempts were made to help by providing mental health services, though few health care workers on the front lines had time to access these services and most looked to family, friends, and team members for whatever support they could give. Attempts, well-intentioned, were made to help by providing "extenders" or redeploying staff. However, more attention needed to be paid to skill set and what roles/responsibilities such people were being asked to assume. For example, taking over communication with families of sick patient requires in-depth knowledge about what is happening, what the treatments are, the response seen, and its implications. Such communication requires a high level of knowledge and skill, and cannot be ascribed to just anyone (without specific training – training that was not going to be provided) without creating problems. Many health care workers felt devalued by such well-intentioned plans and even more devalued when those recruited to help were better financially remunerated for less knowledge, skill, and responsibility. Once again, the concept of "resilience" was used, this time for health care workers. Initially, it was used as a compliment, then a rallying cry, then transformed into an obligation to help those worse off, then, finally, as an expectation. Many workers have left health care or have left departments key to the response to the ongoing pandemic. These same departments are key to health care systems' recovery and efforts to help patients who have been waiting far too long for help. While everyone in health care understands the choice to leave, the result is more work and greater expectations (from self, the organization, and the public) to meet the very real health care needs of the population. As I write this chapter, we are in the midst of a human resource crisis in health care. It could have been both anticipated and avoided if there had been society-wide public campaigns (similar to recruitment efforts for the Armed Forces in times of need) to recruit and train those with an interest in health care. The crisis could have been mitigated if there had been a way of truly streamlining recognition of the qualifications of international health care workers currently living (and unemployed) in countries that were different from those in which they trained.

Earlier, I wrote that the pandemic was the first time everyone was directly asked to help their health care system. But what has the health care system's response been to the reciprocal question, "How are you helping us?" Perhaps my next statement will be seen by many as controversial; however, I believe that the health care system has contributed to the polarization of society by asking society to bow to its needs during this pandemic without sufficiently considering how it could also meaningfully mitigate the suffering of the people it serves, people beyond those immediately struggling with acute illnesses, in particular (and so narrow in scope), and those struggling with the virus itself. Planning has been, in large part, reactive and not proactive in nature. Prevention and mitigation of spread during each "wave" of variants has, in large part, been exactly the same. There have been no concurrent plans on how to balance the needs of the health care system to serve those affected with the virus while also responding comprehensively to those in need of help from other illnesses. Nor have there been systematic efforts to balance the needs of health care systems with the harms that restrictions cause to those within society, many of whom have lost everything they have worked for. If the pandemic has taught us anything, it's that reactive silo planning alone will never succeed in responding to human needs. And the trade-off, the price, will be counted in the divisions in society, in families, in the loss of civility, in the creation of the many faces of "us" and "them"

As a health care professional, I find the hardest part of this pandemic has been to see such potential opportunities to mitigate hardship all around without anyone even trying to think outside the box, trying to create think tanks on how these measures could have been operationalized or could be in the future. The health care system can't do this alone – it needs multilevel cooperation from government, businesses, and industry. But I believe the health care system has to accept responsibility for some of our current societal divisions. I believe it can and should lead the way in the future in discussions to harness societal resources and be part of widespread and better solutions in future pandemics. If some of what I have suggested as proactive measures to harness our power as a collective had been done, perhaps we wouldn't be in such a mess nor so ripped apart today. As a critical care physician who saw the devastation and divisions, who saw the horrors of what the virus can do, who saw the choices made and the measures taken, if I had one wish that could be granted, it would be to see a call to action to critically examine what really happened in the interactions between our health care systems and our societies. It would be an honest and comprehensive exploration of how we could work together to truly integrate *health* into all our lives – and become siloed no more.

PART SEVEN

Lessons and Transformations

This section, "Lessons and Transformations," looks to the future and posits two simple questions: What did we learn from the pandemic experience? And what will we, collectively or individually, take from it? To better address these questions, we included recollections not just from the "usual suspects" (hospital-based physicians or nurses) but also from psychologists, chaplains, and environmental experts.

"Turning Pain into Progress" illustrates the efforts of a clinical psychologist with an expertise in pain to turn the negativity of the pandemic into something positive: initiatives meant to tackle needle phobia, an underappreciated source of vaccine hesitancy in adults. "A Dumpster Full of Flowers" is the recollection of a "travel" nurse/nurse practitioner who was dropped as emergency help into the hot zones of the pandemic, from a near-apocalyptic Manhattan to a grieving corner of Texas. "The Same Room" attempts to make sense of one of the great mysteries of the pandemic: why did some die, yet others survived? "No Visitors" shares the vantage point of a hospital chaplain into the most bittersweet of the pandemic experiences: a "good" final family goodbye. "History Will Judge Us. And That's OK." asks a series of difficult questions: How do we come to a collective consensus on scientific "fact"? How do we respond when that consensus is challenged and perhaps even in error? Are we willing to admit our mistakes, or do we cling to our comfortable dogmas?

32 Turning Pain into Progress

Jody Thomas, PhD
CEO, Meg Foundation; Adjunct Faculty, Stanford University School of Medicine

Submitted 13 December 2022

I'm not here because anyone thinks you're crazy. I'm here because sometime in the last few hours, a lot has happened, and you likely feel like you've entered the Twilight Zone. I'm here to help you navigate that feeling, all the things that are happening right now, and what is going to happen next.
— Me, more times that I can count, to understandably confused and somewhat defensive people who were not thrilled when a shrink showed up in their hospital room after an unexpected diagnosis or life-changing trauma

As a paediatric medical psychologist and expert in medical illness, pain, and trauma, my job has been to help people navigate through the hardest, most vulnerable times in their lives. That time when their child is diagnosed with a brain tumour. That time they have to tell their child that they have been diagnosed with terminal cancer and will not get to see that child grow up. That time when they lose their child in a tragic accident and then have to break the news to the child's siblings. I walk with them on the path of adjusting to the harsh reality of a life-altering disease diagnosis. I am there to help children learn how to live a life of meaning and purpose when they're not really sure whether they are going to make it to adulthood. I am on the floor with them when they are brought to their knees by the crushing grief of losing a child or sibling.

It has been my job to help people in those moments when the whole view of their future vanishes in an instant and they are instead left to pick up the pieces and start rewriting their story. It has been my job to sit there with them in that pain, in that suffering, and be fully present as they are forced by tragedy to completely reorganize the way their world works and learn to cope with the chaos that naturally ensues. Not because they want to, but because they *have* to – there is no other choice.

They have no choice but to unwillingly embrace the overwhelming fear and uncertainty that explodes into their world uninvited. They have no choice but to make it their friend, or at least their uneasy acquaintance. They never asked to be forced to accept and deal with the grief that comes with mourning the loss of what they thought life was going to look like. If I'm boiling it down to its essence, the core of what I do is to teach people to learn to live with fear and uncertainty.

Truth be told, when you think about it that way, it's a really fucking weird job. And during the pandemic, it got a whole lot weirder. It put me in a peculiar position of being uniquely prepared for the bizarro world that we all unwillingly but inescapably entered in 2020. When the pandemic hit, fear and uncertainty came down like a sledgehammer on all of us. Let's be honest, since the start of this madness, we've all been marinating in fear and uncertainty.

As much as my 25 years of professional experience has taught me, I can honestly say I wasn't ready for this. No one was. Not my psychologist colleagues, not anyone. How could anyone be? I wasn't ready to have the whole world fall apart all at once. People pointed out that my job has made me accustomed to tragedy, uncertainty, and teaching people to cope under incomprehensible stressors. And that is true – it is "up my alley." Adjusting to massive life changes is in my wheelhouse. But I sure as hell wasn't ready to have everyone need to do it *at the same time*, all while I was struggling to do it myself. It is one thing for a limited number of individuals to have their world rocked by vagaries of existence, but it is another to have it happen to everyone all at once. We were all riding the tsunami together. Yet, at least at the beginning, we weren't riding it so much as we were under it.

Here is the other, stripped down, core principle of my work: human beings survive the unthinkable by learning to make meaning from their experience. It is a uniquely human capacity to create meaning from the absolute horror that happens to us. Let me be crystal clear: this is *not* the same as "everything happens for a reason." That is a philosophy to which I not only whole heartedly *do not* subscribe but indeed find stunningly offensive. No one should be told their suffering is part of a grand plan. No one should be told there is some sort of "good reason" their child is dead or has some horrific, painful illness. I have borne witness to more situations than I care to count where well-meaning but out-of-touch people say things like "everything happens for a reason" to make themselves feel better. This inane phrase exacts a very high price from the suffering person on the receiving end of the misguided comment.

There is no "good reason" that, as of writing this chapter, over a million Americans have died from COVID-19. There is no good reason that millions more people have been left physically, emotionally, psychologically, and financially devastated. That said, getting through any massive trauma is a whole lot easier when you are able to find some sort of meaning in it, and in doing so, learn to live with fear, uncertainty, and grief. When we do, it opens up windows of opportunity for joy, happiness, and healing that so many people in horrific situations often forget exist.

So, what potential meaning lies in the insanity of the pandemic times for medical providers? What can we do with all the suffering we have witnessed? The suffering that those on the front lines have endured for far too long? I am not arrogant enough to tell you exactly what that is. That is up for everyone to decide for themselves. Years of experience have taught me that you cannot decide anyone's meaning for them. That is a task we must each do on our own.

That said, apparently I am arrogant enough to offer a possibility: long before COVID, our patients were doing battle with fear and uncertainty every time they walked through the doors of a medical facility. While we were all going about our usual professional days, it was there – the frightening monster in the corner menacing our patients – while many times we barely gave it a thought. It wasn't anyone being unfeeling or negligent – it was just that we were used to our world. It was a world we knew well and felt comfortable in, and it was easy to forget that our patients are often visitors in a foreign land, not necessarily aware of the customs and the language. By the very nature of the day-to-day-ness of it all, we likely rarely noticed the monster in the corner.

But what about now? We all understand the burden of fear and uncertainty in a way we never knew before the pandemic. That monster invaded our world so thoroughly it was impossible to ignore. We now know what it is like to be in that wildly uncomfortable space of being so very acutely aware of fear and uncertainty.

So let us embrace that. Remember that. Take a mental note of what we've been through and then decide what we as individuals and a field are going to do with that. And then consider the possibility of using that experience. Play with the notion that getting to know that monster so well opens up new opportunities for how we can relate to, and be empathetic with, our patients. We can surely understand them in a way we never have before.

We did not ask for this disaster, and God knows there is not a universe in which I would sign us up for it. But we might as well get something out of it. Personally, professionally, and just as human beings sharing this very messed up planet in this very challenging period of time.

So what meaning did I find in the COVID muck, you may (or may not) ask? As an expert in pain, coping, and medical adherence, I and my colleagues knew COVID had the potential to be a turning point. When it became clear that vaccines were going to be the key to the path out of pandemic hell, there were a lot of us in the field who realized that compliance and uptake was going to be a major uphill battle.

We have spent decades beating the drum about the high prevalence of needle anxiety and the very clear massive (and massively under-recognized) negative impact on medical adherence as well as personal and public health outcomes. Needle anxiety is a health care–changing issue for 63 per cent of kids, 50 per cent of teens, and 25 per cent of adults. Those numbers are staggering. What has made that all the more frustrating has been the historical underuse of simple, research-proven strategies to manage pain and anxiety around needle procedures. Best practice guidelines that have decades of research behind them are simply not followed. Many, if not most, providers don't even know they exist.

It turned out our fears were justified. It was like watching a train wreck in slow motion: vaccines became this bizarrely political maelstrom, and conspiracy theories were birthed seemingly overnight. The research was clear that, hiding in the middle of the chaos, was the fact that needle anxiety was and is a major barrier to vaccine uptake, but very few were going to openly admit that. We live in a world where it is more socially acceptable to say that you believe Bill Gates wants to microchip you or that you "don't believe the science" than it is to admit you are afraid of needles. It's ridiculously hard for people to admit that they aren't actually terrified of the vaccine, but the idea of having it injected into their arm is unbearable.

I so strongly believe in this needle anxiety as an issue that I am the chief executive officer (CEO) of a non-profit organization dedicated to empowering people around pain and medical anxiety. We create free pain management tools and resources based on cutting-edge medical science, designed to turn information into life-changing action. We knew this was our moment. If we were ever truly going to get people to care about this issue, now was the time.

So, on top of the tools we already had for kids and families, we launched a brand-new campaign targeted to help the *one in four* adults with enough needle anxiety to change their health care decisions (including the decision to vaccinate). We even created a coping plan tool for teens when they deemed our other materials too "babyish."

To generate more impact quickly and effectively, we supported other good work and partnered with organizations big and small. We worked with everyone: from universities encouraging students to vaccinate, to community health groups looking to increase vaccination rates in Black and LatinX populations, to major hospitals and health care systems, to national organizations like the American Academy of Pediatrics.

I'm pretty thrilled to say our work garnered national and international attention. Appearances on podcasts, blogs and articles, and interviews on major news outlets helped us get these tools into the hands of people who needed them. I even became a "trusted messenger" for the *We Can Do This* campaign for the U.S. Department of Health and Human Services and did press events with the U.S. Surgeon General.

Though it was utterly exhausting, every word written or spoken, every email, every meeting was an opportunity to feel like I was actually *doing* something that helped. It was a time when I often felt helpless and like I was bathing in the frustration of trying to deal with lockdown/remote school/physical separation from friends, family, and my patients. I cannot overstate how good it felt to feel like we were doing something that got needles in arms, people protected, and all of us that much closer to whatever was becoming the new version of normal.

Here's one last thought to consider. Another core tenet of my work is this: we are all stronger than we think we are and capable of more than we thought possible. Most unfortunately, learning that lesson nearly always requires very bad things to happen. We don't have to love (but sadly must accept) that the process nearly always really, really sucks. But we can embrace that underneath the suffering are opportunities for wisdom, growth, joy, and finding strength we never knew existed. It is safe to say that, over the course of the journey from hell we have been on since 2020, LESSON LEARNED.

33 A Dumpster Full of Flowers

Ingrid Duffy, RN, FNP
Freelance Nurse Practitioner, Denver, Colorado

Submitted 30 June 2022

My nursing career began almost 30 years ago when nurses traditionally wore white. A colour traditionally symbolizing cleanliness, honesty, innocence. Over the years, the white uniform has mostly disappeared, along with the innocence. In the Emergency Department, we were eventually given the option to wear burgundy scrubs to alleviate the inevitably frequent task of removing blood stains from our "whites." However, as the footwear requirement remained a mandatory white, burgundy scrubs could not fully erase the events of a rough shift. Even if I wanted to forget a particularly gruesome event, there would be some spot on my shoes that would bring it all back. Sometimes I'd find myself looking at a stain on my shoes and thinking about a tragic event, and realize that the shoes were too new to have that particular person's blood. But then, whose blood was I staring at? Time for a new pair of shoes.

I was between jobs at the beginning of COVID-19 when I received a text looking for nurse practitioners to help in New York City public hospitals as they were rapidly becoming overrun with overwhelming volumes of critically ill COVID patients.

Having a desire to help, as well as being in need of a job, I answered the text and was informed that I was to report to Manhattan by 10:00 p.m. the next evening. I was then provided with a plane ticket and a brief list of items to bring, including a stethoscope, N95 masks (if you could find them), face shields, and uniforms. No white, just solid black scrubs and black shoes.

The airport was eerily empty. There were only five other passengers on a plane with a seating capacity of roughly 150 headed to New York City (NYC). Each of us sat silently with our masks on in separate corners of the aircraft. While I was waiting at baggage claim in another nearly empty airport, a middle-aged man with a strong Middle-Eastern accent approached me and fumbled through several ID cards to show that he was, in fact, an Uber driver. He helped drag my bags to his car while explaining he already had a family member in the hospital with COVID. And while he had great concern (he said "terrified") that he was putting himself and his family at risk by mingling with the public, he had to do so as he was the sole provider for his family of five. With few cars on the road due to the lockdown, the drive from La Guardia to my hotel near Penn Station was quick, pausing only for traffic lights and emergency medical services (EMS) vehicles. The trip ended with expressions of concern for each other's safety and the health of our loved ones, a fist bump, and a gift of one of the scarce, sacred N95 masks that I had brought.

By 10:00 p.m., I had checked into my room with instructions to meet in the ballroom the next morning at 6:00 a.m. dressed for work.

With 1050 rooms at full occupancy, the ballroom of the New Yorker on Eighth Avenue was a sea of nurses, nurse practitioners, and physician assistants, all masked and dressed in black. The three huge antique chandeliers in that room had illuminated countless gatherings since they were installed in 1930, but I'm guessing none quite like this one.

That evening those of us assigned to the night shift would return to the lobby where we would sign in before boarding our bus to work. As I walked through the revolving brass Art Deco door, I briefly fantasized that I was about to hail a cab and say something like "Forty-Eighth and Broadway please" or give the name of an upscale restaurant so popular the cab driver wouldn't need an address. But as I completed my half-circle and stepped outside to hail my imaginary taxi, I could see only tour buses lining both sides of the streets surrounding the hotel. Each bus had a plain white piece of paper with a hospital name printed in Helvetica taped inside its front window.

This fleet of tour buses had been designated to take us to one of eleven of NYC's public acute care hospitals. My bus was to bring roughly thirty of us to Brooklyn for our night shift. The streets were still empty that first evening, except for the police, EMS, and us. By the end of the week, our nightly commute was dominated by tour buses coming from at least ten other hotels like the one where I was staying. More buses, more nurses, more nurse practitioners (NPs), and more physician assistants (PAs). When we got close enough to another bus, I checked out the scrubs. All black. That was the first time in my life that the word "dystopia" truly seemed to apply.

By the end of the first week, many tears had been shed on our bus. Tears for patients we had lost or were about to lose, tears of fear and exhaustion, and tears of helplessness. It was as if, in addition to strenuous and stressful work, we had also been holding the tears of patients' families and loved ones who were unable to visit or to sit with the sick and dying.

My work group consisted of six NPs assigned to work the night shift in the emergency room (ER). Upon our arrival, it was clear that the ER was operating at more than double its normal capacity. So many patients occupied the open floor plan that only a thigh-width space remained between beds and stretchers.

It didn't take long to recognize that, while our group of NPs helped to fill in this unit's provider staff, there were only four remaining nurses available on this shift to take care of eighty very ill patients. Many of the full-time staff were missing due to contracting COVID themselves – a frightening realization. It's hard to work in any hospital without at least considering your own mortality. Or the mortality of someone you love. And in order to be effective, you need to be able to put some of your emotions on hold. But with this disease, before any treatment, before any vaccine, I faced a new feeling – fear. Before, there were always occasional body fluid exposures from a potentially infected patient or the occasional angry patient or family member who tries to rush in with a weapon to settle a score. But this was different. I was afraid of being in that bed, being on that stretcher, with no family permitted to visit. And with very little hope of survival. I started imagining that I could see the virus in the air. If a ventilator circuit was open, I'd see a cloud of deadly virus coming out of the tube. Fear can save you from making a careless mistake. It can make wearing a mask, gloves, and gown for hours more tolerable. It can keep you sharp.

Within the first half hour of my first shift, one of my ventilated patients' blood pressure and heart rate began to drop, quickly and continuously. My autopilot kicked in. I began chest compressions and called a code. When you call a code in a hospital, within minutes you are usually surrounded by a host of other trained professionals and all the equipment and medicine you might possibly need. This time was different. As I looked around, I could see that there wasn't anyone available to assist with this patient, as there were two other patients currently being intubated and yet another receiving chest compressions. What momentarily captured my view were the faces of the other patients.

So many feverish patients were coughing, lying in beds within inches of other people who were just as sick or even sicker. Terror filled their eyes as they watched intubation after intubation and code after code – terrified that their turn to be placed on a ventilator was next. And when that time came, would a ventilator even be available? If you've never been starving for oxygen, it can be hard to imagine. You could try having someone hold you under water or pinch your nose and cover your mouth too long. It is terrifying. But to watch it happen to someone next to you while it is happening to you at the same time, I just can't imagine. It was hard to witness.

As a nurse, you see lots of pee and poop (and worse). So much that you might think it doesn't bother us. But, given a choice, less bodily fluid outside the body is better than more. And this was more. So many spilled bedpans and urinals that the floor was slippery with urine. Staff had started throwing disposable pads over the puddles so we could continue to run from patient to patient without slipping in urine.

As the nights wore on, a disturbing trend would befall a portion of the patients. In addition to fever and shortness of breath, they would develop raging diarrhoea. As they could see how busy the department was, some patients would attempt to ambulate to the restroom on their own. Typically, it was upon the return to their stretcher that they would decompensate, eyes wide and gasping for air, ultimately crumpling to the floor in need of intubation or chest compressions.

A 75-year-old Spanish-speaking gentleman, I will call him Mr. Valdez, conveyed to me that, although he had a high fever, shortness of breath, along with feeling awful, he wanted to be cured as quickly as possible so he could return to work. Of no surprise, testing revealed that he too had COVID. I initiated treatment based on the current hospital protocol. By morning, he had decided that he had received ample treatment and would like to go home so as to make room for someone else. I saw that a lot. Very sick people trying to give up their bed to someone they felt needed it more. Via an interpreter, I explained that he was still too sick to leave at this point and that he should not go to work with a COVID diagnosis. I managed to convince him to stay, hoping he would soon get a room upstairs in the hospital proper. I was not convinced he'd make it home. I couldn't really be sure he'd make it to the bathroom and back.

On my way in to work the following night, I ran into my Mr. Valdez. The bus had dropped us off a block or so away from the hospital because our driver couldn't navigate the street. It was too narrow due to a line of waiting ambulances along both sides of the street, waiting in line to drop off more patients. Sadly, I knew that the only way beds would become available was if someone else didn't make it. But there was Mr. Valdez, walking away from the hospital! Google translate at the ready, I walked right up to him and asked how he was doing. We had a fairly long conversation through my smart phone and some exaggerated gesturing. He thanked me for taking care of him, but he could clearly see that there were few, if any, people leaving the ER alive, and he had decided that he wanted to die at home in the company of his family. He said he had signed out against medical advice and only had to walk six blocks to get to his house. My worry for him, and a need to save at least *one* patient, compelled me to pull out my tools and check his oxygenation while standing in the street. It was 85 per cent. I tried to look less concerned than I felt. We exchanged an "air-hug" and a fist bump, and he continued his walk home.

I have worked in other emergency rooms, and it is not uncommon for there to be a group of people with nowhere else to be but to hang around the grounds of the hospital, typically near the outside of the Emergency Department. They are not patients but rather people looking for a place to get out of the weather or maybe find a meal. While gathering supplies for our next intubation, I met one of these people. His name was Jon. He was a tall man with a blond beard, standing hunched over. He was holding himself up with one of the rolling supply carts that store things such as IV catheters, tubing, alcohol preps, and syringes. His eyes locked on mine as he rifled through the cart, grabbing syringe after syringe, shaking each one at me and then throwing it on the floor. "See these?! They're empty! Can you help me and put some drugs in here?" he groaned loudly through his mask.

Confused, I looked around for someone to escort Jon out, but only one security officer was working that night, and he was not available because he was helping an exhausted morgue attendant whom I'm pretty sure was having the busiest night of his career. I grabbed Jon a sandwich, guided him back outside, and explained that, due to COVID, it would be safer for him to be on the streets.

An average hospital morgue can hold around fifteen bodies. Until recently, funeral homes would pick up the deceased within a day or two. But funeral homes throughout the city were also full. So that night the officer and the orderly were moving the "deceased overflow" outside to a refrigerated truck. As I hurried back inside, a television in the waiting room broadcast the words of a local funeral director: "When you overwhelm the health system, you also overwhelm the death system." Pretty succinct summary, if you ask me.

Later I met Michael. He was only 32. He told me that he was the youngest of six children and also that he was the only son. Together we cried as he told me about his parents and his sisters, and how worried they were about him and how much they loved him. His oxygen saturation continued to drop. Eventually his hunger for air had reached a point where, as terrifying as it had been watching the decline of the other patients around him, he realized the only way he could fill his lungs with the comfort of oxygen was to accept intubation. His eyes said, "Do whatever you can. Please don't let me die." It was hard for him to cry as he was struggling so much to breathe. Between gasps, he did manage to get across that he was crying because he couldn't say goodbye to his parents or sisters, or tell them how much he loved them. Through our tears, he signed the consent form. My chest clenched as I fought to stay composed enough for the upcoming procedure. We didn't have much time. The sedation was pushed, and Michael was placed on life support. My gown, gloves, mask, and face shield were soaked and steaming from sweat. I could taste my own salty tears.

Serendipitously and just in time to prevent an untimely emotional unravelling, I looked up to see a woman wearing black boots and cut-off shorts. She started screaming as she ran through the unit with a kitchen knife buried to the handle in her right thigh. Her blood discoloured the urine puddles as she ran to the med room and barricaded herself inside. It appeared her instinctive plan was to replenish her blood loss with a couple litres of apple juice, which she had spotted on the counter next to the med cart. I watched the juice spill down her face and shirt as she guzzled, and all I could think was, "She's going to be fine, but someone better get her an N95."

The current demographic for this ER consisted of a single diagnosis: COVID. If possible, all other emergent patients were diverted to other facilities so as to reduce their exposure to COVID. But Jon staggered into the ER to beg for needles, drugs, or both every 3 or 4 days. It certainly was unusual to have someone freely wandering about the department in this manner, but it was an unusual time. I came to wonder if his routine visits weren't a direct result of his dealer having COVID.

Just before sunrise, the buses would arrive to take us back to our hotel. It could take up to an hour for everyone to get to the bus after finishing up their shift. On the way to find a seat, I'd pass nurses who were so exhausted they were already asleep. Some were crying, praying, or both, while others were on the phone with their loved ones/families. Myself, I would usually just stare out of the window as a dystopian view of Brooklyn and Manhattan passed by.

People in masks stood waiting on markers painted 5 feet* apart in front of the few open stores and bodegas. Other long lines curved around city blocks with those awaiting their turn in white COVID testing tents. Many municipal services were on hold. Each day, the view

---

* 1.5 metres.

included fewer people and more overflowing trash cans. Eventually, the cans became completely obscured by additional bags of trash. Once in a while, a windy day would bring the reappearance of the cans as masses of paper and trash blew down the streets into eventual piles against the sides of buildings, parked cars, and deserted subway entrances.

One morning as our bus pulled in, facing north on Eighth Avenue, we noticed the beginning of a mural on the side of a tall building across the street from our hotel. Several platforms covered with tarps protecting what I imagined were buckets of paint and other supplies hung from the top of the building. Each morning, as I would drag myself back towards the rotating hotel door, I would make a mental note of the progress of the mural. Trying to imagine the final picture helped me to disengage from work. While getting dressed for work, it gave me something to look forward to instead of another bleak evening bus ride to Brooklyn.

My sanctuary, a room on the thirty-fifth floor of the hotel, had an outstanding view of the Empire State Building and Madison Square Garden. After twenty-one shifts, I was able to spend my first full night there. Unable to sleep, I stared out of the window expecting to watch the colourful light display from the Empire State Building. However, that night's display was only a single red circling light, much like what one would see on the top of an ambulance. A symbol of a city under siege. Those who could leave were gone, and those who were left were calling for help. I guess the help was me.

Downstairs, the hotel's restaurants and bars were closed. It was strange seeing only limited hotel staff and weary medical personnel dressed in black wandering around this classic property in Manhattan. One day, I noticed that counsellors had been added to the team staying at our hotel. They stood out because they were some of the very few people in the area wearing street clothes.

I had been working hard to keep myself tightly wound emotionally. If I fell apart, I wouldn't be able to make myself get back on the bus for another round of force-fed helplessness. I established a daily ritual of dodging the counsellors. In order to avoid contact, I would conveniently keep my face pointed upward to check out the progress of the mural. If a counsellor spoke to me, they'd get an elbow or fist bump, and I'd keep moving. It was as if a plain-clothes emotion patrol had set up checkpoints between the lobby and the buses. Their purpose was sound, and I'm sure quite needed. But if I tapped into all of the sadness, fear, and rage I was concealing from myself, it would release a geyser I was afraid I couldn't control. As the daily bus boarding and deboarding wore on, I continued to sneak past by staring upward, slowing my steps only enough to focus on what had been added to the mural but not enough for an actual conversation. Emotions weren't going to make any of this easier.

I think I let one counsellor introduce themselves once. That was enough. From then on, I would simply nod or smile and take peace knowing they were there watching out for me. My compartmentalization skills were in full swing.

My partner flew to NYC with my favourite seasoned pot roast and some Gulf shrimp in his backpack. He got a room a couple blocks away from mine and prepared a home-cooked meal in a Hell's Kitchen hotel with a hotplate. We took turns eating to minimize exposure risk. Even while wearing masks in each other's presence, it was as close to normal as I'd felt in weeks. Several of my newly acquired COVID NP friends shared stories of smuggling spouses, sneaking visits. My need to feel close to someone was more powerful than ever. Gloves and masks and social distancing can wear on you. But I know what I'd seen just hours before. And if the man I love got this disease, how could I not be responsible? So, we had adjoining rooms. And wore N95s when we were together. He fell asleep in his bed while we were up late talking, so I went to my adjoining room. I left the door open so I could hear him breathing. When I woke up in a few hours, he had snuck into my bed and was spooning me, mask and all.

After a couple of months, our NP group was reassigned to the Internal Medicine Department to cover the inpatient floors. With all of the patients infected with COVID, the unit looked much like the ER except now each patient would have their own room. At first take, it was an improvement. However, it wasn't long before most of these patients had to be intubated. With the intensive care units (ICUs) being full, we had little choice but to convert this general inpatient unit into a temporary ICU. Several other units followed in succession and were converted to ICUs as well.

Our staff physician, who had volunteered to take leave from her family practice in order to help in the hospital, was the only provider present who was fluent in Spanish, which meant that she would be the one to call family members when someone passed away. Some mornings, she was tasked with calling up to a dozen families before starting her day taking care of her patients who were still struggling to stay alive.

Somehow, I thought that moving to an inpatient unit would mean that the patients would be more stable. However, the codes and intubations continued as they did in the ER. After one of these codes, I recall a nurse asking me to check on her patient across the hall while she prepared the lifeless body of the patient we had been trying to resuscitate for transport to the morgue. I walked across the hall and found her other patient crumpled on the floor in the bathroom doorway – pulseless, next to her cell phone. Her resuscitation was also unsuccessful.

Another common occurrence was calls from friends and family members trying to reach their sick loved ones. One morning around 2:00 a.m., I answered a randomly ringing portable phone. It was a young man calling to speak to his sister who had been recently moved out of the ICU and transferred to the inpatient unit. He said he had been calling her cell phone but was not getting any answer. She was sitting peacefully, partially upright in her bed, breathing on her own but barely responsive. She seemed barely alive. Her brother requested a video chat so he could see her. I tried to prepare him by explaining her condition and started the call on her cell phone. He did not, however, prepare me for the group of fifteen to twenty family members, including her school-aged children, who were also with him on the call. Their reaction to seeing their mother in this state is an image that still haunts me. A reminder that the victims of this disease weren't just the ones in the morgue.

Months later, I was reassigned to work with the Laredo (Texas) Fire Department. Initially, I was relieved. I didn't want to set foot inside another hospital. However, during my first week, one of the fire department's captains succumbed to COVID. We, the contract staff, were to help cover dispatch while the fire department family would attend their fallen brother's funeral.

When I arrived at work, they had just finished washing and waxing various department vehicles to be driven in the funeral procession. Each vehicle had a large black bow fastened onto its grill. Each firefighter and paramedic was wearing their badge with a black ribbon across it.

It was January, 9 months since this whole COVID thing started and 9 months since visitors of any kind were allowed in the hospitals. This funeral was the closest I had been able to be to a family grieving the loss of one of their own. Up until this point, no families could come to visit a loved one in the hospital. As we covered Central Command from the fire station, we watched the funeral procession on one of the many large TVs while we took 911 calls. Even though we had never met the captain, tears rolled down our faces as we watched the graveside ceremony. The chief stepped onto a podium. "On behalf of the Laredo Fire Department, I extend my deepest condolences … He will be greatly missed by his fellow brothers and sisters. I ask that we keep him in our thoughts and prayers, that we honour him for all the contributions he made attempting to stop the spread of this virus. May God continue to bless and keep His protective shield on all those who are in the front lines helping others during this time." The captain was 45 years old. He had 25 years of service with the department. In short, he had been in this family since he was 20.

With everything on lockdown, I had a hard time finding a place to clear my head. I took to taking walks in cemeteries some mornings after work. Outside, I didn't have to wear my mask, and somehow, being near those crying for someone they had lost made me feel more connected. Perhaps it was a way for me to show respect to the patients and the families of those I couldn't save. It was a place I could anonymously grieve with them. On many of my walks, I'd stop to pay my respects to the fallen captain.

Each gravesite was ornately decorated with brightly coloured flowers. Row upon row of bright colour, row upon row of sorrow. Conveniently, I was already appropriately dressed in black. I wound around towards the other side of the cemetery where I noticed the grounds keepers had been clearing sites of old flowers and preparing spaces for new burials. Dozens of wheelbarrows containing old bouquets were scattered throughout the grounds, all leading to an overflowing dumpster of flowers.

I wish I could say that my black scrubs protected me from the stains of my experience.

34 The Same Room

Hassan Al-Habeeb, MD
Critical Care Medicine Consultant and Neuro Critical Care Consultant, Riyadh National Hospital, Riyadh, Saudi Arabia

Submitted 14 February 2023

In the last quarter of 2020, deaths due to the coronavirus were at their peak. Seeta, a woman in her 60s with leukaemia, fell ill. Her body was emaciated, and she was overwhelmed by pain. Exhausted by cancer, which weakened her immunity when COVID-19 attacked, she quickly became seriously ill. It took only 2 days for her to need the intensive care unit (ICU). Her two daughters were constantly by her side.

Seeta's health turned from bad to worse. We took all the measures we could, but they were in vain. The two girls were looking at me with sad and broken looks, the effects of sleeplessness and tiredness clear on their faces. All the vital signs indicated that Seeta's body could give no more and that she was about to die. Here, the doctor must exert self-control, must try not to fall apart from sadness when he sees loved ones waiting to hear the news, waiting to hear joyful news, not news that brings unhappiness and grief.

I don't know why I carry the intensive care patients' stories home. Sometimes I get up at night and contact the ICU: "Was such and such an investigation performed?" "Has the patient been given a dose of such and such medication?" Maybe it's the nature of the medical profession in which care never ends. Sometimes I think it's simply because medicine is greater than the limits of any work, for caring transcends time. Sometimes I think maybe the memories linger with me as my way of honouring each person I care for. What is certain is that stories like this one will be forever etched in my mind, will forever be part of me.

I met with Seeta's daughters. I held myself together while I was with them, wishing so much that I could have done more. I broke the devastating news. It was only 2 days after she had been admitted to the ICU. The two girls entered their mother's room, where she was lying on the ICU bed. They stayed until she had breathed her last. One of them hugged her and said brokenly, "Mom, where did you go?"

We lived through the loss of so many lives, so many people held dear. Yet what will always haunt me about this story is that the attending physician who had been treating her in the clinic for the last few years was also infected with COVID. He was admitted into the same room she was in.

That was where the doctor and his patient shared the same room.

He survived.

35 No Visitors

Rev. Kristel Clayville, PhD
Former Hospital Chaplain; Lecturer, Technology Ethics and Health Humanities, University of Illinois, Chicago

Submitted 4 January 2023

The incoming page simply read "5–2077." I knew what that meant. I was the only chaplain at the hospital from 7:00 a.m. to 7:00 p.m. on Sundays, so I quickly finished up my visit in the Emergency Department (ED) and called 5–2077 for more details.

The voice on the other end sounded tired.

"Security. West Lobby."

"Hi, this is the chaplain. You paged?"

"Yeah. I've got two for the eighth floor."

"I'm in the ED, so I'll be there in about 10 minutes."

As I suspected, two family members had arrived for an end-of-life visit with a COVID-19 patient, and I was needed to escort them to one of the closed COVID units. It was the first summer of the pandemic, and I had not yet been on the closed COVID units. I had talked to patients from these units on the phone before they were intubated, and I'd helped them fill out Power of Attorney paperwork via FaceTime. And I had seen COVID patients in the ED, but so far, I had not been on the closed unit.

The closed COVID units were created in March 2020 to handle the anticipated influx of COVID patients. It involved moving in modular room dividers, closing off corridors, creating more negative air flow, and constructing liminal areas for putting on personal protective equipment (PPE) and for decontamination. The medical staff on these units didn't go anywhere else in the hospital, were always in full PPE, and it was still assumed that they would get COVID. The staff who would replace them when they did get sick were under orders to remain at home and wait to be called in.

As a chaplain, I was used to being with patients and families at the end of life. It was one of the things we were called on to do most frequently, but since the pandemic began, that work had mainly been relegated to bereavement phone calls. Patients of all kinds were dying without family present. News stories ran on TV and in print about patients dying alone. On one shift, I even fielded a phone call from a concerned citizen about how horrible the situation was. She wanted to know if her prayer group could bring the chaplains any kind of gear that would make it safe for us to sit with dying COVID patients since their family members were not allowed to visit. Hunting gear? Modified tarps?

Given the external and internal discontent with the "No Visitors" policy, the hospital changed it: two visitors would be allowed for end-of-life visits. Chaplains would meet the visitors as security to escort them to see the patient. The absence of visitors was sad and created ethical problems, but now the presence of visitors was foreboding. Two by two, every set of visitors meant that a patient was dying. I started to dread seeing visitors lined up at the security desk in the lobby.

I had taken several sets of visitors up to the COVID units previously. In the elevator, I'd prepare them for the PPE area and inform them that I wouldn't be going on the unit with them. Later, I'd meet them on the other side of the decontamination area to escort them back to the lobby. PPE was still very much in short supply, and the hospital had to use some of it for family members for these end-of-life visits. That was one reason that I didn't go on the unit. Also, no one had asked for a chaplain; we were the escorts by default, but it wasn't clear to me that any particular family wanted a religious professional to be part of their last visit with their loved one. So I would give the visitors directions and help them with their PPE, and then manoeuvre myself through the corridors to the decontamination area and exit.

But this Sunday was different. When I got the page to call 5–2077, I was already wearing an N95. There had been a cardiac arrest patient in the ED, and his entire family had tested positive for COVID. Given the PPE shortages, once I had put on an N95, I wore it for the rest of my shift.

When I got to the security desk, there were only two women waiting.

I introduced myself, "Hi, I'm Kristel. I'm a chaplain here, and I'll be taking you to the eighth floor. Who are you here to see?"

One of the women spoke, "Mrs. Williams. My mother," and pointing to the other woman, "Her grandmother."

"OK. I'm glad you are getting to see her." I gestured towards the elevators, and we all walked towards them.

Pointing to my face, the granddaughter asked me, "Will we get a mask like yours when we get up there?"

"Yes, you'll get a mask like this, a protective gown, gloves, and goggles too. You'll have all the things you need to be safe while visiting your grandmother." As I answered her question and reassured her of the safety that PPE provides, I decided to escort this twosome all the way to the door of Mrs. Williams's room. After all, I was already wearing an N95, which was the most scarce element of PPE.

Because of my previous experiences with patients on the unit, I had imagined that this mother and daughter would go in and visit a patient who was intubated and sedated, and could not talk to them. Every patient I had talked to on the phone on these units had ultimately been intubated. Much of what we talked about was their fear of that procedure and also their fear of never waking up again. Did they want the last thing they saw to be a team of doctors and a tube? But even during these conversations, the patients would be gasping for breath, and without exception, when I looked at their charts a couple of days later, there would be a notation that they were on a ventilator.

Still, I understood why this mother and daughter would want to visit under those conditions. Mrs. Williams had probably been admitted through the ED, and they hadn't seen her for days, maybe weeks. They had probably fielded calls from doctors updating them on her condition and possibly a call from a chaplain as well. On the ethics committee, we had tried to figure out how to tell patients coming to the ED with mild COVID cases that seeking treatment meant being alone and that if treatment didn't work, they would die alone. The alternative would be to try to make do at home and try not to infect their family members. There were no good choices, and we didn't come up with good ways to communicate the stakes of being admitted to the hospital with COVID. But the stakes were stark: if treatment failed, then they would die alone. And yet, it is still unethical to suggest to sick people that they not seek treatment for any illness, much less COVID.

In the liminal space between the elevator and the COVID unit, Mrs. Williams's daughter, granddaughter, and I put on our PPE, our paper and plastic armour to protect us while we were on the unit.

As we approached her room, we could see through the room's glass doors that Mrs. Williams was sitting up in bed, and she wasn't on a ventilator. When her daughter and granddaughter came in, she greeted them with a big smile, and they started talking! I don't know what they talked about – I stayed outside the room and looked in through the glass door and windows. They laughed a lot. A nurse came over to look in, and I asked him about the patient's condition. He said that, when the doctors told her they didn't think intubation would help her, she chose palliative care, and because she did, she got to have an end-of-life visit that she was awake for.

It was a heartwarming story. The hospital had helped Mrs. Williams make a decision about how she wanted to die, and she was getting to actively say goodbye to her daughter and granddaughter. It was the best possible outcome, and yet I was so sad. The longer I looked at the trio laughing and enjoying being together, the sadder I got. Don't get me wrong. I'm glad that they got that time together. I just kept thinking that, when her family leaves, she knows that she is going to die alone. Not exactly alone, because there will be nurses and doctors, and maybe a chaplain. But when her daughter and granddaughter walk out, she knows that she'll never see them again. And they know that they will never laugh with her again or see her smile. There was some closure for these three people, but there was no uncertainty about what comes next. And uncertainty leaves room for hope.

It was the best possible ending – a meaningful and intentional goodbye – and my eyes were full of tears, so full that they had escaped my eyelids and were running towards my N95 mask. That had me a little panicky about how effective a wet N95 might be, so I headed for the decontamination area. The visitors would find their way there because they always did, and I would meet them on the other side.

36 History Will Judge Us. And That's OK.

Joe Vipond, MD, CCFP(EM), FCPC
Emergency Physician, Calgary; Co-Founder of Masks4Canada and ProtectOurProvinceAB; Co-Founder of the Canadian COVID Society (https://covidsociety.ca)

Kashif Pirzada, MD, CCFP(EM)
Emergency Physician, Toronto; Co-Founder of Masks4Canada; Co-Founder of the Canadian COVID Society

Submitted 16 June 2022

The COVID-19 pandemic catalysed an unprecedented explosion of health care and public health advocacy. With government policy often being written from scratch, typically as the science was being elucidated, there was and continues to be ample opportunity for various voices to weigh in, often on all sides and often through all forms of media, social or otherwise.

Several proposed methods of managing the spread and treatment of COVID-19 have elicited polarized reactions. Ivermectin is an essential element of COVID-19 treatment or is dangerous and unscientific quackery. Vaccines have the potential to be dangerous, and their use should be decided by the individual, or vaccines are safe and need to be mandated to protect vulnerable citizens. Masks are a simple and effective tool to prevent transmission, or they are dangerous, interfere with breathing, prevent appropriate childhood development and socialization, and shouldn't be used.

There are prominent voices from medical, social, and political perspectives advocating for each side of these positions. Both sides think they are on the side of what is good and true, and want policymakers to adopt their position. They care. Everyone! Listen to me! I'm right!

How can policy leaders tell which of these options they should follow with such impassioned advocates on either side?

First, and the most obvious, is science. The scientific method is still the best means we have for ascertaining the truth about a topic. While not every individual scientific paper is accurate, overall, science collectively gets closer to ascertaining the truth as evidence is gathered and assessed rigorously. For example, science shows that the evidence supporting ivermectin in COVID-19 treatment is lacking, and true risk of harm exists.

Not every issue has a perfect "right" answer, however. Arriving at the "right" can be more than just balancing the scientific benefit and risk. Values may need to guide our decisions. Anti-vaxxers believe that their right to avoid vaccination based on their personal beliefs and values is inalienable and that this choice shouldn't have consequences on their engagement in society. Others feel that protecting society, and its most vulnerable, means that participation in society should be contingent on keeping others safe through vaccination. So, do we value collectivism or individual rights? Since the end of the Second World War, the Western world has edged increasingly towards supporting individual rights. But with COVID-19, and especially with the climate crisis, we simply will not win unless collective action is prioritized.

Similarly, a frequent division is status quo versus new ideas. "We've always done it this way" is often seen as the path of least resistance for many reasons, and not just for medicine. Erring on the side of inaction often seems safer and more comfortable psychologically than erring on the side of action. What happens if we are wrong seems less of an issue if we did nothing than if we did something and contributed to harms. Pushing for something new seems dangerous as it means stepping into the unknown. In medicine, we can see this outlook in the very slow rate of adoption of new knowledge in clinical practice. And often, the overly bureaucratic systems we've built include people who may not benefit from any kind of significant change.

For every advocate wanting to change the world, there's an equally passionate advocate trying to keep it the way it is. Yet the only way to progress as a society, especially in dire times such as these, is to quickly evaluate and implement new ideas and new methods. It is to embrace nimbleness and flexibility by quickly developing, evaluating, and implementing new ideas, grounded as much as possible in emerging science. We should adapt to new knowledge with speed and agility as unravelling scientific enquiry reveals an ever-increasing number of the pieces of the puzzle before us.

Yet the most powerful differentiator between divisions, in our minds, is history, which will be the ultimate judge as to the appropriateness of positions taken. For example, think of Ede Flórián Birly,[1] who is not a household name. He was the professor of obstetrics in Budapest in the early 1800s who believed that childbed fever (a significant cause of early maternal mortality) was due to unclean bowels and preferred purging as a method of treatment. We are certain that he cared about his patients and strongly believed that he was acting at the era's highest standard.

He was wrong.

A man called Ignaz Semmelweis[2] challenged the status quo, supposing dirty hands were the source of childbed fever. And over time, history has determined that washing hands is indeed a good thing to do for childbed fever and beyond. Thus, it is Semmelweis's name we remember, not Birly's. The history of medicine is rich in the stories we need to continue to learn from.

We now stand at the precipice of another great controversy: the mode of transmission of the SARS-CoV-2 virus, the pathogen causing COVID-19. We have been vocal advocates for the fact that it is predominantly an airborne/aerosol-transmitted virus rather than the accepted paradigm of many members of the respected Canadian medical establishment that it is primarily transmitted via contact/droplet means.

This argument is not an academic one. The paradigm chosen mandates the public advice, public policy, and workplace safety requirements given by our leaders.

The status quo asserts contact/droplet transmission. Despite the scientific evidence that has emerged to the contrary, it is adamantly upheld by many of our colleagues – virologists, infectious disease specialists, and public health specialists who "own" the field and whose voices have been providing most of the guidance in this pandemic. Others within these fields may feel compelled to "toe the line" set by some of these prominent and indeed highly credentialed voices, tacitly taking a vow of silence lest they face potential scrutiny and reputational and/or career damage. Both insiders and outsiders may feel they have no right to challenge the authority of those recognized as experts. However, increasingly, there is an overabundance of scientific evidence reinforcing the airborne transmission route, while there is a distinct paucity of literature supporting surface contact/droplet spread.

Being an advocate, a role that health care professionals are taught to embrace, means stepping forward, exposing yourself to challenge, and sometimes even to ridicule. But with ongoing hospital outbreaks, the persistent daily death counts around the world, and the threat not only of more COVID-19 waves but also of pandemics from other respiratory pathogens, this work matters. We need to seek truth and have open discussions about the emerging science so we can best mitigate the spread, the death, and the increasingly worrying spectre of long COVID.[3]

Where is the truth? Science will eventually reveal it. With every wave, increasing evidence of our failure to fully understand the pathology, the politics, and the human psychology of the pandemic is evident. History will judge us. And we are OK with that.

The piece above was adapted from an op-ed the two of us co-wrote (but never published) in late autumn 2021. In and of itself, it is a piece of historical writing as the pandemic continues. We were confident that, with increasing publication of scientific papers recognizing the importance of airborne transmission and recognition by such austere bodies as ASHRAE (American Society of Heating, Refrigerating and Air-Conditioning Engineers), the CDC (Centers for Disease Control and Prevention), and PHAC (Public Health Agency of Canada), we seemed to be on the cusp of science protecting us and our fellow citizens.

We were naive.

It was to be expected, we suppose. After the 2003 SARS (severe acute respiratory syndrome) outbreak, Justice Archie Campbell in Ontario led an independent commission, releasing a report in 2006 to explore ways future pandemics should be better handled.[4] Two broad themes came out of it: use of the precautionary principle to guide policy and treatment of future pathogens as airborne from the outset. Both lessons from this 2006 SARS report were ignored and, indeed, actively opposed throughout the early COVID-19 pandemic by leaders in public health and infection control. Part of the report discusses the differences between how Vancouver and Toronto initially managed the influx of SARS into their hospitals. Vancouver used airborne-appropriate personal protective equipment (PPE) such as N95 respirators early on during the SARS epidemic. Toronto started with contact/droplet precautions, only later adopting similar airborne precautions, with the delay causing much more illness and death. The resistance to learn from these historical lessons continues today.

Since our original authorship, there have been significant attempts to rewrite history to denigrate the airborne paradigm.[5,6] The "droplet contingent" – deeply entrenched in academia and in international health organizations – have been busily nominating each other for major awards, lending a thin veneer of legitimacy to their position. Significant administrative complaints have been filed against multiple advocates of airborne precautions, stifling their voices.[7,8]

Major media outlets continue to interview many of the same few players, seemingly without ever checking back to see if their guests' previous predictions bore out over time. "Minimizers," those who think many if not all aspects of the COVID-19 pandemic have been overblown, have an outsized voice in Western media, despite being wrong time and time again. As the pandemic evolves, the pundits' takes continue to underestimate the danger of emerging variants,[9] focus on acute illness, and forget the unknown potential of each in causing long COVID, already causing significant global cognitive and physical disability.[10] The promotion of overconfidence, devoid of the precautionary principle, in prevention and control of transmission, overconfidence in sterilizing (transmission-halting) vaccines, downplaying the impact of COVID-19 infections on kids and the risk of in-school transmission, and prematurely predicting, repeatedly, the end of the pandemic all increase the pandemic's impact on global health and its duration.

Masking, always a needlessly hot source of division and a political hot potato, is no longer mandated in any venue in Canada, including health care facilities replete with vulnerable patients. Indeed, it is becoming rarer to hear of a politician or public health official donning one or to see a public health advice advocating for mask use. Masks are becoming increasingly absent and continue to be predominantly of the surgical or cloth varieties as opposed to respirators, which are specifically designed to better mitigate airborne transmission. If there are any COVID-19 mitigation measures, they focus on contact/droplet precautions: hand sanitizer, bins for sterile and used pens at counters, and store signs encouraging patrons to cough in their elbow and to stay 2 metres* apart. While these methods are possibly effective to help limit the spread of some non-COVID-19 pathogens, they are not key methods to prevent airborne transmission.

In hospitals, we have recurrent outbreaks on the wards infecting the vulnerable when they are in our care.[11] Incredibly, despite 3 years of recurrent failings to stop outbreaks, there has been no reconsideration of whether the protections in place are adequate in many centres. If we consider how other well-recognized airborne pathogens are managed, we see there is a difference. Even the suspicion of tuberculosis (TB) will land a patient and their health care team in full airborne precautions:

---

* 6.6 feet.

a room with negative pressure isolation, N95, and full PPE for their health care providers. Yet TB, depending on where the infection is located and the pathogen burden a patient is experiencing, may not in fact be readily transmissible, and the infection control measures taken may be more than required. Indeed, hospital outbreaks of TB are very rare, and repeated hospital outbreaks unheard of. If there are repeated outbreaks of TB or measles (also an airborne pathogen), one would expect some reconsideration of the adequacy of safety protocols. Yet COVID-19 hospital and long-term care outbreaks have resulted in severe illness and deaths among patients and likely will result in more patients and staff struggling with long COVID. If investigations have occurred, they certainly have not resulted in any substantial changes in approach to prevent future events. From our perspective, it has been frustrating that infection prevention and control leaders seem to accept staff infecting patients and vice versa as inevitable. It is an ominous change to accept infectious disease transmission in hospitals as A-OK.

Expert opinion, political expediency, unwarranted optimism, and citizen fatigue are winning over science and the precautionary principle, even as new waves appear on the horizon.

Even worse, there seems to be a move to dispense with any attempt to mitigate transmission at all.[12] A strategy that now mainly relies on vaccines to protect people, despite many people of various ages not having received boosters or even first doses, runs the risk of increased viral transmission and of new variants further hampering the effectiveness of current and developing vaccines. We are in a new phase where it appears to be more widely permissible, even perhaps encouraged, to be infected in the illusory pursuit of what is now widely acknowledged to be unattainable herd immunity.[12] So why bother with masks, ventilation, filtration, or even teaching people about the ideal mask to use when many of the powers that be have decided, in an unwritten policy, that everyone is going to be infected, in fact possibly multiple times annually? And, by the way, forget the risk of long-term consequences such as long COVID[10] and staffing crises caused by both acute and chronic COVID-19 illness.

There are numerous reasons why we believe that this approach is the wrong direction for our leaders to have led: accelerating variant evolution, recurrent pressure on our health care systems, ongoing hospitalizations and deaths among the immunocompromised (and immunocompetent, too), the impact of long COVID on individuals and society,[10] and increasing evidence of the failure of this strategy from an economic perspective, as hospitals, flights, education, and other services are in the news daily with cancellation woes and systems failures.

On so many levels, it was to be expected. Mitigating airborne transmission is hard: it takes money to upgrade ventilation, to install filtration systems, and to maintain these tools. There is intellectual doubling down, as it is increasingly challenging to reverse the initial position that SARS-CoV-2 is spread via droplet/contact transmission. Reversing the stance on transmission would be acknowledging wrongdoing and the subsequent preventable infections and deaths that resulted from this "expert" advice. But it is deeply disconcerting to see institutions such as universities, establishments dedicated to truth and higher learning, awarding and supporting influential individuals who have not admitted to their errors, especially in light of the now vast evidence supporting airborne viral transmission.

This situation points to a greater problem: we were wrong to look to a fixed group of establishment experts to guide us during the pandemic. If you look at the underlying skills that lead to a successful career in academia, there is very little overlap with skills that ensure success in a fast-evolving, world-threatening scenario. There needs to be mental agility, an ability to consider one's own biases, the ability to chart a safer course with limited information, and the ability to admit error and alter course when the evidence suggests so. The unfortunate defensive, siloed, and "empire-building" nature of most academic and national/international health organizations has worked very strongly against the public interest throughout this crisis.

A recurrent issue through the pandemic has been the call for more randomized controlled trials (RCTs) to guide policy. RCTs are viewed as the highest level of evidence in medicine as the human body is a complex system that requires very exacting methods to avoid bias in clinical trials. By double-blinding subjects and researchers to the intervention used and randomizing subjects to one of two or more arms of the trial, this bias is better mitigated through RCTs to allow for a result closer to the "truth." But there are problems with relying on this form of evidence generation during a pandemic: RCTs take time, which we often do not have when making policy decisions, and they are not necessarily an appropriate method to find truth for non-pharmaceutical interventions (NPIs), such as masks.[13] For NPIs, other research methods, such a materials science, computer and physical modelling, and laboratory work are better scientific methods to find truth, as evidenced by the absence of RCTs for evaluating helmets, seat belts, parachutes, or any number of engineered safety systems. Similarly, RCTs should not be the standard we seek to be applied to safety systems such as ventilation and filtration, or masks, during a pandemic.[13]

So, what is to be done? In a perfect world, we can imagine world and public health leaders having an epiphany in one of the next few waves that current practices are not having the desired outcomes, and efforts are made to pivot to sensible transmission mitigation, emphasizing airborne precautions. We could begin by dusting off the 2006 SARS Commission report and applying its lessons on the precautionary principle, in addition to using our newly acquired knowledge of airborne transmission. This approach would mean education programs explaining to the public and organizations how to understand airborne pathogen spread and how to prevent it: starting with high-quality (well-fitting and filtering) masks and respirators in indoor public spaces, particularly during times of high community transmission; preferentially socializing outdoors; improving ventilation through heating, ventilation, and air conditioning (HVAC) repairs and upgrades, and opening windows and doors where safe to do so; monitoring carbon dioxide to assess adequate ventilation in enclosed spaces; adding high efficiency particulate air (HEPA) or equivalent filtration systems to those spaces that require it, such as poorly ventilated spaces.

We also need to rely less on narrow fields of expert opinion and more on a broad swath of experts from all backgrounds of science, engineering, humanities, bioethics, and more. In particular, we should incorporate the expertise of engineers, whose background in the physical sciences and modelling can help inform mitigation strategies for complex problems such as pandemics. We also need input from occupational hygienists, many of whom devote their careers to understanding and educating others on the function of PPE like respirators.

Lastly, we need to rediscover the ability to engage in large, society-wide, meaningful projects together. Examples could include the enormous effort behind the Apollo project, tens of thousands of engineers working towards a common goal; the fight against fascism in the 1930s and 40s that took a united, total effort by the free world; the introduction of universal health care in much of the developed world. The fight against an incredibly contagious, harmful airborne pathogen will need something on this level.

Human systems rely on humans to function, and as we have seen, both are fallible, particularly at times when radical shifts in emergency management systems are required. Science has been an incredibly powerful tool for humanity because it provides us with an investigative road map to reveal the truth throughout complexity. But we know that rigorous science takes time and that the precautionary principle is an appropriate guiding star as science catches up to uncover the truth. By using precaution with what we do not yet know, and science with what we now know, we can extricate ourselves from this pandemic while better preparing ourselves for the next.

History will judge us. All of us. It's time to learn from it too.

Note: The above was written in the summer of 2022 and represents our views at that time. We hope it is now hopelessly out of date.

REFERENCES

1. Ede Flórián Birly. Wikipedia. Last edited 4 June 2024. Accessed 14 June 2024. https://en.wikipedia.org/wiki/Ede_Flórián_Birly
2. Ignaz Semmelweis. Wikipedia. Last edited 11 June 2024. Accessed 14 June 2024. https://en.wikipedia.org/wiki/Ignaz_Semmelweis
3. Government of Canada. Post COVID-19 condition (long COVID). Modified 28 May 2024. Accessed 30 July 2024. https://www.canada.ca/en/public-health/services/diseases/2019-novel-coronavirus-infection/symptoms/post-covid-19-condition.html
4. Campbell A. *Spring of Fear*. The SARS Commission: final report. Vols. 2 and 3. Commission to Investigate the Introduction and Spread of SARS in Ontario. The Honourable Mr. Justice Archie Campbell, Commissioner. Ontario Ministry of Health and Long-Term Care; December 2006. https://www.archives.gov.on.ca/en/e_records/sars/report/index.html
5. Conly J, Fisman DN, Prather K. Is airborne transmission an important and mitigable aspect of the COVID-19 pandemic? a panel discussion. University of Calgary Department of Community Health Sciences and the O'Brien Institute for Public Health Seminar Series webinar. 9 April 2021. Accessed 26 September 2023. https://www.youtube.com/watch?v=2mh0BXX2Gr8
6. Greenhalgh T, Jimenez JL, Prather KA, Tufekci Z, Fisman D, Schooley R. Ten scientific reasons in support of airborne transmission of SARS-CoV-2. *Lancet*. 2021;397(10285):1603–5. https://doi.org/10.1016/S0140-6736(21)00869-2. Medline: 33865497.
7. Heller D. Medical whistleblower calling out COVID incompetence risks deregistration. *Independent Australia*. 14 July 2022. Accessed 28 July 2024. https://independentaustralia.net/politics/politics-display/medical-whistleblower-calling-out-covid-incompetence-risks-deregistration,16550
8. Swannell C. AMA Victoria to call for royal commission into AHPRA [Australian Health Practitioner Regulation Agency]. *InSight+*. 18 July 2022;(27). Accessed 28 July 2024. https://insightplus.mja.com.au/2022/27/ama-victoria-to-call-for-royal-commission-into-ahpra/
9. Mahindra AS. COVID-19 deaths skyrocket in the UK: know the symptoms, precaution measures. *Times Now*. 4 September 2023. Accessed

28 July 2024. https://www.timesnownews.com/health/covid-19-deaths-skyrocket-in-the-uk-know-the-symptoms-precaution-measures-article-103345495
10. Mazer B. Long covid could be a "mass deterioration event." *The Atlantic*. 15 June 2022. Accessed 28 July 2024. https://www.theatlantic.com/health/archive/2022/06/long-covid-chronic-illness-disability/661285/
11. Alberta Health Services. *Acute Outbreaks in Alberta: Novel Coronavirus (COVID-19)*. Alberta Health Services. Updated 19 September 2023. Accessed 28 July 2024. https://www.albertahealthservices.ca/assets/info/ppih/if-ppih-covid-19-acute-care-outbreaks-list.pdf
12. Howard J. *We Want Them Infected: How the Failed Quest for Herd Immunity Led Doctors to Embrace the Anti-Vaccine Movement and Blinded Americans to the Threat of COVID*. Redhawk Publications; 2023.
13. Oliver M, Ungrin M, Vipond J. Masks work: distorting science to dispute the evidence doesn't. *Scientific American*. 5 May 2023. Accessed 28 July 2024. https://www.scientificamerican.com/article/masks-work-distorting-science-to-dispute-the-evidence-doesnt/

PART EIGHT

Those Left Behind

This section, "Those Left Behind," addresses one of the sad realities of the pandemic: all of the resources dedicated to the care of those infected with COVID-19 came at a cost. Funds usually dedicated to public services were diverted; programs and resources previously available were shuttered; and too many were left to "fend for themselves." "The Other Epidemic: Overdose Crisis" describes the lesser publicized tragedy of the pandemic years: the boom in opioid and other substance abuse and the resulting carnage. "Accessing Mental Health Services: An Expanding Public Need" recounts the challenge in combating one of the most awful dilemmas of these times: the need for mental health services had never been higher, yet the barriers to access never so high nor the constraints to their delivery so intractable. "From the COVID-19 Ashes: A Journey in Life Transformation" tells a story of loss and eventual triumph. The loss of employment due to the economic and social disruption caused by the pandemic was a condition suffered by millions, with a toll measured not only in billions of dollars but also in untold damage to the sense of self and worth. Happily, some have been able to recover from this loss stronger with a renewed (or redirected) sense of purpose. "Leading from the Ground: Families Supporting Families and Children with Disabilities" recounts the struggle faced by families of children with disabilities during the disrupted COVID years and the necessity for such families not only to band together to support each other but to actively advocate for resources and better public awareness of the challenges faced by these individuals and their families.

37 The Other Epidemic: Overdose Crisis

Meaghan Reaburn, PharmD, BScPhm, RPh
Clinical Pharmacist Lead, Manager, Quality & Risk, Canadian Mental Health Association Waterloo Wellington

Submitted 14 October 2022

The "Walking Dead." A once engaging individual, joking and kibitzing with those around them, now sits "lifeless," "blank." The overdose crisis is a reality now more than ever, taking the lives of countless individuals, leaving behind remnants of a life lived. The unprecedented population-level anxiety and isolation created during the pandemic gave rise to the perfect storm whereby substances took hold. Substance users were forced to use alone, compounding an already risky practice. Substances became the driver in many individuals' lives, other basic needs taking a back seat.

The data detailed herein is reflected in the report titled *Changing Circumstances Surrounding Opioid-Related Deaths in Ontario during the COVID-19 Pandemic*, prepared for the Ontario Drug Policy Research Network, Office of the Chief Coroner/Ontario Forensic Pathology Services, and Public Health Ontario.[1]

The research speaks volumes about the increase in opioid-related deaths. An opioid-related death is defined as "an acute intoxication/toxicity death resulting from the direct contribution of consumed substance(s), where one or more of the substances was an opioid, regardless of how the opioid was obtained."[1(p4)] Data from the Office of the Chief Coroner/Ontario Forensic Pathology Services looked at the period between February 2020 and December 2020, and found that the opioid-related deaths in Ontario increased by approximately 79.2 per cent. Overall, there was a 60 per cent increase in opioid-related deaths in 2020 as compared to the previous year. The largest increases were seen in Toronto, Ottawa, Peel, Region of Waterloo, and Sudbury. The report found the rate of overdose deaths more than doubled in fifteen of thirty-four public health units across Ontario.

The age groups identified as being most affected by fatal overdoses were individuals between the ages of 25 to 44, with a 61.4 per cent increase in deaths, and those aged 45 to 64, with a 119.5 per cent increase in mortality. Among women, a 43.6 per cent increase in opioid-related deaths occurred compared to a 93 per cent increase in men between February 2020 and December 2020. The vast majority of opioid-related deaths have been deemed accidental. Marginalized individuals have been affected to a far greater degree. Some of the programs designed to help the homeless during the pandemic were in fact harmful to this group of individuals, noted in data from the Office of the Chief Coroner showing an increase in overdose deaths at hotels and motels that were being utilized as COVID-19 isolation services.[1(p14)]

Contributing factors to the provincial increase in opioid deaths were deemed multifaceted, detailing changing access to health care services, changes to more toxic unregulated drug supply, changes in supports for substance users, increased anxiety and isolation, and early release of individuals from prisons.

When looking at primary substances related to the overdose crisis, fentanyl alone was found to be a direct contributor to opioid-related deaths, while all other opioid use decreased – including heroin, oxycodone, and morphine. An increasingly toxic drug supply was identified throughout the pandemic. Considerable variability in the prevalence of fentanyl in local drug supplies was linked to unreliable strength in batches of drugs purchased on the street. Disruptions in access to prescription opioids early on in the pandemic may have created a shift to reliance on access to opioids through unregulated drug supply. An attempt to mitigate this issue was introduced through legislative changes, which gave pharmacists the ability to adapt or renew prescriptions for controlled substances. This measure was taken to facilitate continuity of care for clients who may not have been able to see their primary care providers for renewals.

Ethical dilemmas arose throughout the pandemic with the integration of safe supply on-site in some shelters in Ontario. Multiple risks were brought to light. A key detail voiced by substance users themselves was that an environment had been set up with a "lack of need to hustle." Substance users found that they lacked motivation and did not need to do anything other than use their substance of choice. They were able to stay in one place with access to all of the basic necessities of life; an environment was created wherein they did not have the need to identify any other goals or motivations that would enable them to be active members of society. Safe supply within the shelter environment proved harmful where safe supply, food, shelter, health care, and medication were provided all in one location, the resultant outcome being that clients never left the shelter and overdoses occurred outside of the 9 a.m. to 5 p.m. safe supply hours without clinical staff for monitoring. Other identified risks included shelter staff observing clients using unregulated substances along with safe supply, some clients turning to the use of harder substances due to exposure to other substance users on-site, and drug dealing on-site. An environment was thus created where staff did not feel equipped to care for clients overdosing outside of safe supply hours, and a dichotomy of philosophy prevailed in which clients could access safe supply while living meaningful lives versus clients appearing as the "living dead," sitting motionless most days in a drug-induced fog.

The need to have clear boundaries and a separate site for provision of safe supply were identified by staff as key components of programming moving forward. Shelter staff identified the need for further collaboration and decision-making with regard to goals and direction for facilitation of the safe supply program. Individuals who were once described as engaged members of society with cyclical substance use have now become "zombies," barely able to look after the most basic activities of daily living. Individuals are found lying on the floor defecating themselves, being too high to care about the basic activities and necessities of daily living.

Looking at a broader scope of outcomes when implementing safe supply will be useful in informing best practices going forward. One of the goals is to create a safe environment for substance users where all individuals can have a good quality of life and be active members in their communities.

Harm reduction strategies were put in place during the pandemic, including naloxone distribution, low-barrier supervised consumption and treatment sites, legislative changes to enable pharmacists to adapt or renew prescriptions for controlled substances, and technology for drug checking to curb fatalities by overdose. Yet these measures were not enough.

The data shed light on the absolute necessity of investing in programming to support those who use substances. These programs include appropriate set-up and location of safe supply sites, consumption and treatment sites, and an increase in services that address harm reduction and housing.

As per the Drug Strategy Network of Ontario, some of the proposed solutions to combat the overdose epidemic include the following:

1 Declare the overdose death crisis an emergency under the Emergency Management and Civil Protection Act and create a provincial task force to address the crisis;
2 Expand and remove barriers to evidence-informed harm reduction and treatment practices throughout Ontario;

3 Eliminate the structural stigma that discriminates against people who use unregulated substances;
4 Increase investments in prevention and early intervention services that provide foundational support for the health, safety, and well-being of individuals, families, and neighbourhoods. This proposal could entail extended hours of safe supply and consumption and treatment sites, utilizing public health guidelines to continue to facilitate support, and evidence-based treatment for individuals during a pandemic.[2]

Much has been learned so far throughout the pandemic with regard to the overdose crisis. The significant isolation created during the pandemic escalated an already risky practice. How do we look to mitigate the impact should future pandemics arise, utilizing public health guidelines to still maintain personal connection, hope, and support to our most vulnerable? The hope would be that the insights gleaned be utilized to further develop priorities, policies, and practices that protect the lives of this group of individuals and quell the overwhelming loss endured due to this epidemic.

REFERENCES

1. Gomes T, Murray R, Kolla G, et al; Ontario Drug Policy Research Network; Officer of the Chief Coroner of Ontario/Ontario Forensic Pathology Service; Public Health Ontario. *Changing Circumstances Surrounding Opioid-Related Deaths in Ontario during the COVID-19 Pandemic.* Ontario Drug Policy Research Network; 2021.
2. Drug Strategy Network of Ontario. *Solutions to End the Drug Poisoning Crisis in Ontario: Choosing a New Direction.* Drug Strategy Network Ontario; 2022. Accessed June 2022. https://www.drugstrategy.ca/uploads/5/3/6/2/53627897/dsno_policy_solutions_final_2022-04-20_v2.pdf

38 Accessing Mental Health Services: An Expanding Public Need

Troy Rieck, PhD, C.Psych
Canadian Mental Health Association, Waterloo-Wellington, Ontario

Submitted 3 October 2022

"We can't keep going on like this." "This is bullshit." "What's it gonna take for something to change?!" These are but a few expressed sentiments heard during the pandemic, which has since been accepted as endemic. Understandable feelings of fear, exhaustion, anger, sadness, loneliness, despondency, and general psychological pain have reared an unwanted soggy mess of intra- and interpersonal turmoil among many members of our communities. While these sentiments have been attributed to the negative impact of the COVID-19 pandemic, they have subsequently been expressed towards our mental health system.

For context, it may be helpful to share some understanding as to who I am and where the impressions I'm sharing in this essay are coming from. While primarily working as a clinical and forensic psychologist in a well-established community mental health agency, I also maintain a private practice and provide consultation work for other leading mental health care organizations in my local community. As well, I have achieved competency in industrial/organizational psychology (more simply, business/work-related psychology), which has bolstered my appreciation for broader system-level implications. While my initial interests were to help high performers become better at their respective activities and achieve their dreams (whether it be in business, sport, or life), my usual day-to-day attention has shifted to supporting efforts to provide the best care possible to those who are most in need of mental health services. Well, who is most in need? I will answer this question further along, including the implied triage-related language ("most" in need), but it is safe to say that the pandemic has affected us all.

As identified in the Chief Public Health Officer's report on the state of public health in Canada 2020,[1] the pandemic posed an unprecedented threat to the well-being of Canadians. It was identified as a severe global health emergency, which resulted in strict confinement conditions, lost jobs, bankrupt businesses, closed schools, and a decline in economic growth and risk for recession. The report also clearly noted that the impact of the pandemic was unequal. More colloquially, we can simply say something to the effect of "the rich got richer, and the poor got poorer." Regarding impact, there was an exponentially more negative impact on those who are marginalized and disadvantaged, as they already had reduced resources (for example, psychosocial, material, biological, health behaviours, and system access). Canadian research by Dozois[2] and Mental Health Research Canada[3] revealed that experiences of high to extremely high anxiety quadrupled and that high degrees of depressive symptoms more than doubled. This research also expressed anticipation that depressed affect would worsen in the context of ongoing isolation and distancing, identified an increase in alcohol and cannabis use, and noted that the perceived quantity and quality of mental health support had decreased since the onset of the pandemic. Further Canadian research by Gadermann and colleagues examining the impacts of the pandemic on family mental health[4] found that, regarding parents with children at home, there was deterioration in their mental health, increased alcohol consumption, increased suicidal ideation, and increased concern regarding domestic violence; nearly a quarter of the parents perceived their children's mental health to have worsened as well. The negative impact of COVID has most obviously been identified as having negative impacts on physical health, but the broader ramifications of the pandemic clearly include a negative impact on our mental health – the extent of which we have yet to understand as concerns of an "echo pandemic" have persisted.

During the throws of the pandemic, hospital staff and units, and related health care professionals, were (at times) redeployed to make way and attempt to support the physical needs of those who contracted COVID. As the physical needs of those afflicted increased, the capacity for hospitals to manage people with significant mental health needs decreased. Triage factors certainly came into play. Community organizations who typically would not be relied upon to try to stabilize people struggling with significant mental health difficulties (Tier 5 – severe and complex patients/clients; for example, high risk for suicide, acute /chronic and atypical psychotic experiences) started to be viewed as a primary option. Inpatient admissions for severe mental health issues appeared to decrease due to alternate needs/demands. Consequently, as there was an increase in the need for mental health supports and services due to efforts to adapt to the effects of the pandemic, so too mental health services needed to try to manage more acute severity of mental health issues in the community. Further complicating this experience, which was notably scary for many community mental health services providers who were not accustomed to managing such risk in the community (feeling the increased pressure of the importance of their interventions as well as not having been well trained to manage such risk), concerns about contracting COVID resulted in a significant shift in how services were delivered: providers would only see people in person if they were high risk and it was absolutely necessary.

As a proxy for in-person connection, what was once developed and used primarily for supporting remote patients/clients, telemedicine (treatment by phone or video), quickly became the norm. The transition to online virtual platforms was rather astonishing as mental health care providers mobilized to find ways to continue to work with people in need. Consistently, colleges of various disciplines (nursing, psychology, physicians, pharmacists, social workers, psychotherapists) scrambled to establish respective guidelines and suggested best practices to approach virtual delivery of mental health services. Indeed, guidance on approached work with patients/clients was a moving target as the pandemic progressed, which unfortunately did not help to assuage the ongoing confusion and discrepancies among the practices of various mental health care providers. Sadly, this situation was challenging for both the patients/clients and the practitioners themselves as they tried to do their best to meet the respective needs but also needed to make personal judgment calls on how to approach their work (sometimes in ways that were different from their colleagues). Additional lack of consistency in this regard simply added to the confusion about how, and in what way, patients/clients might receive services, piling on further inconsistency and unknowns in an already anxiety-provoking environment. Aligned with this challenge, mental health service providers were also working on their own to manage the shared experience of ambiguity that all members of society experienced throughout the pandemic.

Anxiety, in the context of ambiguity, will (often) fill the space. In other words, anxiety thrives in the context of the unknown (or what is perceived to be uncertain/unstable). For some mental health care providers and patients/clients alike, this anxiety resulted in running on adrenaline and a wide variety of coping strategies in an effort to manage our experiences until some semblance of consistency could be seen. Unfortunately, many of these "coping strategies" are such that they are not meant to be used for a long period of time (for example, externalized coping efforts – seeking things outside ourselves to help, like alcohol and drugs). Furthermore, the adaptive coping strategy of connecting with friends and family who have been positive influences in our lives was quickly torn away from us, beyond the use of phone, email, and/or virtual means. As well, distance from our colleagues and usual routines was markedly disrupted. Talk about a paradigm shift. Many mental health care providers were fearful to work in person (some still are), and the pendulum has since shifted to anxiety about seeing others in person and what that might be like (akin in some respects to social anxiety), which has further debilitated return to in-person work. People have also become accustomed to online work and their pandemic-established routines, which are once again being disrupted for change. While other businesses are demonstrating success in shifting to virtual work primarily (for example, banking), and despite some promising evidence that telehealth can be effective (see, for example, a study by Fernandez and colleagues[5]; and studies by Lin, Fernandez, and Bonar[6]; Lin, Casteel, and colleagues[7]; and Lin, Heckman, and Anderson[8]), this evidence is not accurate for all populations being served. People experiencing severe and complex mental health concerns have been identified as facing additional barriers (navigating technology, access to internet, access to devices, limited finances, safe/confidential space). Furthermore, while some may prefer virtual sessions, it is hard to put a price on the value of being able to see the mental status of someone in person to best assess their current functioning. Not surprisingly, lessons learned from quality-of-care reviews (following sentinel or adverse events that occurred during the pandemic) consistently identified COVID as a factor that disrupted processes set in place for supporting people who were at risk for dying by suicide or significant deterioration.

The pandemic further highlighted the difficulty of integrating care through coordination of information, particularly through electronic platforms. For example, lag time for uploading documentation into a system or sharing of information to relevant community partners was challenging. Needless to say, this problem is something that was previously challenging as privacy officers (and their respective organizations) did not come together to establish a shared understanding of circle of care, how to accept collateral information from other service providers and families, and how to ensure smooth transition of services (for example, shared discharge planning). While my understanding is that such difficulties are being discussed at various tables across the province (speaking specifically in Ontario), the pandemic certainly highlighted various gaps in our system that warrant further clarification and shared dedication towards resolution. Much like marriage and family counselling efforts, so too will the multifaceted dynamics need to be considered, as well as the fostering of trust among agencies and additional perseverance to try to understand each other. As one of my own highly respected colleagues likes to say, we are "better together."

I hope that my ramblings have elucidated some of the experiences that are learnings and areas of opportunity with respect to mental health care in our communities. The pandemic has been a magnifying glass for the system, a cause of increased and likely ongoing mental health needs, and, I hope, also an impetus for action.

REFERENCES

1. Chief Public Health Officer. *From Risk to Resilience: An Equity Approach to COVID-19*. The Chief Public Health Officers report on the state of health in Canada 2020. Public Health Agency of Canada; 2020. Accessed 20 July 2024. https://www.canada.ca/en/public-health/corporate/publications/chief-public-health-officer-reports-state-public-health-canada/from-risk-resilience-equity-approach-covid-19.html
2. Dozois DJA. Anxiety and depression in Canada during the COVID-19 pandemic: a national survey. *Canadian Psychology*. 2021;62(1):36–42. https://doi.org/10.1037/cap0000251
3. Mental Health Research Canada; Health Canada. Mental health during COVID-19 outbreak: poll #5 of 13 in series. Mental Health Research Canada; 2021. Accessed 20 July 2024. https://www.mhrc.ca/s/MHRC-Poll-5-Final-Public-Release.pdf
4. Gadermann AC, Thomson KC, Richardson CG, et al. Examining the impacts of the COVID-19 pandemic on family mental health in Canada: findings from a national cross-sectional study. *BMJ Open*. 2021:11(1):e042871. https://doi.org/10.1136/bmjopen-2020-042871. PMID: 33436472.
5. Fernandez E, Woldgabreal Y, Day A, et al. Live psychotherapy by video versus in-person: a meta-analysis of efficacy and its relationship to types and targets of treatment. *Clin Psychol Psychother*. 2021;28(6):1535–49. https://doi.org/10.1002/cpp.2594. PMID: 33826190.
6. Lin L, Fernandez AC, Bonar EE. Telehealth for substance-using populations in the age of coronavirus disease 2019: recommendations to enhance adoption. *JAMA Psychiatry*. 2020;77(12):1209–10. https://doi.org/10.1001/jamapsychiatry.2020.1698. PMID: 32609317.

7. Lin LA, Casteel D, Shigekawa E, et al. Telemedicine-delivered treatment interventions for substance use disorders: a systematic review. *J Subst Abuse Treat*. 2019;101:38–49. https://doi.org/10.1016/j.jsat.2019.03.007. PMID: 31006553.
8. Lin T, Heckman TG, Anderson T. The efficacy of synchronous teletherapy versus in-person therapy: a meta-analysis of randomized clinical trials. *Clinical Psychology: Science and Practice*. 2022;29(2):167–78. https://doi.org/10.1037/cps0000056

39 From the COVID-19 Ashes: A Journey in Life Transformation

Dorrette Ruddock, RN
Medical Surgical/Neuroscience Intensive Care Unit, Toronto Western Hospital, University Health Network

Submitted 6 July 2022

Practically and approximately, 2 years ago COVID-19 transformed our lives. Some experienced death and family sadness, while others found new life, like a breath of fresh air. The latter is what happened in our family. Let me tell you, it has truly been a whirlwind of change, if I can use such an analogy.

Unfortunately, things did not go well at first. At the inception of the pandemic, my husband was laid off from his job as a cook in a hotel kitchen, where he had been employed for 20 years. COVID has taught us so much, mainly how integral and important family is. When all was locked down, all we had was family. A few days after my husband lost his job, Sasha, our second daughter who is social media–inclined and very savvy, approached her Dad with a challenge. She said, "Daddy, I know that there are a lot of my friends who are locked in because of COVID restrictions and are now unable to use Uber Eats or go to the restaurant. I know they love food, but they are all facing a challenge in the kitchen because they can't cook. Why don't you and I start a cooking tutorial via YouTube?"

Deddy's Kitchen, sharing my husband's and our family's love of Jamaican cooking, our culture, traditions, and recipes, was formally started within a few weeks of the start of the lockdown. Our daughter Sasha is such an inspiration to us, and we appreciate so much that, as a young lady, she took time out of her busy schedule to help her parents. Her vision and creativity is extraordinary. My family was thrown into the spotlight overnight.

Yet soon thereafter, right at the pinnacle of the lockdown, my husband, daughter, and I got infected. My daughter and I had minimal symptoms, but the story was very different for my husband. With no treatments available, we were at home using herbal remedies for symptom relief. These remedies did not help him though. On the Thursday night of that week, I went to bed and awoke in the night with an unshakeable feeling that I must take my husband to the hospital in the morning. Waking up early on Friday morning, I asked him how he was, and he said, "Not good." We immediately helped him get ready to go to our nearest hospital.

I took my husband to the Brampton Civic Hospital Emergency Department, where he was immediately admitted to the intensive care unit (ICU) and placed on high-flow oxygen. He had an arduous time. He was placed on all the medications available – these were mainly steroids – but his oxygen saturation was not improving. I have always had a very strong faith; my belief in God has always helped me in times of trouble, in times of need. But I was so worried. I had already seen the havoc and destruction COVID could cause when, as a nurse, I cared for people in the ICU. I was so afraid of losing the man I love. This period of time was one of the longest and hardest that I have ever lived.

Then one evening, an exceptional nurse was assigned to care for my husband for a few shifts and decided to prone him (have him lie on his stomach) for most of the 24 hours that make up a day. At this time, proning patients was not being done routinely as its benefits were not fully appreciated. The nurse helped my husband prone over a 48-hour period, and ever so slowly he started to turn the corner. His oxygen saturation started to improve, and he started to feel better. He was discharged from hospital after 2 long weeks.

My husband was isolated for another 2 weeks at home. Post isolation, he started to exercise again, and his physical strength started slowly to improve. Within a month or so, he was back taping *Deddy's Kitchen*. His love of cooking, his laughter, and his joy in the family's participation in choosing recipes and filming each episode are contagious. What started as a challenge in a moment of adversity has transformed our lives. *Deddy's Kitchen* has become an international sensation. We have had the opportunity to meet such amazing employees from YouTube and Google. My husband doesn't need to return to being a chef in a hotel restaurant; he has now had the opportunity to retire. Now we all get to spend more time together enjoying sharing our love of food, family, and culture with friends and followers around the world. We were awarded the YouTube Plaque for 100,000 subscribers, and at present our subscribers are over 300,000 and growing.

As an ICU nurse myself, I worked on the front line for the entire pandemic, and I am still at it. I have seen and encountered many things, but I still give thanks. Because of our faith in God and our belief in our Heavenly Father, I believe my husband has been given another opportunity. At this time, I am getting teary eyed because writing this chapter has uncovered such deep memories of such a trying and challenging time. This particular verse of the Bible (NKJV) came to have even deeper meaning for us: "I can do all things through Christ who strengthens me" (Philippians 4:13).

It is so easy to feel overwhelmed when life throws unexpected hardships our way. I wanted to share our story, to remind us all of how lives can be unexpectedly transformed after what seemed like the worst of times. Despite all we have lived through, COVID has taught me and my family that it's so important not to lose hope, so important to keep yourself open to new opportunities – just look at *Deddy's Kitchen*!

40 Leading from the Ground: Families Supporting Families and Children with Disabilities

Tina Trigg, PhD
Associate Professor of English, The King's University, Edmonton, Alberta; Canada Board Director, President, and Past President, Inclusion Edmonton Region

Submitted 27 September 2022

The year 2020 is a time period many would like to forget with the stasis, uncertainty, and fear that accompanied the onset of COVID-19. Isolation and loss of routine was difficult for most and utterly debilitating for others. As a parent and advocate for individuals with disabilities, the consistent invisibility of this part of our community in policies and practices was more than theoretical. I watched in horror as triage protocols put my daughter – and thousands of other children – at risk by deeming her less likely to receive care and by restricting the presence of a support person should she be hospitalized. I listened with growing alarm as policymakers cut educational support staff and shifted schools online, while parents tried to modify our own employment by working from home, changing hours, or increasingly, leaving jobs to provide caregiving and support for children learning online. Scheduled activities were cancelled, venues shuttered, and – for a time – even playgrounds were cordoned off with yellow police caution tape. Life felt surreal. People were told to stay home with the inequitable assumption that home was a safe place for everyone. Families of children with intellectual disabilities were no different – we, too, were exhausted, bewildered, and isolated – and in the middle of all this upheaval, many of us had to navigate additional vulnerabilities: physical, emotional, social, and financial.

As global data emerged, the level of risk for certain populations to develop severe or fatal outcomes from the COVID virus became a more clearly defined spectre. My family grappled with the terrifying reality of a five-to-tenfold increased likelihood of hospitalization or death for one of our children. As national and international experts pored over emerging information and conducted experiments, families struggled with clearly communicating the fluctuating recommendations on face masking, social distancing, and surface or airborne contaminants. Children could no longer welcome a friend with a hug or even a fist bump; human touch was suddenly forbidden, and faces were confusingly hidden behind masks or contained in two-dimensional frames on computer screens. For children with reduced verbal articulation or developmental delay, these were formidable barriers to communication, and for all children, these barriers severely restricted and redefined play. The world shrank (for all of us) as we stepped apart. It seemed everyone was struggling (admittedly or not), and a few months into the pandemic, now recognizing we were confronted with a long-haul social challenge, the essential question became, How then do we live?

This was a question that needed to be answered both personally and in community, for one thing was clear: we cannot live well in isolation. As trauma and crisis psychologists reminded us, there are helpful and harmful ways to respond in times of crisis; we needed to choose the helpful responses for ourselves, our families, our communities. Moreover, experts affirmed that times of uncertainty create a tremendous need for trusted leadership that provides practical steps and restores hope. Awareness of this need to lead confronted me every day in the eyes of my two children – in the wariness that thinly disguised their fear and the grey cloud of defeat that rolled in with yet another cancellation notice. People withdrew either in fear or out of self-defence to avoid further pain or disappointment, and mental health made headlines. But how do we lead when there are no clear answers and we too feel knocked down flat on our backs? We lead from the ground – however we are able.

◆◆◆◆◆

When March 2020 brought global shutdown, the sudden halt resulted in extensive cancellations, not only for individuals but for organizations – particularly community groups and non-profits that rely on volunteer labour. Inclusion Edmonton Region is one such organization: a grassroots non-profit family-based advocacy organization in Alberta,

Canada, that supports persons with developmental disabilities to lead meaningful lives fully included in all aspects of community life. No stranger to crisis, Inclusion Edmonton Region is composed of families who regularly face discrimination and systemic barriers to inclusion; many families, including mine, find the organization in a time of personal crisis, identify with its values and vision for social change, and become supporters of the community-based movement for inclusion. Importantly, the organization is made up of and serves people at all ages and stages of life – from infancy to old age. As a family-based advocacy organization, Inclusion Edmonton Region seeks to affirm and empower individuals with intellectual disabilities, their families, and allies to enjoy fully inclusive lives through the lifespan in community – home, school, work, and recreation. In a necessary effort to prevent viral spread, pandemic restrictions severely impacted these same areas. Not one of them looked the same as before, and families struggled with navigating all of them. Here, then, was part of an answer to how we, as families, could lead to provide practical steps and restore hope: in shared vulnerability and fully prepared to make mistakes together, we could lead from wherever we were – including from the ground – in the stuff of everyday life at home, school, work, and play.

This realization provided the board of directors with a framework. The changed realities of a global pandemic created other significant limitations: reduced timelines (8 months rather than 12), meeting format (virtual rather than in person), and perhaps most importantly, personal capacities (fragile, variable, and unpredictable for everyone). Leadership demanded honouring all of these limits – and with as much grace as possible. Moving forward required creativity, strategy, and teamwork, but remaining dormant in the face of desperate need was just not an option for an organization that believes in possibility.

A key goal of Inclusion Edmonton Region in that first year of COVID was to remain true to our inclusive vision in a sustainable way; that is, we vowed to be realistic about capacities and still be relevant to emerging needs during the unusual, ever-changing demands of the pandemic. Taking our focal areas of home, school, work, and recreation, we reimagined a full-day in-person advocacy workshop into two half-day virtual workshops. These sessions targeted two areas of urgent concern for families of individuals with disabilities: education and financial support. Children with disabilities had been largely overlooked and sidelined in the emergency online learning of spring 2020; as fall loomed, the ongoing uncertainties of how to access and sustain inclusive education in the face of a full year of unpredictable shifts to online learning filled many families with unease. The Advocacy 101 workshop sought to dispel some of that fear by clarifying current legislation and family rights; the goal was to provide strategies and resources for inclusive education advocacy and to counter misinformation. Despite extensive research evidence that all children have improved social and educational outcomes in inclusive mainstream classrooms comprised of same-age peers, families of children with disabilities are regularly pushed towards segregated programs – even when we explicitly request inclusive education. The pressure to segregate only increased during the pandemic as families were strongly encouraged to choose online learning or home schooling to limit viral exposure – despite the considerably increased risk to mental health posed by ongoing isolation. Consequently, this expert-led workshop sought to equip families to be confident advocates for their children's learning before the school year began, to weigh personal risks – both short- and long-term, physical and mental – and to connect families to the broader movement for inclusion.

Beyond school age, families of individuals with disabilities faced increasing stress and difficulty accessing provincial funding for support needs – needs that were changing alongside social policies. Closure of schools, clubs, workplaces, recreation facilities, sports fields, community groups, and places of worship meant a consequent removal of supports normatively provided in those spaces; instead, individuals with disabilities were at home 24/7. In a seemingly untenable situation, families were increasingly stressed by a lack of available personal support workers and, at the same time, by the additional exposure risk they brought every time one stepped into our homes. The pandemic intensified already escalating problems that confronted families seeking to secure or sustain government support to cover extraordinary expenses. Clearly, there was room here for providing practical steps and restoring hope – for leadership (if imperfect) – as we all navigated this time of crisis. Hence, Inclusion Edmonton Region organized an expert-led half-day virtual workshop on navigating financial support that filled to capacity, showing the urgent need for clear information, practical strategies, and in-depth resources, as well as for hope and solidarity. While staggering the two virtual events a few months apart was more work administratively and required extra time as well as significant recasting of content, the changes also increased the ability of more community members to attend and from a broader geographical area. Considering the urgency of issues, level of stress, and broad impact of the content, the unforeseen benefit of reaching more families was definitely worthwhile.

While these two sessions were aimed at practical issues and obstacles, a movement for inclusion is driven by a progressive vision for social change, equity, and dignity for all persons. Hence, as the calendar flipped to 2021 with no end of the pandemic in sight, we recognized how easy it could be to lapse into "January blues." For families struggling with ongoing isolation, restrictions from travel or gathering for festivities, loss of loved ones, and perhaps a frightening feeling of stasis and uncertainty, Inclusion Edmonton Region sought to provide a safe space to acknowledge that grief together and – within all the different limitations we have – to plan for leaning in to a full, meaningful life. Led by experienced facilitators in small groups, "Living Inclusive Lives in the New Year" was an opportunity to gather virtually with our membership to collectively refresh our vision (in a challenging time) by networking, sharing stories/strategies/goals, and to offer some resources to support both creating and sustaining fully inclusive lives in every aspect of our communities. Of the three major events, this New Year gathering required the most vulnerability to organize and to attend; sharing our deep sorrows requires a level of trust and intimacy that is difficult to achieve in a timed, online meeting with people you know only a little – or perhaps not at all. With appropriate guidelines to ensure that verbal participation at any point was voluntary and all voices were respectfully heard, many of those attending were surprisingly open. People seemed hungry for meaningful connection and to be able to share in a non-judgmental space what has been difficult in order to make room for choosing one tangible step to move (even just a little bit) towards what is good – whether at school, home, work, or in recreation. No one had magic solutions, but the range of participants drew on hard-won experience; we could offer one another affirmation in the face of discouragement, new ideas to tailor or try at different life stages, and strength to keep investing in a community where everyone belongs.

It was a session that reminded us of the need for human relationships that connect beyond the surface and of the essential truth of human agency: even within limits, we have choice. As concentration camp survivor Viktor Frankl asserts in *Man's Search for Meaning*, "everything can be taken from a [person] but one thing: the last of the human freedoms – to choose one's attitude in any given set of circumstances, to choose one's own way."* While we cannot dictate what life will bring, we can

---

* Frankl VE. *Man's Search for Meaning*. Lasch I, trans. Beacon Press; 2014:62. Frankl's *Man's Search for Meaning* was originally published in German in 1946; the first English translation was published in 1959.

choose how we face it and what we focus on; our attitude determines our actions and what we imagine is possible. We are each called to lead – even in the darkest days – and to do what we can, knowing our capacities will change and we might not always predict how. To do the little we can is better than choosing to do nothing. This stark reality and the ongoing need for self-compassion may be among the most important truths COVID has exposed.

Nonetheless, the pandemic brought many unbearably difficult circumstances to families; some policies starkly discriminated against persons with disabilities – often by overlooking additional vulnerabilities and so literally not seeing them. Inclusion Edmonton Region worked at a local level to partner with families of children with developmental disabilities, always seeking to connect individuals who share a vision for the broader social movement for inclusion. Similarly, we partnered with Youth @ the Table through Volunteer Alberta to bring young people onto our non-profit governance board to hear their voices, and we supported the provincial work of Youth for Inclusion that seeks to develop leadership in youth for building fully inclusive communities. If anything, the pandemic revealed how interconnected we are as humanity, yet how easily we also draw boundaries and simply fail to see others. Thus, while local work may appear autonomous, it is actually enabled by provincial, national, and international advocacy organizations concurrently working for meaningful change and social justice in their respective spheres. In the case of Inclusion Edmonton Region, these direct partners are Inclusion Alberta, Inclusion Canada, and Inclusion International. These larger-scale organizations work tirelessly to advocate for families and children with developmental disabilities on individual, social, and systemic levels.

During the pandemic, all levels of engagement have been necessary to protect adults and children with disabilities. Mental health risks – at levels of isolation regularly experienced by individuals in the disability community – were now being felt by the general public and so were raising considerable alarm. General unemployment rates made headlines as they inched upwards – though never above single digits – despite the brutal fact that individuals with intellectual disabilities in Canada experience ten times that rate of unemployment as a norm, not resulting from a pandemic. Disabled citizens in Canada were the last to receive federal pandemic-related financial relief – and only after a strong national advocacy campaign. Public health measures were equally problematic: large-scale, highly public, and controversial campaigns were needed to advocate for changes to COVID vaccine prioritization and to triage protocols in order to address increased vulnerabilities in persons with disabilities. Securing these protections was the result of intense provincial and national advocacy campaigns successfully undertaken against discriminatory systems and policies fuelled by unconscious bias that devalues persons with disabilities.

Within this context, every piece matters. To affirm and equip families with current, correct, clear information is essential; to empower families to become strong advocates for their children with disabilities creates a committed network of like-minded persons working for social justice in our own community: this is local-level work where families support families. A successful movement for inclusion requires all levels of engagement, and we all have a role to play – if we so choose – at home, work, school, and in recreation to ensure every person has an equal right to belong in our communities. We need not settle for less. Believing in possibilities for a better world, we lead from the ground – or wherever we are.

Organizational websites for further information:

Inclusion Alberta (https://inclusionalberta.org)
Inclusion Canada (https://inclusioncanada.ca)
Inclusion Edmonton Region (https://www.inclusionedmonton.org)
Inclusion International (https://inclusion-international.org)
Volunteer Alberta (https://volunteeralberta.ab.ca)
Youth @ the Table / Y@TT (https://youthgov.volunteeralberta.ab.ca/)
Youth for Inclusion (https://inclusionalberta.org/what-we-do/youth-for-inclusion/)

PART NINE

Reconsider/Reflect/Revisit/Return

Our collection ends with "Reconsider/Reflect/Revisit/Return," two essays that grapple with the long-term effects of the pandemic on our collective psyche and try to account for the losses suffered and damage done. "How COVID-19 Made Salient the Need to Reconsider the Relationships Between Health Care Providers, Their Family, Friends, Co-Workers, and the Public" puts forward a hard, hard truth: that the pandemic forever altered the relationships between health care workers and the lay public and those within the various elements of health care itself, the consequences of which will only be evident in years to come. "Science and Truth During and After COVID-19" acknowledges one of the great losses of the pandemic – the wider public's loss of faith in the integrity of science – and details the ongoing struggle over what "truth" means in the current public domain and who gets to define it. The conflict over the nature of science, truth, and meaning not only underpinned the societal fracturing of the past 3 years but looms large over our collective future, be it a united or a fractured one.

41 How COVID-19 Made Salient the Need to Reconsider the Relationships Between Health Care Providers, Their Family, Friends, Co-Workers, and the Public

Matyas Hervieux, BSc (Hons), DHS, MA, MD, CCFP(EM)
Department of Emergency Medicine, University Health Network, Toronto

Submitted 24 February 2023

I worked, and continue to work, throughout this pandemic on the front line as an emergency room physician in urban, rural, and remote hospitals across Canada. To understand the effect that the COVID-19 pandemic has had on my relationships with family, friends, the public, and other health practitioners, I think it is important to understand the relationship I had with these groups before COVID and to look at how they have changed since the pandemic started.

Perhaps a good place to begin is to consider the well-known lines of the British poet Thomas Gray, who wrote in his "Ode on a Distant Prospect of Eton College":

> where ignorance is bliss,
> 'Tis folly to be wise. (stanza 10)

Over the years, these lines have resonated with me at times when I have been confronted by the burden of having medical knowledge, that is, "wisdom," when others around me have enjoyed the "bliss of ignorance" that comes without having medical training. Perhaps the most painful example of this burden was when I listened to an oncologist tell my mother she had metastatic triple-negative breast cancer – which I knew to be a death sentence – but then I had to be careful to demonstrate optimism in front of my mother and family members as she sought to fight the odds and seek "curative" treatment. After my mother's death, I often reflected on the burden that medical knowledge places on its practitioners in general, and on me in particular, especially at that time.

Although I call it a burden, the benefits of medical knowledge and being trained about the scientific method obviously come with considerable privileges and advantages. In many ways, being a physician among non-medical family and friends puts us in a truly privileged position. Most importantly, we have the advantage of understanding complex medical knowledge, and we understand how to advocate within, access, and navigate a complex medical system when our family and friends, or we ourselves, fall ill.

We are also trusted to be involved in the most intimate details of our loved one's lives, oftentimes in situations when they are most vulnerable and scared. Usually when other important family members' and confidantes' opinions are devalued, our opinions are respected, relied upon, and trusted. The fact that our experience and expertise give our opinions more weight in the health decision-making of those in our personal networks provides us with a sense of control and agency that makes it easier for us to cope when one of our loved ones is struggling with illness. This agency, in turn, can lend us confidence that most of the time medical decisions made by our loved ones will go the way we feel will give them the best chance at a good outcome. This realization helps diminish some of the anxiety we otherwise would feel if decisions were made that did not accord with our perspective.

Ultimately, the extent that we are affected by family's and friends' medical decision-making is directly related to how close we are to those individuals and how a change in their health status or death might affect us emotionally, financially, and so on. But the decisions made by our family and friends, except in rare circumstances, do not affect or risk our own personal physical health and safety (a reality, which, as discussed below, has changed dramatically since the onset of COVID).

It is true that the "burden" of having medical wisdom, at times, is exhausting and intrusive. We are not infrequently solicited for medical opinions on our days off, during a shift, or from random people we meet at a social gathering. At times, we are called upon to take the lead in managing our family's and friends' health care, including speaking with other medical professionals who are caring for our loved ones, even if our specialty has nothing to do with the specialty of the other provider! Yet even though at times it can feel intrusive to be solicited for help, upon reflection, most of us realize that we should be quite honoured to be called upon by those in need and that we have the connections to help them access care in a timely manner. We should be grateful that our medical "wisdom" commands respect and appreciation, and helps those we care about access appropriate and timely care.

Yet being a physician when a family member faces illness is a challenging and difficult role, made increasingly so in proportion to the closeness of the relationships and the severity of the illness. At such times, we must navigate our own emotions and grief while trying to remain supportive and optimistic: we must be "ignorant" and "wise" at the same time. My mother's journey with cancer hit me hard; physicians are human, and to see someone you love struggle with serious illness, face difficult decisions, and have a poor outcome is never easy. It is perhaps harder in some ways as we cannot unlearn what we have been taught: there is no possible moment of refuge in ignorance.

Clearly, the same burden of medical knowledge pertains to the relationships we have with our patients. Our jobs demand that we must see people at their most vulnerable, provide hope when we can and inspiration even at times when the odds are stacked against our patients. We must negotiate the burden of medical knowledge with the awareness that medicine is not an exact science and that, no matter how bleak a prognosis, we must help our patients live the best lives they can.

Fortunately, patient-centred decision-making has softened some of the burden placed on practitioners as we navigate the process of medical decision-making with our patients. We now routinely inform patients about the uncertainty of many medical procedures and the unpredictability of the outcomes of those procedures; rather than advising patients on what to do, we assist patients in making their own decisions.

This patient-centred approach has had clear benefits for patient autonomy. But it also has clear limitations for patients, the most important of which is that it is simply unfair to expect patients – who need to make complex life-altering or life-ending decisions for themselves or their dependents – to somehow be able to understand the medical knowledge and to develop the critical appraisal skills that come with scientific training to make a truly informed decision. Nonetheless, we trust that our experiences and medical training will help bridge the gaps in our patients' understanding about the medical scenarios that confront them.

In short, even before the pandemic struck, the role that physicians play in medical decision-making had changed: our voice may carry considerable weight, but our opinion ideally should be weighed against the expectations, goals, and needs of a patient, their family, and other resources when making medical decisions. It is ultimately the patient who will make the final decision. We simply hope that – regardless of whatever resources the patient may access – our opinion carries enough weight to steer a patient in the direction that will give them the best chance of a good outcome.

For these reasons, after my mother died, I was grateful to return to providing medical knowledge to those whose decision-making would not have such a profound impact on me personally. Unfortunately, the COVID pandemic hit not long after my mother died. For the first time in a long time, I was thrust into the throws of "ignorance" along with everyone else regarding COVID because the information was simply not available to provide certainty on how to protect ourselves, our loved ones, our patients, and our communities from this deadly virus. Like the population in general, our ignorance surrounding COVID's transmission, treatment, and long-term effects was not blissful: this ignorance was terrifying. All any of us could do was to engage with emerging information and try to appraise it and make informed decisions about what to do to protect ourselves, and those around us, from COVID.

Luckily, as medical professionals, most of us have been trained to engage with and interpret emerging scientific research and discourse, so we can quickly sift through, and act upon, the emerging body of knowledge pertaining to the COVID pandemic. Although we understood that there would be no double-blinded randomized control studies to rely upon, we are trained to understand the strength and weaknesses of emerging cohort studies, case studies, and the reliability of expert opinions. And even though this emerging information (especially in the early stages) was extremely limited and often speculative, we were able to formulate educated opinions and implement practices that we had some confidence in.

Arguably, the ignorance surrounding COVID was all the more terrifying for front-line workers, who were expected to continue to work and to risk our lives and personal safety with limited knowledge, limited supplies, and limited support. As we health care providers attended Town Hall meetings and engaged with emerging clinical evidence, some of this ignorance dissipated, and we began to understand the importance that public health measures such as mask mandates, lockdowns, and other restrictions would play in mitigating the effects of this pandemic, in general, and would help to keep us safe in our workplaces, in particular. And by "flattening the curve," we hoped that these interventions would give our already-stressed health care system a fighting chance by avoiding the onslaught of sick people that so alarmingly overwhelmed the Italian and New York health systems.

These initiatives were key elements that needed to happen to protect all of us from COVID, especially when no vaccines were available.

Unfortunately, as scientific research and vaccines emerged that promised to help guide us safely through the pandemic, we were simultaneously bombarded with a cacophony of pseudoscientific voices that challenged emerging empiric evidence. The challenge that this pseudoscientific discursive presented was that it offered non-factual but plausible alternatives to a scientific approach that appealed to a wide range of followers, who included not only anti-vaxxers and so-called freedom fighters but also a surprisingly significant proportion of the population.

That scientific research and pseudoscientific misinformation were emerging and being disseminated at the same time meant that, for laypeople, the idea that they should privilege emerging scientific knowledge over pseudoscience and speculation was not so clear cut. But as "team members" and advocates for their own health, laypeople felt empowered to engage with emerging "health information" and make their own decisions about health practices and policy, even though it was impossible for most of them to differentiate science from pseudoscience or mere opinion.

Thus, the pandemic presented new epistemological dilemmas for society: How do laypeople discern what is valid research and what is mere speculation or even quackery? What kind of importance do laypeople put on quantitative research versus qualitative research? Do laypeople rely more on persuasive stories and opinion pieces or on evidence-based research when making life or death decisions?

Historically, laypeople have been trained to trust scientific information that has been around for long periods of time; the longer a treatment has been around and worked, the more reliable and trustworthy it would appear. Laypeople have never truly been given the opportunity or training to understand that it is the methodology which produces scientific research that gives this research credibility and that the methodology behind this research is what justifies implementing treatments/public health measures/and so on. It is the implementation of this research over time that confirms the research has real-world applicability and builds trust in the research, especially for laypeople.

With COVID, for the first time, many laypeople were being asked to blindly trust the scientific process without an understanding of the methodology that goes into these processes and without years of lived experience with similar forms of therapy. For example, the public were being told that novel mRNA vaccines were safe because scientists assured they would be safe; at the same time, the public were simultaneously being bombarded with information stating the dangers of this science from naysayers. Clearly, the novelty of these vaccines made them seem precarious, especially to populations who gain trust with medical interventions once they have been implemented and stood the test of time to ensure safety (for example, recall thalidomide). For these reasons, public education focused on demystifying the science behind the vaccines' production with the hopes that, if the public understood the methodology, they would change their perception about the safety of these vaccines. This strategy required an epistemological shift within the public domain that was surprising effective. Yet, for many, vaccines continued to be viewed as unsafe and risky – which they may be – perhaps especially to those inclined to anxiety, doubt, conspiracy theories, and in those populations with justifiable distrust of institutions based on historical abuse.

Another epistemological shift during the pandemic was in how the public appraised the effects of COVID and COVID-related deaths. For example, much of the public learned the term "comorbidity" for the first time. The public somehow concluded that, if someone had a comorbidity and died of COVID, the death was a result of the comorbidity and not COVID.

Likewise, if a patient died of COVID, we were immediately asked if they were vaccinated or not, with the implication that it was partly the patient's fault for their poor outcome. Yet, even if an unvaccinated person was more likely to became severely ill or die of COVID – which of course they are – the fact that COVID was responsible for this outcome was also not immediately accepted. As clinicians, we were constantly grilled about the comorbidities of the unvaccinated, with the implication that we were withholding information about these comorbidities simply to make the risk of being unvaccinated appear greater than it actually is or, alternatively, to make COVID appear more virulent than it really is.

Thus, another important epistemological shift that has come out of the pandemic is that much of the public no longer trust information provided by health care providers. It is assumed that health care providers withhold information to suit our own agendas and that the public has the right to openly challenge us and our experiences. While health criticism is not only important but necessary, the constant scepticism of our front-line experiences made it clear to us that, to many, our experiences were not important or respected. Rather than attempting to understand these experiences and support us through the loss we were witnessing, we instead experienced scrutiny that magnified our horror as we witnessed people from all walks of life succumbing to this virus.

Trust in health care professionals in general, and emerging scientific information regarding COVID in particular, was eroded further by the surprising number of health care practitioners who spoke out against restrictions, who wrote prescriptions arbitrarily for mask exemptions, and who rejected the importance of vaccinations. For laypeople – and for health care providers who were less confident in the science – the harm that these dissident health care providers caused cannot be overstated. By rejecting clear scientific evidence and encouraging the public to ignore public health measures, these irresponsible providers made scientific research appear arbitrary and mutable, undermined the voice of health care providers *en masse* by making us appear ignorant and driven by subjective bias, and sent mixed messages to laypeople who were seeking clear direction. And their dissidence gave fuel to conspiracy theorists, pseudoscientists, anti-vaxxer groups, and the like, which meant that, from the public's perceptive, the voice of health care providers appeared fractured and unreliable.

Another factor that caused health care providers to lose our credibility in the public eye was the unscientific response of politicians and public health authorities to the pandemic. The fact that politicians and public health authorities rejected clear scientific research that demonstrated the importance of restrictions, mask mandates, and other measures further undermined our credibility in the eyes of the public. As we advocated for such measures, we were met with further scrutiny and scepticism.

Combined, the above factors meant that the nature of the relationship between health care providers and our populations changed in significant and important ways throughout the pandemic. Indeed, prior to COVID, despite the limitations of the patient-centred model, the opinion of a physician still had significant influence. However, with COVID, there was no way to reconcile inconsistencies presented by patients whose preferences were to avoid mask mandates, who requested mask exemptions, or who refused to be tested for or accept that they or their family members had COVID once they tested positive. Instead of working collaboratively with us, a small subset of patients became abusive to clinicians, targeting us verbally and physically, and staging protests, which included invasions of hospitals by maskless protesters. One of my worst experiences was being berated by a family whose mother was dying of COVID. They were so convinced COVID was a hoax that they imagined me to be pretending their mother had COVID, and in doing so, I was not even trying to find and treat the real cause of their mother's suffering. If you take a moment to imagine how they must have felt, however mistakenly, you will easily be able to imagine how they treated me. This situation was made even more horrible and tragic by the realization that their own unvaccinated status would mean their mother would die without them by her side and that, in their eyes, we had killed their mother by failing to investigate her illness and treat her appropriately.

If it was not salient before COVID, the fallacy that the patient-centred model allowed for informed decision-making was laid bare during COVID. The emerging pandemic patient-centred model taught patients to devalue our suggestions, to engage with "the literature," and to formulate their own opinions about COVID, even though they were not given the tools to appropriately discern science from pseudo-science or information from misinformation; the consequence of our hands-off approach to advice-giving was that those who could not critically appraise information were subject to misinformation that would not only risk their health but jeopardize the health of the entire population. Moreover, the fact that so many people were unable to access their primary care providers – who are supposed to act as a stop gap for this type of misinformation – meant that the public had no objective and trusted voices to help them sort through what was science and what was misinformation.

Perhaps it is necessary, but there is an irony that our desire to empower and protect patients by encouraging them to be their own decision-makers ultimately left our entire society vulnerable to those generating misinformation about COVID, mandates, and vaccinations. Moving forward, we must reconsider how we are going to train the general public to be able to engage in the critical appraisal they need to protect themselves, and those around them, from such manipulation. We must also consider the ways we failed the public by limiting access to primary care providers when, arguably, many patients needed these providers the most.

Equally problematic is that the pandemic made it clear that a surprising proportion of the population does not have any interest in trying to think critically and scientifically. Critical thinking in general, and scientific thinking in particular, is inconvenient because it obligates the thinker to look at the evidence, its sources, and its biases and to weigh the evidence on the strength of the methodology that created it. It is not important, and in fact it is deleterious to the scientific method, if you have a desired outcome or finding you are hoping for: you need to remain objective and let the evidence guide your decision-making. Unfortunately, during the pandemic, it became clear that personal behaviour, public opinion, and public health policy were being informed by people's preferences. It was people's desire to not have mandates, to congregate, to unmask, and to refuse vaccinations that was guiding decision-making rather than evidence.

It was demoralizing as a clinician to learn how solipsistic and self-oriented a subset of our population had become or perhaps always were. That intelligent people were unwilling to follow mandates, for example, was not only intellectually disheartening but it was personally upsetting. First, it was disheartening because it was clear that self-oriented decision-making was not going to simply have an impact on the individual making the decision; rather, the consequences of this type of decision-making would impact the health and well-being of all our citizenry. It seems that many people in Canada have forgot this basic premise: to live in a democracy means that you do not have the right to do whatever you want whenever you want; instead, you give up some individual freedoms for the protection and benefit of all of us. Thus, the point of our socialized health care system, and our democracy, is that we accept that resources are limited and must be shared, and that it is each of our duty and obligation to behave in ways that ensure these resources are not squandered needlessly or overwhelmed; we must act responsibly and with a social conscience as individuals, which means our wants and freedoms come second to following public health policies that protect all of us. Sadly, many in our society have forgotten this fact, have never known this fact, or have absorbed too much of the liberal individualism south of our border and mistakenly believe freedom and democracy mean having whatever you want whenever you want it. For these reasons, the pandemic has caused disillusionment among many of us who see this type of movement towards liberal individualism to be not only uncivilized but also a real threat to social medicine and our democracy.

Second, and most disturbing to me, was the fact that, for the first time in my career, the medical decisions of my patients, friends, and family had a direct impact on my own health and well-being, as well as on my ability to work to help others in need. Indeed, as front-line workers throughout the pandemic, we worked for more than a year without vaccinations, and those members of the public who decided to act in irresponsible ways were directly jeopardizing the health and safety of every front-line worker and thereby indirectly jeopardizing the health and well-being of our loved ones and our patients.

It was disheartening to have family and friends who ignored mandates and eventually declined vaccinations because of personal preference, misinformation, and concerns about civil liberty. For the first time, as a physician, I experienced my professional opinions being discarded and dismissed in favour of misinformation and twisted science, even among those close to me. It was painful to witness one of my colleagues lose both parents to COVID just weeks before they were to be vaccinated due to exposure that was likely attributable to family members. It was similarly troubling that, as physicians, we were continually following protocols and procedures – not just at work but decontamination procedures when arriving at home – to protect our family and friends only to realize that, when our loved ones had the opportunity to protect themselves and us (and all those we care about), many chose to engage in high-risk behaviour that jeopardized their health and well-being and that of their family on the front line!

It was depressing to witness unmasked people in public, to hear stories of grandparents contracting COVID because they were asked by their children to provide childcare for their grandchildren, or to hear the stories of those who presented to the Emergency Department with COVID who had contracted it because they attended superspreader events during lockdown. These patient stories were painful reminders of how a subset of our population simply did not seem to care about the impact their decision-making would have on society, their loved ones, or front-line workers. It is still troubling to reflect on the myriad patients I saw during this time whose surgeries and procedures had been unnecessarily cancelled because of successive outbreaks of COVID that were completely preventable. The choices based on misinformation of our families, friends, and politicians translated into far too many heart-wrenching preventable severe illnesses and deaths.

The pandemic also changed the nature of the relationships many of us have with our colleagues and workplaces. It was demoralizing to listen to the complaints of co-workers who were under threat of being fired, or who were fired, because they declined vaccinations. It seemed shocking that anyone working in an emergency department would be willing to put everyone in that department at risk because of a lack of social responsibility predicated on personal preference, misinformation, fear, and so on. It was shocking that these individuals seemed oblivious to the potential harm their choice to avoid vaccination could cause to the rest of us and that they thought we would support their solipsism.

It was frankly horrifying to witness colleagues providing disinformation about COVID, championing conspiracy theories, or expressing xenophobic attitudes towards China. I suppose that Canadians do not tend to engage in deep political discussion at work, but the polarizing aspects of COVID, mandates, and the like made these conversations common, and it became salient how far some health care providers' political views seemed to deviate from scientific data and were predicated on narcissism, ignorance, or self-interest. The morale of our workplaces has never been so significantly undermined by the differences arising from many of these polarizing conversations.

Equally upsetting was witnessing health care providers showing up to work sick. Even now, workers routinely show up to work with colds, sore throats, or other respiratory symptoms, and these workers have not tested themselves for COVID because it is "just a cold" or because they do not want to have COVID and alter their schedules. Front-line workers routinely become ill because of colleagues who deny their symptoms or fail to understand that their mild symptoms could lead to severe symptoms for someone else.

I struggle when I realize that front-line workers are attending social events and superspreader events without wearing masks. I have felt the pressure to take my mask off in these events because I feel like the world has moved on from COVID, that everyone is choosing to be "blissfully ignorant," and I cannot. On the one hand, I realize that, at some point, we must move on. But, on the other hand, I feel that front-line workers should be the ones holding the line and protecting ourselves and our patients until this pandemic is truly over. Do I choose bliss or wisdom, ignorance or folly? I am still uncertain where I stand on this issue.

For all these reasons, for many front-line workers, COVID has affected our relationships with our family, friends, co-workers, and the public. Many of these relationships have become strained, and many front-line workers have simply given up and left their jobs. Those who remain have, to a large extent, stopped educating others about COVID because we no longer want the arguing, scrutiny, and disrespect that ensues. Perhaps the accusations of impropriety for any number of outlandish claims, such as falsely inflating COVID numbers or falsely attributing patients' deaths to COVID to make more money on death certificates, has taken its toll. Perhaps we are exhausted and feel defeated. There seems to be reluctance to share our ongoing experiences about COVID and COVID-related deaths because we don't want the scrutiny. Perhaps we have succumbed to the strain of having been harassed, demeaned, and even threatened in our workplaces by anti-vaxxers, conspiracy theorists, and "freedom fighters" who want to pick fights with health care workers.

In sum, this pandemic has taught many of us something that, in different ways, we had already feared: that a surprising number of people do not understand the work we do as front-line workers and that the risks to our safety are not fully appreciated. Society has moved on, stopped wearing masks, and acts like the pandemic is over because most seem to feel invincible, because they have either already had COVID, or because they are not worried about getting COVID due to vaccinations and the circulation of weaker variants. The impact that not masking or taking other measures continues to have on the front line, our hospitals, and our surgical wait times no longer appears to be a concern to the general public but only to those who need to care.

These experiences have taught us that we need to understand the fragility of respect for others in face of humankind's need to seemingly hear and believe what they want to believe. Yet, in the face of the appeal of disinformation and the existence of such disrespect, perhaps the most important question that arises from this pandemic is, What risks should we, as physicians and health care workers, be willing to take for others?

I am still grateful when I am out in public and I see someone wearing a mask, even if that mask offers that individual little protection. I imagine that those wearing masks are trying to send a message to front-line workers to let us know that somebody cares and that somebody still is making an effort to protect all of us.

The questions for us all are these: Is it acceptable for us, as health care providers, to allow ignorance to undermine our health care system and social democracy? Do we not have an obligation to educate the public? Should we not be advocating for schools to teach critical thinking so that our society does not continue to fall prey to misinformation? What is the obligation for the members of society at large to address these issues? Should we not all be alarmed about how our complacency is damaging our relationships with each other? Should we not be concerned about how our own protectionist attitudes are infringing on others' rights and undermining a convivial society? Is there no longer a place for duty and social responsibility in our society? Or do personal preferences and individual entitlements trump everything?

What I am slowly having to come to terms with is that it feels as if, in the pandemic milieu, people have given up: that "ignorance is bliss," and it truly is a "folly to be wise." Wisdom puts you at odds with your family, your friends, your community, and your co-workers.

If I could do it all again, sometimes I think I would prefer to be ignorant of the experiences I have had during the pandemic: I wish I had not seen pregnant women on ventilators; healthy people dying; those suffering from long COVID, myocarditis, or pulmonary embolisms; or experienced my own thrombotic event. I wish I had the "ignorant" optimism of a layperson who, once vaccinated, had the false security that they were protected from this deadly virus or who believed that, if they contracted COVID once vaccinated, they would pose little risk to their loved ones, co-workers, and others. I wish I could delude myself into believing that the choices I make do not negatively impact our society at large and our health care system in particular. But the sad reality is that we live in a world of sweatshops, corporate greed, social inequities, and child poverty in even the richest of countries; the self-interested choices we make every day impact the quality of life of other people, but we are, fortunately, not usually able to see that impact. COVID made salient that, even when confronted with the potential harm our decisions may cause to others, many of us make those decisions anyway.

If the burden of my medical knowledge is, at times, too much, then reflecting on the reality of the world as it is, at times, seems equally unbearable. But it is at times like these that we must reflect on our decisions and their outcomes. We must advocate for all people to re-engage with the social contract, put our self-interests aside, and commit to the well-being of one another.

Again, I am drawn to the wisdom of another poet, Alexander Pope, who, despite my atheism, summarized my feelings on this matter precisely in his 1733 "Essay on Man" when, in the last stanza of Epistle III, he wrote:

> Man, like the gen'rous Vine, supported lives;
> The Strength he gains is from th' Embrace he gives.
> On their own Axis as the Planets run,
> Yet make at once their Circle round the Sun;
> So two consistent Motions act the soul,
> And one regards *itself*, and one the *Whole*.
> Thus God and Nature link'd the gen'ral Frame,
> And bade Self-love and Social be the same.

42 Science and Truth During and After COVID-19

Peter G. Brindley, MD, FRCPC, FRCP
Professor of Critical Care Medicine, Adjunct Professor of Anesthesiology, Adjunct Professor, John Dossetor Health Ethics Centre, University of Alberta, Edmonton

Submitted 5 September 2022

At the time of writing (autumn 2022), a very real, very horrible war is still raging in the Ukraine. By contrast, look back over COVID-19 during 2022: what we North American doctors and nurses often gratuitously called "conflict" more often occurred in the comparative safety of cyberspace. It's important not to conflate literal and figurative war. Regardless, what this physician – and others who tried to engage the wider public during COVID – discovered was that, during any fight, "truth" can be the first victim, and "science" can be readily weaponized.

I became one of those talking-head doctors who went on TV and radio hoping to reassure and recommend. In order to do so, I found myself in parallel discussions about two issues: what truth is and is not; what science is and is not. I frequently failed, and therefore, among my many COVID lessons, I came to appreciate how science, truth, and the scientific method is regularly under attack. The following "science primer" is because I still long for a shared understanding and hope for détente. It is also because medicine's information war is far from over.

Previously, combatants might have argued that God was on their side. Now, in a reputedly secular time, it is about claiming to "own the truth" and "follow the science." The problem is that untruths – and

---

This chapter is adapted from "Science and Truth during the Covid-19 Pandemic" by Peter G. Brindley, published in *BMJ*, 2022;379:o3070. https://doi.org/10.1136/bmj.o3070 © 2022 BMJ Publishing Group Ltd. All rights reserved.

junk science – can become accepted as "gospel" merely by being repeated ad nauseum or found online. This fact is especially concerning when the internet can spread nonsense at least as fast as hard-won truth; or, as Brandolini's law cheekily states: it takes far more work to dispel BS than to produce it.[1] We titular academics might assume that our singular mission is to seek out new knowledge. By contrast, COVID taught us that it takes considerable effort just to hold our ground. While it is impossible to fully police the internet, we clinicians and scientists also need to walk the beat.

We need to engage because the "truth" is less owned by experts and reputable peer-reviewed sources. The internet has democratized communication but can also be – hyperbole aside – a disinformation superhighway and worldwide web of lies. Personalized search algorithms mean that, with a few innocent clicks, different people end up not only on different pages but in different realities. Without action, we run the risk of parallel "truths" on parallel tracks. This issue matters mightily because medicine is among the most searched and debated topics online, with an estimated 500 million daily tweets and 3.5 billion daily Google searches.[2] "Truth" refers to how closely something approximates reality and accuracy. Truth is not about popularity, convenience, allegiance, or political tribe.

"Science" is best understood as an intellectual and practical activity that deliberately studies the world, primarily through observation and experimentation. Each word of this definition matters, whether it be "deliberate" (rather than random) or "observation" (rather than just opinion). Carl Sagan – one of the first scientists to understand the need to engage with the public – added that science is not "static knowledge" but rather "a way of thinking" and an "ongoing commitment."[3] In other words, it is a philosophical pursuit by which we inch towards an ever more confident truth. Science is as much a verb (how you think) as a noun (what you believe).

The nuance of the scientific method is lost in angry tweets. It can also be lost in our schools, and universities, if students are conditioned to cram in, and spew out, what they believe to be eternal truths. "Truth" and "science" come from a lifelong commitment to the highest level of evidence, not from cherry picking favoured observations. Science really is a "discipline" in that it takes hard work and self-control. Its beating heart is the scientific method, which involves making observations, forming hypotheses, fashioning predictions, conducting experiments, and objectively analysing results. It must be iterative and plausible, and if the best evidence does not support the hypothesis, then it is rejected. People might like a politician's exaggerated certainty, but humanity is better off inching towards a more robust scientific truth.

Science is not owned by any group, and there must be room for diversity. Moreover, something does not qualify as "science" simply because it is published somewhere, or because somebody with a science degree said so. While we must remain open to plausible (that is, testable and rejectable) ideas, that does NOT mean that *nothing* is truly known, and *anything* is equally likely. The scientific method dispassionately advocates for the truth and, therefore, must throw out failed or highly unlikely ideas. It means trying to disprove what we might want to be true. This is why the truth can change overtime, even if that idea seems counterintuitive at first.

Science may turn some people off because findings need to be accurate more than expedient. Moreover, questions beget questions, and hence, when scientists reply "well, it depends" or "further study required," they are being diligent not difficult. Others may feel let down by what they fallaciously assume is confusion, rather than just complexity. Science is hard work, truth is nuanced, and almost all humans (including clinicians) would rather have it easy. Because science should not care whether we *like* its answers, it can seem elitist and exclusionary. Instead, it should be a defence against propaganda and a way to protect the vulnerable and disadvantaged. We need the scientific method because we can all be willfully blind,[4] especially when other answers are comforting or self-serving.

Importantly, science is worth the time, funds, and sweat. For example, scientific discoveries have saved billions of lives, and from 1900 to 2015, global life expectancy has more than doubled to well over 70 years.[5] Science has propelled us into space, cured disease, and catalogued all recorded wisdom. It's impressive stuff, but we need to acknowledge its shortcomings. In addition to not necessarily teaching us HOW to live, science has wrought plenty of harm. In a (literal) vicious cycle, war advances science, and science advances war. In other words, the terrible Ukrainian carnage is fuelled by mad science (the spectre of nuclear fission bombs), not just mad politics (the threats of Vladimir Putin). Accordingly, we should not be surprised if others do not automatically share our scientific fervour. And that is before we even accept that science – not just politics – has plenty of putative scammers, scoundrels, and downright scumbags.[6–10]

Sam Kean's recent book, *The Icepick Surgeon*,[6] reveals how often scientists can twist a noble pursuit into a sinister obsession. Kean shows how naked ambition can push rational people to cross ethical and legal lines, all in the name of science. Examples include – but are in no way limited to – the origins of science in the transatlantic slave trade, grave robbers supplying anatomists, and Edison marketing the electric chair. Importantly, though, Kean makes it clear that science's sins are not all safely buried in the past. We can likely connect the medical abuses of Tuskegee and Nazi Germany with vaccine hesitancy and icepick lobotomies with mistrust of modern mental health care. In other words, science is as noble or as fragile as the people who wield it. That is why the following caution, often attributed to Einstein, states: "Most people say intellect makes a great scientist. They are wrong: It is character."

One of science's recent bête noires was Elizabeth Holmes, the former chief executive officer (CEO) of Theranos.[9] Wearing a reassuring white lab coat, she promised easy, cheap, needle-free clinical diagnoses. We collectively bought the hype so willingly that this university dropout raised $800 million and created $9 billion of liminal value. In short, hyperbole sells, and "science" polishes the sales pitch. Even here, however, science is the solution: in the form of *better* science. Scepticism (not nihilism or cynicism) is central to science. True scientists do not ask if an idea appeals. Rather, they ask, "Is it too good to be true?" – which brings this epistemological discussion all the way from the Ukraine to the comedian podcaster and self-admitted non-scientist, Joe Rogan.

During COVID, some scientists penned an open letter urging Spotify to crack down on Rogan's "COVID-19 misinformation."[10] This letter followed Rogan's interview with Dr. Robert Malone, a scientist critical of mRNA vaccines, and Rogan's pro-ivermectin stance. The scientists hypothesized that Rogan's podcast created "a false sense of balance," "a sociological issue of devastating proportions," and "a menace to public health." These words are heavy criticism for podcasting and initially seem contradictory to the call to engage. However, there is every reason to believe that influential figures can morph public behaviour far more than scientists can. For example, estimates are that $150 million was misspent on ivermectin by US insurers alone.[11] Clearly, no one person is to blame, and clearly Rogan and Holmes are not Putin. The point, instead, is that, whether we are discussing COVID, cyberspace, or the Crimea, the truth often takes a beating, and it is our duty to protect the innocent.

REFERENCES

1. Brandolini's law. Wikipedia. Accessed 22 July 2024. https://en.m.wikipedia.org/wiki/Brandolini%27s_law
2. Brindley PG, Byker L, Carley S, Thoma B. Assessing on-line medical education resources: a primer for acute care medical professionals and

others. *J Intensive Care Soc*. 2022;23(3):340–4. https://doi.org/10.1177/1751143721999949. Medline: 36033246.
3. Carl Sagan. Wikipedia. Accessed 24 July 2022. https://en.m.wikipedia.org/wiki/Carl_Sagan
4. Heffernan M. *Willful Blindness: Why We Ignore the Obvious at Our Peril*. Walker and Company; 2011.
5. Desjardins J; World Economic Forum; Visual Capitalist. These discoveries saved billions of lives. *World Economic Forum*. 28 March 2018. Accessed 22 July 2024. https://www.weforum.org/agenda/2018/03/the-50-most-important-life-saving-breakthroughs-in-history
6. Kean S. *The Icepick Surgeon: Murder, Fraud, Sabotage, and Other Dastardly Deeds Perpetrated in the Name of Science*. Little, Brown and Company; 2021.
7. Wise J. Boldt: the great pretender. *BMJ*. 2013;346:f1738. https://doi.org/10.1136/bmj.f1738
8. Paul E. Marik. Wikipedia. Accessed 22 July 2024. https://en.wikipedia.org/wiki/Paul_E._Marik
9. Bilton N. Exclusive: how Elizabeth Holmes's house of cards came tumbling down. *Vanity Fair*. 6 September 2016. Accessed 24 July 2024. https://www.vanityfair.com/news/2016/09/elizabeth-holmes-theranos-exclusive
10. Bond S. What the Joe Rogan podcast controversy says about the online misinformation ecosystem. *NPR*. 21 January 2022. Accessed 22 July 2024. https://www.npr.org/2022/01/21/1074442185/joe-rogan-doctor-covid-podcast-spotify-misinformation
11. Chua K-P, Conti RM, Becker NV. US insurer spending on ivermectin prescriptions for COVID-19. *JAMA Network*. 2022;327(6):584–7. https://doi.org/10.1001/jama.2021.24352. PMID: 35024763.

Afterword: Where Do We Go from Here? A Time to Reflect, a Time to Heal

Laura A. Hawryluck, MSc, MD, FRCPC
Professor, Critical Care Medicine, University of Toronto

15 February 2023

It is not the critic who counts; not the man who points out how the strong man stumbles or where the doer of deeds could have done them better. The credit belongs to the man who is actually in the arena, whose face is marred by dust and sweat and blood; who strives valiantly; who errs, who comes short again and again, because there is no effort without error and shortcoming; but who does actually strive to do the deeds; who knows great enthusiasms, the great devotions; who spends himself in a worthy cause; who at the best knows in the end the triumph of high achievement, and who at the worst, if he fails, at least fails while daring greatly.
– Theodore Roosevelt, "Citizenship in a Republic," address delivered at the Sorbonne, Paris, 23 April 1910

There is no good reason why we should fear the future, but there is every reason why we should face it seriously, neither hiding from ourselves the gravity of the problems before us nor fearing to approach these problems with the unbending, unflinching purpose to solve them aright.
– Theodore Roosevelt, Inaugural Address, 4 March 1905

After every life-changing event, whether it be one in an individual life or one that leaves none of us untouched, it is important to look critically at what we have been through – what went well, what did not – in order to learn and, in time, hopefully, to heal. *Pandemic Voices* is our attempt to explore some of the most challenging moments of the pandemic, the innovations, the stories of lives saved, the stories of lives lost, and the prices paid. In sharing the heartbreaks, the triumphs, and the scars left behind, these stories from the front lines reflect on the societal divisions that came into being and the need to recognize that, fundamentally, we are and will forever be more similar than we are different. Therein lies our strength; therein lies our humanity. These stories from the front lines illustrate that, if the COVID-19 pandemic has taught us nothing else, it has shown us the need for, and the strength of, living in kindness and empathy for one another.

Yet for all the stories captured in this volume, there are many more left untold. As we continue to live with COVID-19 and anxiously watch its steady mutation and the rise and fall of "variants of concern," we desperately hope that none of them will ever again be able to achieve the heart-wrenching destruction we saw during the peak of the Delta wave. In every country, we have lost far too many lives to this virus.

However our journey with COVID-19 progresses, in time there will be other new emerging infectious diseases that will threaten us and those we love. Surveillance, early detection of suspicious symptom clusters, big data, and artificial intelligence may allow us to detect these emerging threats sooner and to better control and contain them. The speed and innovation of medical science in developing vaccines and other ways to mitigate the impact of COVD-19 has demonstrated our collective progress compared to our efforts combating the viral pandemics of the past. Yet ironically, the very speed of development led to distrust and division. It is certain that the science has not been perfect: it almost never is. What should be certain and clear to everyone is that it will continue to improve and that it will be shared openly and equally no matter who you are or where you live.

We do not know what the future will bring, but we do know that there are already powerful lessons we can learn from sharing our collective lived experiences in this pandemic. And if we listen to the lessons learned, together we can build a better path forward. We want to thank all of our authors for their insightful and invaluable contributions. We want to thank all of our readers. Help us all do better. Help us all move forward.

Glossary

adult respiratory distress syndrome (ARDS): A very severe acute lung injury that results in life-threatening respiratory failure. People with ARDS need to be treated in the ICU on a ventilator because their lungs are failing and oxygen supplied by masks is not enough to keep them alive. The illnesses that can cause ARDS may be from a direct insult to the lungs or from severe illnesses outside of the lungs due to the body's response to such illnesses (e.g., life-threatening infections, pancreatitis, severe brain injuries, to name but a few). The severity of ARDS is assessed by the PaO2/FiO2 ratio, the amount of help the ventilator needs to give, and the compliance of the lungs (which can be measured on the ventilator).

aerosol generating procedure (AGP): A treatment procedure that creates aerosolized particles, which can spread through the air and infect those near the patient receiving treatment. AGPs include procedures such as intubation (putting someone on life support), bronchoscopy (looking into someone's lungs with a camera), and suctioning (inserting a small, long plastic tube through the breathing tube to help remove phlegm).

benzodiazepines: A class of medications used to sedate patients in the ICU to keep them comfortable and help them breathe in synchrony with the ventilator (e.g., midazolam/versed).

bronchoscopy: A procedure that involves looking into someone's lungs with a camera, potentially taking samples of phlegm to send to the lab to see if there is any infection (known as bronchoalveolar lavage or BAL), and suctioning up phlegm to help clear it, if it is blocking the airways.

central line: A large intravenous line inserted into the larger core veins of the body so that life-support medications that are hard on smaller veins (such as adrenaline) can be given safely. The veins in which these lines are placed include the internal jugular in the neck, the subclavian under the collar bone, and the femoral vein in the upper leg.

chief resident: A hospital-based title given to a physician who is still in training and is designated as the lead physician within their particular field of training at the hospital they are working at.

code blue: An emergency call indicating an adult cardiac arrest (i.e., it indicates a situation is occurring where someone is at imminent risk of, or has already, stopped breathing and/or whose heart has stopped). Hospitals have different colour-coded emergency call systems for crisis situations that are called "code" situations. These codes are called over the public broadcasting system overhead and through the "code team" (a team of health care workers who respond to the crisis).

code pink: An emergency similar to a code blue, but in a child.

CPR (cardiopulmonary resuscitation): A set of treatments that follow algorithms defined and updated by the American Heart Association, which include chest compressions, medications such as adrenaline, potentially defibrillation (as done with automated external defibrillator [AED] machines), and intubation.

critical care nurse: A nurse who has specialized in critical care nursing by taking additional training to provide care for patients on life support. Critical care nurses may also have received further training and work as members of the Critical Care Rapid Response Team. They may also be known as an ICU nurse.

critical care physician: A physician who has completed a second subspecialty in critical care medicine. Their first subspecialty could have been obtained in adult or paediatric anesthesia, internal medicine, surgery, neurosurgery, or emergency medicine. They may also be known as an intensivist.

critical care rapid response team: An ICU team that supports other hospital teams in caring for acutely deteriorating hospitalized patients by helping stabilize them on hospital units and/or increase the monitoring they receive and/or facilitating their admission to the ICU. It may also be called a Rapid Response Team.

critical illness: Any illness that is acutely life-threatening and requires life-support treatments.

diptheria: A bacterial infection of the mucous membranes of the nose and throat that can worsen to damage other organs, such as heart, kidneys, and nervous system, and can be deadly.

edema/oedema: A medical term that means swelling of tissues. The term is often used to indicate swelling of skin, which happens frequently in severe illnesses and is a very common problem in patients with life-threatening illnesses being cared for in the ICU. The difference in spelling is only reflective of North American vs British spelling.

endotracheal tube: A hollow plastic tube with a small inflatable balloon on its end that is usually inserted through a person's mouth into their windpipe. Once the balloon is inflated, it creates a seal, which allows the tube to be connected to the ventilator (breathing machine).

extracorporeal membrane oxygenation (ECMO)/extracorporeal life support (ECLS): A machine that can replace the lungs and/or heart in very carefully selected patients whose lungs and/or heart have failed to the point that life-supporting medications alone are not enough to keep them alive. Such machines can only be used on a temporary basis as a bridge to recovery or to transplant in some situations, and because they are so invasive, the risks of complications are high. While these machines may be life-saving, that is only true when people for whom they are used do not have a lot of other organ systems that are failing either on an acute or a chronic basis.

fellow: A physician who has completed their residency and is in their final years of training to become a subspecialist in their field of study (e.g., an ICU fellow is in the final stages of training to become an intensivist).

Food and Drug Administration (FDA): An agency in the United States that is responsible for protecting the public health by ensuring medications are safe and effective in treating the illnesses they are being used for.

hospitalist: A physician whose clinical practice is exclusively hospital based. Such physicians are generally specialists in internal medicine and, in some locations, may be trained as family physicians.

hypoxemic: Someone whose blood oxygen levels are low. Since the body's organs depend on oxygen to work and survive, the lower the level of oxygen in the blood, the more critically ill that person becomes, and the more likely they are to need a ventilator and ICU care. If they remain severely hypoxemic on a ventilator, they are in a very critical situation and are less likely to survive.

infection prevention and control (IPC or IPAC): A hospital-based health care professional team that is responsible for assessing and initiating professional practice measures to reduce the risk of transmission of infections in hospitals.

inotropes: A class of life-supporting medications that help the heart to beat more strongly when it is failing.

intensive care unit (ICU): A specialized hospital unit where highly trained health care professionals, the equipment (including ventilators, central lines, specialized monitors), and the medications to treat patients with life-threatening illnesses are located. These units are the only areas in any hospital that can provide ongoing care for such patients. They often, but not always, have rooms that can be negatively pressurized (i.e., rooms designed to clear aerosolized infectious particles from the air).

intensivist: A physician trained in critical care medicine who treats people with life-threatening illnesses. They may also be referred to as a critical care physician.

intubation: The act of inserting an endotracheal tube to connect a person to a ventilator.

life support: A group of treatments that aim to keep people with critical illnesses alive. They include ventilators, medications that raise (and sometimes lower) blood pressure, medications that help the heart beat more strongly, medications that control abnormal heart rhythms, and machines such as dialysis, which replace the function of organ systems that have failed or support those that aren't working properly.

mechanical ventilation: See ventilator.

nosocomial: An infection acquired while in hospital.

occupational therapy/occupational therapy team: A team of health care professionals who work with patients to assess them for and teach them how to use assistive devices to increase their mobility and ability to perform activities of daily living.

ORNGE: The name of the Ontario Canada critical care patient transport team. The paramedics who work with ORNGE are highly trained to resuscitate and care for critically ill patients on life support and transport these patients to hospitals throughout the province to ensure they receive the care they need.

paediatric intensive care unit (PICU): an ICU that cares for children with life-threatening illnesses.

PaO2/FiO2 ratio: A ratio showing the level of oxygen in arterial blood divided by the concentration of oxygen being supplied to the patient. A lower number means a more severe lung injury. A number less than 150 signifies a very severe lung injury.

PCR (polymerase chain reaction test): A test to detect a virus's genetic material (DNA) and identify whether it is present or not.

personal protective equipment (PPE): Equipment worn to protect health care workers from exposure to infectious diseases. PPE can vary depending on whether the need is to protect from pathogens that are airborne or those that are acquired from contact/touching infected surfaces. In the COVID-19 pandemic, PPE included masks, face shields/eye protection, gowns, and gloves. The type of masks, which one to wear and when, and the types of gowns were a source of tension in many centres and in many countries around the world. PPE was not available everywhere, and shortages were very common, especially early on in the pandemic. Even the differences in appearance of gowns with the same protection properties gave rise to stress and conflicts.

pertussis: The illness known as whooping cough, which is caused by a bacterial infection.

physiotherapy/physiotherapy team: A team of health care professionals skilled at providing and designing exercises that help increase strength and mobility. Provided by physiotherapists, such therapies – in particular early rehabilitation and mobilization (ERM) – are crucial in regaining strength after serious injuries and illnesses. Physiotherapy plays a very important role in helping people recover from life-threatening illnesses when they are in the ICU. They help strengthen people so they can breathe without the help of a ventilator, help them regain abilities to sit in chairs, walk, and begin their (usually prolonged) journey to recovery during their hospital admission and beyond.

prone position: Lying on one's stomach for 12 to16 hours at a time. Such positioning helps improve a seriously and/or critically ill patient's ability to breathe and was/is used extensively in caring for COVID-19 patients in hospital.

proning: Assisting a patient to lie on their stomach in bed. Such a manoeuvre helps improve a critically ill person's breathing and increases their blood oxygen levels.

propofol: A medication commonly used in the ICU to sedate (put patients to sleep) in order to intubate them and to keep them comfortable and help them breathe in synchrony with the ventilator.

rapid response team: An ICU team that extends beyond the walls of the ICU, whose goal is to identify critically ill patients in the hospital and either stabilize them on the hospital unit that is currently caring for them, move them to an area in the hospital that can monitor them more closely, or facilitate rapid admission to the ICU. Such a team has been shown to improve outcomes of hospitalized patients by rapidly responding to their deteriorating situation and preventing in-hospital cardiac arrests. This team may also be known as a Critical Care Rapid Response Team.

renal replacement therapy (RRT): A continuous form of dialysis used in people with acute kidney failure in the ICU. This way of providing dialysis is designed to be easier for the body to tolerate by causing less blood pressure instability.

resident: A physician in training within a designated field of clinical medicine. Once medical school is completed, a physician is given the designation of resident during their clinical training. This training is known as residency.

respiratory therapist: A highly skilled health care professional who is trained to recognize and alleviate respiratory distress and to manipulate therapies from oxygen delivery systems to ventilators to help stabilize patients with life-threatening illnesses. They are not available in every ICU worldwide – typically they work in North American ICUs. In other centres, ICU nurses and intensivists will manipulate the ventilator settings.

RT-PCR (reverse transcription polymerase chain reaction): A different method to identify the presence of a viral infection by producing its DNA from an RNA source.

sedation: A combination of sedatives and narcotics given intravenously in the ICU to keep patients comfortable while they are on a ventilator.

self-proning: The ability of a patient to lie on their stomach without assistance from the health care team. Self-proning was commonly done in patients struggling with COVID-19 infections in hospital unit settings.

sepsis: A life-threatening illness that is caused by the body's response to a severe infection. It may cause a shock state and is then called septic shock.

shock: An acute life-threatening state in which a patient's organs are not receiving enough blood supply to function normally.

speech-language therapy/speech-language pathology team (SLT/SLP): A team of health care workers who are responsible for evaluating a person's ability to swallow and for giving guidance in how to do so safely. They assist in assessing a patient's ability to communicate and provide guidance and aids to facilitate communication with health care team members as well as with the patient's family and friends.

telemedicine: Medical consultations and guidance provided via various confidential, private, and secure web-based platforms.

vasodilators: A class of intravenous medications that decrease blood vessel tone and lower blood pressure when it is too high. These medications may also, in some situations, help the right side of the heart when it is failing. They need careful monitoring, tailoring, must be adjusted to a patient's needs, and can only be given in an ICU. They are usually administered through central lines.

vasopressors: A class of intravenous medications that increase blood vessel tone (causing an increase in blood pressure) and the heart's ability to beat. These medications need careful monitoring, tailoring, must be adjusted to a patient's needs, and can only be given in an ICU. They are usually administered through central lines.

ventilator: A machine, also called a breathing machine, that helps a critically ill patient breathe when they can no longer breathe on their own (i.e., when their lungs are failing). A critically ill patient may need a ventilator for a number of different reasons, including but not limited to lung problems, heart problems, severe infections (sepsis), and severe brain injuries. A ventilator can be invasive (when a person is attached to it through an endotracheal tube) or non-invasive (when the connection is via a mask interface, e.g., BiPAP). Non-invasive ventilators are not able to provide as high a level of support as invasive ones.

Contributors

Sabrina Agnihotri, MD, is a postgraduate year five (PGY5) psychiatry resident in the Department of Psychiatry at the University of Toronto. At the time of writing the chapter, she was co-chief resident of psychiatry within the University Health Network, Toronto. She has a BSc in psychology and biology from York University, an MSc and PhD from the University of Toronto in developmental neurosciences, and a post-doctoral fellowship in brain injury and health economics from the Bloorview Research Institute. She obtained her MD from the University of Toronto.

Hassan Al-Habeeb, MD, is an adult critical care and neuro critical care consultant, Riyadh National Hospital, Riyadh, Saudi Arabia. After completing his training in anesthesia, he completed a dual fellowship at the University of Toronto in adult critical care and trauma neuro critical care. His expertise and interests include the emerging impact of AI on clinical practice. He is a passionate storyteller and writer, offering a unique blend of professional insight and human experience.

Keith Azevedo, MD, is an assistant professor in critical care and emergency medicine at the University of New Mexico School of Medicine. He obtained his medical degree from the University of Massachusetts, completed a residency in emergency medicine at the University of New Mexico and an anesthesia critical care fellowship at Washington University. He has a specific interest in the use of extracorporeal membrane oxygenation for advanced cardiac and respiratory failure and works part-time as an American Mountain Guide Association–trained rock-climbing guide.

Melissa Begay, MD, is an assistant professor in the School of Medicine at the University of New Mexico. She is a member of the Navajo Nation.

Peter G. Brindley, MD, FRCPC, FRCP, is professor of critical care medicine, adjunct professor of anesthesiology, adjunct professor, John Dossetor Health Ethics Centre, University of Alberta, Edmonton. His academic focus includes resuscitation, crisis management, human factors, and teamwork. He was awarded the Intensive Care Society Senior Fellowship for his international contributions to critical care. He co-founded the *Critical Care Commute Podcast*, which discusses critical care with a wide variety of worldwide experts.

Rev. Kristel Clayville, PhD, is a lecturer in technology ethics and health humanities at the University of Illinois, Chicago. A former hospital chaplain, she also uses her chaplaincy experience and skills to teach ethics and religion in the medical school.

Alvaro Coronado-Muñoz, MD, is an associate professor in the Division of Pediatric Critical Care at The Children's Hospital, Montefiore Medical Center, Albert Einstein College of Medicine, New York. During the pandemic, he was an assistant professor in the Department of Pediatrics, Division of Critical Care, at the University of Texas Health Science Center at Houston. He collaborated remotely with colleagues from Latin America. In particular, he worked with Dr. Jesús Domínguez-Rojas and colleagues in his home country, Peru, on research projects exploring the pandemic's impact on paediatric patients.

Akash Deep, MD, FRCPCH, is the director of the paediatric intensive care unit (PICU) and staff governor at King's College Hospital, London, and professor of paediatric critical care at King's College, London. He is the chair of scientific affairs for the European Society of Paediatric and Neonatal Intensive Care Society (ESPNIC) and chair of the science and education committee of the UK Paediatric Critical Care Society (PCCS). He is the advisor to the UK Sepsis Trust for paediatric sepsis.

Jesús Domínguez-Rojas, MD, is chief of the pediatric intensive care unit INSN, in the Department of Emergencies and Critical Areas, Instituto Nacional de Salud del Niño, Lima, Peru. He is a professor of pediatric intensive care medicine subspecialty, Universidad Nacional Mayor de San Marcos, a researcher of publications on critical children, president of the Oncology Committee of the Latin American Society of Pediatric Intensive Care (SLACIP), and director of Fundamentos Pediatricos Criticos (PFCCS-SCCM).

James Downar, MDCM, MHSc, FRCPC, is professor and head of the Division of Palliative Care, clinical research chair in palliative and end-of life care, and works in critical care medicine and palliative care at the University of Ottawa. He is an adjunct professor at the Australian Centre for Health Law Research at the Queensland University of Technology. He is president of the Canadian Critical Care Society and co-chair of the Pan-Canadian Palliative Care Research Collaborative. In 2021, he received the Award of Excellence from the Ontario Medical Association's section on palliative medicine.

Ingrid Duffy, RN, FNP, is a family nurse practitioner with a background in neuroscience and emergency medicine. After her pandemic experience, she has shifted her practice to geriatrics, palliative care, and hospice with a PACE program in Lafayette, Colorado.

Sabrina Fiorellino, JD, is a serial entrepreneur who founded Fero International Inc. in 2020 after completing the sale of a large private road-building company that she had founded in 2017, which achieved over $80 million in annual revenue. Sabrina also spent 10 years as legal counsel at two large firms on Toronto's Bay Street. During her tenure there, Sabrina supported a large portfolio of clients across diversified industries on various transactions, including capital raises and M&A exceeding $1 billion CAD.

Laura A. Hawryluck, MSc, MD, FRCPC, is professor of critical care medicine, University of Toronto. During the pandemic, she was physician lead of the rapid response team at Toronto Western Hospital. A poet, a writer, and a physician, she believes access to empathic and humane health care is a fundamental global human right. She has received awards for her work throughout her career to improve access to high-quality critical care internationally, end-of-life care in Canada, and for her contributions to both medicine and law.

Matyas Hervieux, BSc (Hons), DHS, MA, MD, CCFP(EM), completed a combined Honours BSc in physiology and psychology, as well as a DHS and MA at the University of Western Ontario. He obtained his MD from McMaster University and completed his family medicine residency and emergency fellowship at the University of Toronto. During the pandemic, he worked as an emergency physician at Georgian Bay General and as a locum at urban sites. He is an emergency physician at the University Health Network in Toronto and in Yellowknife.

Kurniawan Taufiq Kadafi, MD, is a member of the teaching staff in the Pediatric Emergency and Intensive Care Division, Department of Pediatrics, Dr. Saiful Anwar General Hospital, Malang, and Faculty of Medicine, Brawijaya University, Malang, Indonesia, as well as head of the Disaster Management Task Force Indonesian Pediatric Society (2021–24), member of the Strategic Advisor Group (SAG) for the International Pediatric Association (IPA), and member of the Technical Advisory Group (TAG) for the Asia Pacific Pediatric Association. From 2012 until now, he has written eleven books, most recently *Principles for Selection of Oxygen Therapy Modalities in Children* (EGC, 2023).

Gabrielle Karlovich, MD, received her undergraduate degree from Cornell University and completed her doctor of medicine degree at the Cooper Medical School of Rowan University in 2023. She is now a general psychiatry resident at Temple University in Philadelphia.

Philip Knight, MD, MBChB, MRCPH, is a paediatric critical care consultant at King's College Hospital and for the pediatric critical care transport team at Great Ormond Street Hospital, London. He has published on patient safety, paediatric critical care transportation, and the impact of the pandemic on patient care and training future physicians. He is actively involved in developing remote monitoring in critically unwell children and novel methods of vital sign analysis in transport.

Erik Kraai, MD, is an associate professor at the University of New Mexico and was the medical director of the medical intensive care unit during the pandemic. He obtained his medical degree from the University of Colorado and completed a residency in internal medicine and a fellowship in critical care at the University of New Mexico. He has a specific interest in the use of extracorporeal membrane oxygenation for advanced cardiac and respiratory failure.

Gianni Lorello, BSc, MD, MSc (Med Ed), CIP, FRCPC, is an associate professor of anesthesiology at the University of Toronto. He was the inaugural chair of equity, diversity, and inclusion for the Department of Anesthesiology and Pain Medicine and chair of the diversity, equity, and inclusion committee at the Canadian Anesthesiologists' Society. He is a health professions education research PhD candidate at the Institute of Health Policy, Management, and Evaluation at the University of Toronto, learning critical social theory at the Wilson Centre.

Russell MacDonald, MD, MPH, FCFP, FRCPC, DRCPSC, is a professor in the Faculty of Medicine, University of Toronto, and medical director for Toronto Paramedic Services and Toronto's Central Ambulance Communications Centre. He is Canada's first formally trained subspecialist in prehospital and transport medicine, and chairs the RCPSC AFC diploma committee for prehospital and transport medicine. His international leadership was recognized with the Air Medical Physicians' Association Distinguished Physician Award and the Association of Air Medical Service's Board Chairman's Award for lifetime achievement, contribution, and service to the prehospital and transport medicine community.

Sonia Malhotra, MD, MS, FAAP, FAAHPM, is an associate professor of internal medicine and pediatrics at Tulane University School of Medicine. She is the associate section chief of general internal medicine/geriatrics/palliative medicine and director of palliative medicine at the University Medical Center, New Orleans.

Ririe Fachrina Malisie, MD, PhD, is a senior lecturer, teaching staff at the Pediatric Emergency and Intensive Care Division, Department of Pediatrics and Secretary Program of Master Biomedic Science, Faculty of Medicine, Universitas Sumatera Utara, Adam Malik General Hospital, Medan, Indonesia; and senior consultant of pediatric emergency and intensive care at the Indonesian Pediatric Collegium. She is chairperson of the pediatric emergency and intensive care working group of the Indonesian Pediatric Society, a member of the Pediatric Acute and Critical Care Medicine Asian Network, and of education/research committees of WFPICS. Her research focuses on infant and pediatric emergency and critical care in low-middle income countries.

Anthony McDermott, MD, is a facilities manager who was born in Glasgow, Scotland, but has lived most of his life in North York, Ontario. He is married and has been blessed with eight children and three grandchildren. He hopes to retire soon. He loves meeting new people and helping anyone who needs a leg up.

Steve A. McLaughlin, MD, is a tenured professor in emergency medicine at the University of New Mexico. He serves as the chief medical officer for UNMH and is the former chair of the Department of Emergency Medicine. Dr. McLaughlin received his undergraduate degrees in biology and economics from the California Institute of Technology and then attended medical school at Mayo Medical School.

Mervyn Mer, MBBCh, Dip PEC (SA), FCP (SA), Pulmonology subspecialty, Cert Critical Care (SA), M Med (Int Med), FRCP (London), FCCP, PhD, is based in the Department of Medicine, Divisions of Critical Care and Pulmonology, at the Charlotte Maxeke Johannesburg Academic Hospital (CMJAH), University of the Witwatersrand, Johannesburg, South Africa. He serves as clinical head of the adult multidisciplinary intensive care unit at CMJAH and is academic head of critical care at the University of the Witwatersrand. Internationally renowned and highly respected, with a deep love of teaching, he is a hands-on clinician, and his research targets improving sepsis outcomes, particularly in developing countries.

Nathan D. Nielsen, MD, MSc, is an associate professor in the Departments of Internal Medicine and Pathology at the University of New Mexico School of Medicine. He was educated at Stanford University, Duke University School of Medicine, and London School ofHygiene and Tropical Medicine. He is the author of several essays on the effect of the pandemic on health care worker psyche in both the general and academic press.

Pamela H. Orr, MD, MSc, FRCPC, is a professor of internal medicine/infectious diseases, medical microbiology, and community health sciences at the University of Manitoba, Winnipeg. She began her career as a general practitioner in northern Manitoba and the Arctic. Dr. Orr works in education, clinical care, and research locally and internationally, with an interest in rural, remote, and circumpolar health.

Andy Pan, MD, FRCPC (EM CCM), DRCPSC (PTM), is the critical care medical director and a transport medicine physician with ORNGE, Ontario's air ambulance and critical care transport service. He is also an emergency physician (The Ottawa Hospital) and intensivist (Montfort Hospital) in Ottawa. He is an assistant professor with the Department of Emergency Medicine at the University of Ottawa.

Bojan N. Paunovic, MD, FRCPC, is section head of adult critical care in the Department of Internal Medicine at the University of Manitoba, Winnipeg. An adult intensivist with over 20 years of experience in medical leadership, a focus in system redesign, young leader mentorship, and quality improvement initiatives, he is also the provincial medical specialty lead, adult critical care, Shared Health Manitoba; regional medical specialty lead, adult critical care, Winnipeg Regional Health Authority; site adult critical care medical lead, Health Sciences Centre, Winnipeg.

Michael Peddle, MD, FRCPC, DRCPSC, is a Memorial University of Newfoundland and Labrador medical school graduate and completed an FRCP in emergency medicine at Western University. With over 15 years of experience, he specializes in prehospital and transport medicine systems as well as emergency preparedness. He is an associate medical officer at ORNGE, overseeing medical operations, education, and dispatch, and works clinically as a transport medicine physician.

Kashif Pirzada, MD, CCFP(EM), is an emergency physician practising in Toronto with academic affiliations at McMaster University and the University of Toronto. He is a co-founder of Masks4Canada and of the Canadian COVID Society, and a frequent contributor to local and national media on medical and health issues.

Fayez Quereshy, MD, MBA, FRCSC, FACS, is vice-president, clinical, and surgical oncologist and minimally invasive surgeon, University Health Network, Toronto. Both a local and national award-winning surgeon, Dr. Quereshy is an academic surgeon-investigator leading a $340 million portfolio that encompasses internationally recognized programs such as the Sprott Department of Surgery. An associate professor in the Department of Surgery and the Rotman School of Management, he is also the site lead at Toronto General Hospital and a practising surgical oncologist within the Princess Margaret Cancer Centre, focused on gastrointestinal malignancies and colorectal cancer.

Houman Rashidian, MD, FRCPC, practices as a general psychiatrist at Trillium Health Partners in Mississauga, Ontario. He obtained his undergraduate degree in psychology at the University of British Columbia. Thereafter, he completed medical school at the University of Ottawa, followed by a psychiatric residency at the University of Toronto. At the time of writing the chapter, he was a PGY5 in the Department of Psychiatry at the University of Toronto.

Meaghan Reaburn, PharmD, BScPhm, RPh, is the clinical pharmacist lead and manager, quality & risk at the Canadian Mental Health Association Waterloo Wellington (CMHA WW). She completed her undergraduate degree in pharmacy at Dalhousie University and a 3-year doctor of pharmacy degree at the University of Florida. Meaghan's role at CMHA WW includes clinical consultation to community treatment teams, assessment, and facilitation of quality-of-care reviews for sentinel and adverse events, risk management, and policy and medication safety organizational practice development. Additionally, she co-developed CMHA WW's electronic prescribing platform and electronic medication reconciliation process – a one-of-a-kind e-health solution with potential for recognition as a leading practice in Canada

Troy Rieck, PhD, C.Psych, is originally from a small town in Manitoba and has studied psychology at the universities of Winnipeg, Guelph, and North Texas. His areas of competency include clinical/counselling, forensic, and industrial/organizational psychology. His work placements include positions in hospitals, community mental health, and private practice. Currently, his efforts focus primarily on clinical and forensic psychological services in the context of supporting community members who experience a wide range of psychological challenges in the Waterloo Wellington region. He is the professional practice lead supervisor at the Canadian Mental Health Association Waterloo Wellington (CMHA WW).

Scott Roach, PharmD, MBA, is the director of Pharmacy Operations at the University of New Mexico Hospital.

Dorrette Ruddock, RN, started as a general surgery nurse in 1992. After a decade, she transitioned into critical care for the next 23 years, caring for those with life-threatening illnesses. She was proud to be a mentor for new nurses and peers before her well-earned retirement in 2023 from the medical surgical neurosciences intensive care unit at Toronto Western Hospital, University Health Network. During the pandemic, she, alongside her husband and daughter, embarked on a culinary adventure that captured hearts and imaginations: *Deddy's Kitchen*, a YouTube channel, which became a beacon of joy, creativity, and familial bonding.

Preeyaporn (Pree) Sarangarm, PharmD, BCPS, BCCCP, is the pharmacy supervisor of emergency medicine and critical care pharmacy services at the University of New Mexico Hospital.

Louis Skevington-Postles, BSc, MSc, is a paediatric physiotherapist working on the paediatric intensive care unit at King's College Hospital, NHS Foundation Trust, London, England. He has degrees in physiotherapy and sport and exercise science from King's College London and Portsmouth University. His recent publications include research on early rehabilitation and mobilization in paediatric critical care and the development of paediatric point-of-care ultrasound training. His particular interests include complex invasive and non-invasive ventilation and point-of-care lung ultrasound.

Rima Styra, MD, MEd, FRCPC, is professor and director of the Division of Consultation Liaison Psychiatry, Department of Psychiatry, at the University of Toronto. She works as a CL staff psychiatrist at the University Health Network. She has a long-standing interest in the mental well-being of health care workers and has researched the effects of new emerging infectious diseases, such as SARS and COVID-19, on their mental health.

Jody Thomas, PhD, is a clinical health psychologist, founder and CEO of the non-profit Meg Foundation for Pain, and adjunct faculty at the Stanford University School of Medicine.

Homer Tien, MD, MSc, FRCSC, is the CEO of ORNGE, Ontario's air ambulance and critical care transport provider. During the pandemic, he led the vaccination program for Ontario's remote northern Indigenous communities and later chaired Ontario's entire COVID-19 vaccination program. He is a trauma surgeon at Sunnybrook Health Sciences Centre and an associate professor of surgery at the University of Toronto. He was previously a colonel in the Canadian Armed Forces and served overseas in the former Yugoslavia and Afghanistan.

Tina Trigg, PhD, is past president of Inclusion Edmonton Region, vice-president of Inclusion Alberta, and associate professor of English at The King's University, Edmonton. A firm believer in the equal dignity of every human being and the power of collective advocacy to create positive social change, Tina invests in building inclusive community in Edmonton, Alberta, Canada, where she lives with her husband and daughters.

Onion Gerald Vergara Ubaldo, MD, MBA, FRCP, FPSCCM, is an adult critical care specialist in the Philippines. He works as a staff intensivist with the Philippine Heart Center, The Medical City, and Rizal Medical Center.

Joe Vipond, MD, CCFP(EM), FCPC, has worked as an emergency physician for over 20 years and is currently at the Rockyview General Hospital. He is past president of the national charity Canadian Association of Physicians for the Environment. He is also the co-founder and board member of the local charity the Calgary Climate Hub, and during COVID-19, the co-founder of Masks4Canada, the Canadian COVID Society, and ProtectOurProvinceAB. Joe grew up in Calgary and continues to live there with his wife and two daughters.

Jean-Ralph Zahar, MD, PhD, is a professor in the infection control unit, Microbiology Department, Assistance Publique, Hôpitaux de Paris, France. He has been in charge of infectious risk prevention, working in this field for about 20 years, based in Paris, France. After training in intensive care and infectious diseases, he became interested in the spread and control of pathogens, particularly multidrug-resistant organisms. He worked for many years on the appropriateness of antibiotic therapy and led an antimicrobial stewardship. During the pandemic, he was particularly interested in the airborne spread of SARS-CoV-2 in and out of the ICU environment.

www.ingramcontent.com/pod-product-compliance
Lightning Source LLC
Chambersburg PA
CBHW030304080526
44584CB00012B/435